AF412893

# HOSPITAL
# INFECTION
# CONTROL

# HOSPITAL INFECTION CONTROL

## Principles and Practice

### Second Edition


**MARY CASTLE, R.N., M.P.H.**

Infection Control Practitioner
Doctoral Candidate in Epidemiology
University of California School of Public Health
Berkeley, California

**ELIZABETH AJEMIAN, B.S.**

Epidemiology Clinician
Infection Control Consultant
Section of Epidemiology
Hartford Hospital
Hartford, Connecticut



A WILEY MEDICAL PUBLICATION

**JOHN WILEY & SONS**

**New York · Chichester · Brisbane · Toronto · Singapore**

Illustrated by Molly Ross, Denver, Colorado



*Library of Congress Cataloging in Publication Data:*
Castle, Mary.
  Hospital infection control.

  (A Wiley medical publication)
  Includes bibliographies and index.
  1. Nosocomial infections—Prevention. 2. Hospitals—
Sanitation.  I. Title.  II. Series.  [DNLM: 1. Cross
Infection—prevention & control.   WX 167 C353h]
RA969.C24   1987      614.4'4      87-8109
ISBN 0-471-83681-8

Printed in the United States of America

10  9 8 7 6 5 4 3 2 1

# Foreword

The first edition of this book was published in 1980, a year that marked the end of a decade of extraordinarily rapid growth in the discipline of infection control; in 1970 very few hospitals in the United States had infection control programs, but by 1980 most hospitals had such programs. These dramatic changes were brought about by repeated urgings from the American Hospital Association and the Centers for Disease Control but, most importantly, by the mandates of the Joint Commission of Accreditation of Hospitals.

The professional support structure and the educational resources available within the field also grew dramatically in that decade. This was a period of extraordinary growth for the Association for Practitioners in Infection Control, the founding of their Journal, the *American Journal of Infection Control*, and the development of a somewhat parallel organization in hospital epidemiology, the Society of Hospital Epidemiologists of America. Journals, textbooks, and monographs written specifically for the beginning infection control practitioner began to appear, and books such as the first edition of this volume began to fill the educational gap that had been created by the growth of the discipline. The Hospital Infection course offered at the Centers for Disease Control, supplemented by other courses offered by the Association for Practitioners in Infection Control, the Society of Hospital Epidemiologists of America, and several state health departments also helped to close the educational gap.

The years that have elapsed since 1980 have seen less in the way of numerical growth, but much more in expansion of the scientific data base in infection control. This ongoing process was initiated at the Second International Conference on Nosocomial Infections, held in Atlanta, Georgia, in 1980. A number of events and forces have influenced hospital infection control in the intervening years. The introduction of reimbursement systems based on diagnosis, led by Medicare, has significantly changed the character of patients in hospitals, as well as underscoring the importance of infection control. No longer are the costs of nosocomial infection fully reimbursed by the insurers; rather, many of these costs represent real dollar losses. As both hospital admissions and lengths of stay decrease, the acuity of care in general hospitals has significantly increased, and probably infection rates, even at baseline, have increased as well. The acute care hospital of today is moving more and more in the direction of intensive care.

Publication of the SENIC study represents another major landmark thus far in the 1980s, the results of which certainly lend strong support and credibility to the discipline of infection control. The CDC guidelines have evolved into generally superb resource documents for infection control practitioners and, although clearly labeled as "guidelines," seem to have defined standards of care in infection control.

The use of computers in processing infection control data has emerged as a major aid to infection control practitioners, and will continue to be so in the future. The reuse of disposable equipment, already a significant issue at the beginning of the decade, remains a significant challenge as cost-containment pressures mount. Among the major disease challenges of this decade, acquired immune deficiency syndrome (AIDS) must rank as the major challenge that confronts us in the future.

All of these new issues and new findings of the 1980s to date are addressed in the second edition of this volume. The authors have drawn on their years of experience as infection control practitioners, and the book is clearly written *by* infection control practitioners *for* infection control practitioners. As with the first edition, the present volume does not attempt to cover the entire field of infection control, but it does provide an excellent fundamental base of information from which to begin. This base of information, supplemented by the existing resource documents such as textbooks and journals in the field, will admirably equip infection control practitioners for their increasingly important role in contemporary hospitals.

THEODORE C. EICKHOFF, M.D.

*Director of Internal Medicine*
*Presbyterian/Saint Luke's Medical Center*
*Professor of Medicine*
*University of Colorado School of Medicine*
*Denver, Colorado*

# Preface

The second edition of this text, as was the first, is designed as an introduction, a current reference, and a background for infection control practice. Part I outlines the structure of an infection control program and examines the clinical and administrative roles of each person on the infection control team within the hospital organization. Part II deals with the concept of infection itself and how hospitalized persons, subjected to certain risk factors, acquire infections. The most common nosocomial infections and their causes for development and the role of the infection control practitioner in identifying, controlling, and intervening to prevent these infections are discussed. Part III is a series of chapters on different activities of the infection control practitioner and infection control committee, including surveillance, reporting, isolation, and in-service education.

For the beginning infection control practitioner, infection control committee chairperson, fellows in infectious disease who will become hospital epidemiologists, or the student in a graduate program in infection control or a related field, the text can serve as an outline of the components of practice and major facets of concern. It is intended to introduce the reader in a systematic way to the entire scope of infection control as it is defined today. Although the book focuses on hospital infection control, the adaptation of basic principles to long-term care is discussed in Part III. In addition to serving the student in the field of infection control, the text will be useful as a policy base for practitioners and infection control committees. Since there are few texts available on this subject, regulating bodies have in the past provided most of the input into the formulation of policy and practice in the field of infection control. This text will be a useful reference for the experienced practitioner and infection control committee for justification of current practices or as a basis for change.

Largely because of acquired immune deficiency syndrome (AIDS), all infection control policies are being scrutinized for their efficacy. Over the last few years major changes in infection control practice have occurred, and policies will continue to be modified. In response to this, we have made some recommendations for current practice, while acknowledging that more research must be done and further studies initiated before such recommendations can be institutionalized. We hope that this text will provide a meaningful and current reference with which infection control practitioners can verify their priorities and determine new areas to investigate in this exciting field.

The authors would like to thank their families and friends who gave support and encouragement in the preparation of this book.

MARY CASTLE
ELIZABETH AJEMIAN

# Contents

**PART III   SURVEILLANCE, PREVENTION, AND CONTROL OF NOSOCOMIAL INFECTIONS**

# HOSPITAL INFECTION CONTROL

# PART ONE

# STRUCTURE OF INFECTION CONTROL PROGRAMS

# 1

# Introduction to Infection Control

## HISTORY OF NOSOCOMIAL INFECTIONS

Infection has been defined as "the process whereby pathogenic organisms become established and multiply in or on the body of a host" (1). Infection dates back to the earliest forms of life. Microorganisms have always resided on and in the human body, more or less in a balance favorable to both. The upsetting of this balance, with resulting invasion and infection, poses a problem of varying degrees of severity for the host.

Nosocomial infections probably date back to the first hospital, room, or gathering of sick people in a geographic area together. The word *nosocomial* means, strictly, *bedside-associated,* but in practice it also means an association with any institution in which people are gathered and given care. Included in this practical definition would be hospitals, extended care facilities, psychiatric institutions, and outpatient care facilities. Nosocomial infections may have occurred, therefore, the first time one person was cared for by another.

Perhaps the most well-known report of the recognition of and efforts to reduce nosocomial infections dates back to the 19th century. Puerperal sepsis, or childbed fever, was well known in Europe as a fatal disease. In 1843 Oliver Wendell Holmes presented his ideas to the Boston Society for Medical Improvement. He believed that physicians who performed autopsies and then examined women in labor were transmitting this disease from the autopsied body to patients (2). His paper and ideas were not accepted by the other physicians.

Although Holmes and other physicians had arrived at conclusions on the spread of contagion in puerperal fever through clinical observation, it was Ignaz Philipp Semmelweis, a physician in an obstetric ward in a Vienna hospital, who documented this fact and demonstrated convincingly the value of hand-washing. He was concerned that the mortality rate from puerperal sepsis in one section of the hospital, which was operated and staffed by physicians, was 5 times greater than a ward that was operated and staffed only by midwives. He deduced the increased mortality was not caused by overcrowding since the ward staffed by the midwives continually experienced a greater patient population than did the physician-operated ward. His investigation revealed that the physicians performed autopsies and did not wash their hands after leaving the autopsy room to care for patients. By contrast, the midwives had no contact with postmortem examinations and were more careful about personal cleanliness. He found that the mortality rate was greatly decreased in his hospital when physicians rinsed their hands in a solution of chlorinated lime after performing autopsies. Both Semmelweiss and Holmes were unaware that bacteria were being transmitted from patient to patient, and both suffered the disbelief of their colleagues (3).

Many years later Joseph Lister demonstrated the relationship between bacteria and infection and developed the first concepts of antisepsis. Florence Nightingale, Shimmelbusch, and others initiated some of the aseptic techniques that we are still using today–for example, rubber gloves, isolation procedures for infected patients, and hospital ventilation and sanitation. These early infection control practitioners recognized that infection morbidity and mortality rates could be lowered, and they worked to determine how to achieve this goal.

With the discovery of penicillin in 1928 by Dr. Howard Florey in Great Britain and its subsequent manufacture and release in the United States in the early 1940s, the antibiotic era began. The drug was so effective in preventing and treating infections that less emphasis was placed on aseptic techniques. When clinicians determined that many bacteria were developing strains resistant to existing antibiotics and that infections were continuing to occur in spite of the drugs, new antibiotics were sought and developed. Indiscriminate use of antibiotics has led to increased resistance in microorganisms and has changed the microbiologic flora in health care institutions.

Only since the emergence of infection control as a discipline have health care personnel turned their focus back to the use of aseptic practices for the prevention of nosocomial infections and the use of appropriate antimicrobial therapy to deal effectively with these infections.

Through the work of the Centers for Disease Control (CDC), the Joint Commission on Accreditation of Hospitals, and state regulatory agencies, guidelines have been created that recognize, measure, and analyze nosocomial infections. These guidelines also provide control measures in the form of patient care procedures and administrative guidelines for health care institutions. In recent years these agencies have stressed the adoption of programs to monitor nosocomial infections. Now, more and more infection control practitioners and clinicians are looking at established and new guidelines to determine methods that will reduce nosocomial infection morbidity and mortality.

## SCOPE OF THE PROBLEM

Hospitals in the United States admit 40 million patients annually. Two million of these patients, about 5%, acquire a nosocomial infection. Approximately 20,000 people die each year from these infections, and nosocomial infections are a contributing cause of death in 60,000 other patients. However, these numbers may actually be considerably higher since this information is not yet available from extended care, or free-standing outpatient medical and surgical facilities. Estimations have been made that nosocomial infections add 4–13 extra days of hospitalization and cost patients and insurers more than $2 billion each year (4–7).

Despite the changes and improvements in therapeutic measures, including antimicrobial therapy and diagnostic and treatment procedures, the rates of nosocomial infections have remained stable; the population of people at risk has changed, as have the microorganisms responsible for the infections.

In addition to the moral commitment of health care professionals "to do the patient no harm," regulatory agencies are requiring institutions to have programs that deal with nosocomial infections. Because of the outcome of the well-known *Darling vs. Charleston Community Memorial Hospital* case in 1965, health care institutions began to experience additional pressure in the form of possibility of lawsuits related to nosocomial infections (8). In this case, the court awarded damages to a college student whose leg had to be amputated because of an infection that was contracted following treatment of a fracture. The result of this and other court decisions has been to strengthen the guidelines and regulations provided by agencies, thus standardizing the practice of infection control (9).

## INFECTION CONTROL PROGRAMS: THE SOLUTION

Infection control programs have evolved in an attempt to solve the problem of nosocomial infections. The key to the control of infections lies in the institution's Infection Control Committee (ICC), the Infection Control Practitioner (ICP), and the program itself. Each of these essential components of infection control programs is dealt with in more detail in the following chapters.

The remainder of this text covers the nature and epidemiology of nosocomial infections, including specific nosocomial infections in terms of incidence, pathophysiology, means of transmission, and control measures. Finally, certain aspects of the infection control program, such as surveillance, isolation procedures, education, and the investigation of epidemics, is covered in more detail.

The infection control program is the method currently being used to address the problem of nosocomial infections in health care institutions. The purpose of this book is to provide those involved in the planning, implementation, or evaluation of infection control programs with useful information on the current state of the art in infection control practice.

## REFERENCES


1. Landau SI (ed): *International Dictionary of Medicine and Biology*. New York, Wiley, 1986.
2. Garrison FH: *An Introduction to the History of Medicine,* ed. 4. Philadelphia, Saunders, 1929.
3. Semmelweis IP: The etiology, the concept and the prophylaxis of childbed fever. In Murphy FP (translation): *Medical Classics*. Baltimore, Williams & Wilkins, 1941, vol 5, No. 5.
4. Haley RW, Culver DH, White JW, et al: The nationwide nosocomial infection rate, a new need for vital statistics. *Am J Epidemiol* 121 : 159–167, 1985.
5. Haley RW, Schaberg DR, Crossley KB, et al: Extra charges and prolongation of stay attributable to nosocomial infections: A prospective interhospital comparison. *Am J Med* 70 : 51–58, 1981.
6. Brachman PS: Nosocomial infection control: An overview. *Rev Infect Dis* 3(4):640–648, 1981.
7. CDC, Nosocomial infection surveillance 1980–1982. *Morbidity and Mortality Weekly Rep* 32(4SS):8SS, 1984.
8. *Darling* vs. *Charleston Community Memorial Hospital,* 211 NE 2d 253 (Illinois, 1965).
9. Shain M, Southwick AF: State licensing regulations and hospital liability. *Pub Health Rep* 81(7):581, 1966.

# 2

# The Infection Control Committee

## BACKGROUND OF THE ICC

In the mid-1950s health care practitioners became concerned about the drastically increased incidence of staphylococcal infections and their resistance to penicillin. This prompted the American Hospital Association in 1958 to recommend: "that each hospital should establish Committees on Infections, to devote particular attention to infections which are acquired in hospitals so they may be reduced to the lowest level" (1).

Although there have been some minor changes in recommended membership, functions, and responsibilities, the basic idea has remained throughout the development of infection control practice (2). The most current recommendations of the Joint Commission on Accreditation of Hospitals (JCAH) state: "Responsibility for monitoring the infection control program shall be vested in a multidisciplinary committee" (3).

The goal of the ICC should be the reduction of infections occurring within, or related to, the institution. LaForce put it more strongly, stating that his committee's goals were prevention of infections in hospitalized patients and hospital personnel (4). The ICC is able to approach its goal with more or less success, depending on the strength of its chairperson, its membership, its authority, and its functions within the hospital.

## CHAIRPERSON OF AN ICC

The chairperson of the ICC is "an individual whose credentials document knowledge of, and special interest or experience in infection control" (3).

Brachman states the chairperson should also have specific training in microbiology, epidemiology, or infectious disease (5). The JCAH further recommends that the chairperson be a physician; LaForce agrees, stating that decisions are communicated more effectively from physician to physician (4). It is critical that chairpersons have the respect of their peers in the hospital and community. In some hospitals the chairmanship of the ICC is assumed by the hospital epidemiologist who is knowledgeable and trained in hospital infection control; in others there may be some difficulty in finding an appropriate chairperson with all the desired qualities. Chairpersons who are interested in and willing to learn about infection control and have the respect of their peers can be supplemented by ICPs with experience and education in infection control practice.

In the past, hospitals have assigned the chairperson of the ICC to serve a 1- or 2-year term. This caused a problem in terms of development, continuity, and maintenance of an effective infection control program. Additionally, educational programs for ICC chairpersons are only now being developed. Most medical school programs in which infectious disease fellowships are awarded include few internships in infection control practice. Until these educational programs are more widely available, chairpersons of hospital ICCs may not be adequately prepared for the role. It is imperative, therefore, that the developed skills of the ICC chairperson be adequately utilized and that the chairmanship of the ICC not be rotated frequently.

## MEMBERSHIP OF AN ICC

Standards set by the JCAH provide a guideline for selecting members of the ICC. "Its membership shall include representation from the medical staff, administration, nursing services, and where available, the microbiology section of the laboratory. Any individual employed in a surveillance or epidemiologic capacity shall be a member of the Committee" (3). Additionally, the JCAH recommends committee representation from medical, surgical, pediatric, pathology, and obstetrics–gynecology (OB/Gyn) services, and house staff, if present within the medical staff. A liaison between the ICC and the local or state health department is suggested. Representatives from other areas in the hospital, such as Housekeeping, Maintenance, Laundry, Dietary Services, Central Supply, Operating Room, Engineering, and Pharmacy, should be named to serve on the committee as consultants or ad hoc members, to attend as needed.

A closer look at the required members may be helpful. The medical staff representative is essential to "provide direction and strengthen the clinical aspects of the program" (3). The JCAH standards further direct that no policies or clinical decisions can be made except at meetings where appropriate physician members are present. It is clear, in current hospital practice, that any decisions involving the medical management and care of patients will require physician input in order to be acceptable to other physicians. Furthermore, the expertise of the physician-epidemiologist and other involved physicians may be essential in the decision-making process in clinical areas.

A hospital administrator must be a member of the ICC for an effective infection control program. The hospital administration is responsible for the allocation of funds and resources within the institution and thus plays an important role in the functioning of the infection control activities. Without the support of administration it would be difficult to initiate new programs or to maintain the effectiveness of established programs. Brachman and Haley state that infection control programs have flourished where there is administrative support and are inhibited in their development when administrators are reluctant to provide support and resources (6). The hospital administration will be unable to appreciate these needs unless it is actively involved in the ICC. The administrative member should be high enough in the administrative structure to be able to give the committee realistic expectations of the implementation of their decisions.

The administrative member of the committee is also in a position to help in the implementation of policies, programs, and control measures. The administrator is a key person in the communication, implementation, and enforcement of hospitalwide decisions.

Another essential number of the ICC is from nursing service. There is no other group in the hospital that has a more prolonged, intimate contact with patients than nurses. Their role in infection control is very important from the standpoint of infection risks to personnel as well as to patients. The nursing service representative should be high enough in the nursing service structure to be able to speak as a representative and have authority within the nursing department to implement change. This member should also have a genuine concern for infection control and be instrumental in carrying out recommendations of the ICC at the nursing level.

A representative from the microbiology laboratory is also an essential member of the ICC because of the impact of the infection control program on the laboratory. Routine infection control activities as well as epidemic investigations require close cooperation between the ICC and the microbiology laboratory personnel. A certain amount of laboratory personnel time and supplies will be used for infection control activities, and the laboratory representative should be qualified to address these issues.

The remaining member of the ICC is the ICP. The ICP is responsible for the daily activities of the infection control program and thus is an indispensable member of the ICC. This position in the hospital and its impact on an effective infection control program are discussed in depth in Chapter 3.

The ICP is mainly responsible for implementing the infection control program. The ICP was originally described and continues to be the liaison between the ICC and the personnel of all hospital departments.

**Table 2-1**

EXAMPLES OF INFECTION CONTROL COMMITTEE MEMBERS IN THREE INSTITUTIONS OF VARYING SIZE AND AFFILIATION

| *Small Community Hospital or Extended Care Facility (<100 Beds)* | *Large Community Hospital (>250 Beds)* | *University Medical Center* |
|---|---|---|
| Pathologist (chairperson and representative from microbiology lab) | Surgeon (chairperson and represents surgery) | Hospital epidemiologist (chairperson, representative from pediatrics and codirector of microbiology lab) |
| Associate administrator | Assistant administrator | Associate administrator |
| Director of nursing | Director of laboratory | Assistant director of nursing |
| Infection control practitioner | Associate director of nursing | Head nurse, surgical unit |
| Internist | Head nurse, ICU | Infection control practitioner |
| Surgeon | Infection control practitioner | Anesthesiologist |
| Infectious disease physician | Internist | Director of the burn unit |
| Ad Hoc | | |
| Dietary director | Anesthesiologist | Infectious disease physician |
| Houskeeping director | | |
| Pharmacy director | Neonatologist | OB/Gyn physician |
| Central supply director | OB/Gyn physician | Surgeon |
| | Pathologist | Housekeeping director |
| | Infectious disease physician | Employee health director |
| | Ad Hoc | Ad Hoc |
| | Dietary director | Central supply director |
| | Housekeeping director | Dietary director |
| | Operating room supervisor | Pharmacy director |
| | Central supply director | |
| | Employee health director | |

Both small and large committees can be effective or ineffective. In general, smaller committees are more efficient, but the success of the committee depends on its chairperson, its Infection Control Practitioner, its agenda, and the administrative support given the committee.

Since the JCAH requires departmental representation only from medical staff, administration, nursing, microbiology, and infection control–epidemiology, in each hospital there is a considerable amount of freedom in determining the number of additional members and specific departments or areas to be represented on the committee. In some hospitals, additional members have been drawn from Employee Health (2,4), Blood Bank (2), and the Outpatient Department (2). Because of size, however, an ICC with members representing all the suggested departments and areas may have difficulty in finding times suitable to all and in making progress. Copies of the minutes of all meetings can keep them informed of activities of the ICC in which they are not directly related. Sample committee memberships are shown in Table 2-1.

Himmelsbach recommended that the committee members represent those specialties necessary for an adequate evaluation of infections and that the members be people with respect and prestige in the institution (7). Infection control committees will vary from hospital to hospital, but it is important that the members be interested in infection control, knowledgeable in the subject or willing to spend some time to learn about it, and have an administrative position high enough in their respective departments to both speak for their area of expertise and implement decisions made in the committee.

Ad hoc representation from all patients areas can make the ICC large and unworkable. Smaller committees, made up of individuals actively involved in infection control activities, or persons genuinely interested in control of infections may be more effective. These individuals should be high enough in the hospital hierarchy to make decisions and have the capacity for implementation. Representatives from the medical staff should be committed to infection control, support the ICC decisions, and disseminate committee information to members of their medical subspecialties.

## AUTHORITY

The ICC is a standing committee of the hospital's medical staff. Administratively, it must report its activities, findings, and decisions to the medical staff through the executive committee, to the director of nursing service, and to the chief executive officer of the hospital (3) (Fig. 2-1). Carefully written minutes of each meeting must be kept and made available to all members and also to department heads and chiefs of services as needed.

More specific lines of authority need to be drawn up within each hospital, and without the authority to initiate prompt and necessary corrective action, the ICC is an ineffectual group. Generally, the ICC fits into a staff rather than a line position in the administrative hierarchy. The successful functioning of

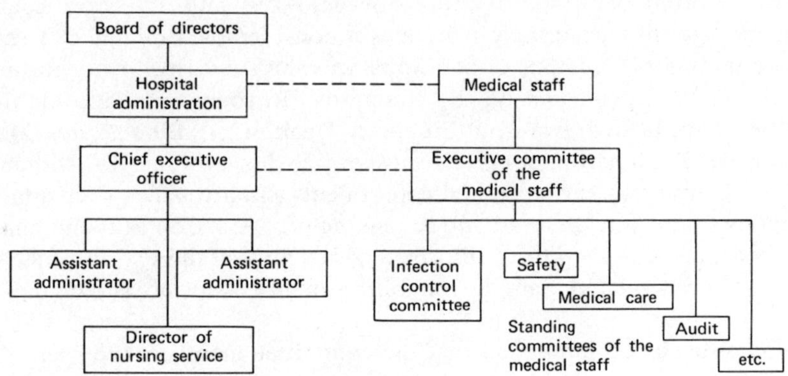

*Figure 2-1*

*The ICC is a standing committee of the medical staff. Its findings and recommendations are reported to the medical staff through its executive committee. The committee is in a staff, not a line, position in the administrative hierachy; the recommendations of the ICC are reported to appropriate members of the hospital administration via the chief executive officer.*

the committee depends on support from the administration and the hospital's board of directors. Specific areas of authority must be delineated in emergencies when critical decisions are needed immediately; for example, if a hospital unit is to be closed during an outbreak of infection. One solution is to give the authority in this case to the chairperson, the appropriate physician (director of the unit in question or chief of the clinical service), and administrator to make emergency decisions in the absence or unavailability of the entire committee. Determining these lines of authority and power in advance and having them approved by the medical staff and hospital administration are crucial early activities of the ICC.

## FUNCTIONS

The ICC gives structure, direction and administrative power to the infection control program. During regular meetings the group serves as a review and recommendation board. Policies, protocols, and results of any surveillance programs are reviewed and recommendations are passed on to other committees, hospital administration, and the medical staff. These review and recommendationfunctions should be examined in greater depth to show the role of the ICC in the infection control program.

## Meetings and Agendas

The ICC is required by the JCAH to meet at least once every 2 months; in order to maintain some continuity, it should meet every month. The agenda and materials should be handed out at least 1 week prior to the meeting and should be appropriate for the level of operation of this committee within the hospital administration. This allows committee members to be well informed prior to the meeting and make appropriate decisions on agenda items.

Daily decisions of the ICP, alone or with the ICC chairperson, should not be made part of the ICC agenda unless they are important as information items.

EXAMPLE. The ICP is consulted by nurses on a surgical floor regarding the appropriate placement of a patient with a wound infection. After talking with nurses and the patient's physician and determining the amount of purulence in the wound, the ICP's recommendation is to place the patient in Wound and Skin Precautions, in a room on the crowded surgical floor with a patient whose wound is nearly healed. This kind of decision should not be brought to the ICC. Even in the event of a disagreement, the ICC chairperson's involvement alone would be sufficient and appropriate. If, however, the question came up repeatedly, the ICP could propose a policy or procedure change to the committee. The Wound and Skin Precautions policy could be modified to specify more clearly the criteria for the placement of patients in this kind of isolation. A change in hospital policy or procedure would be ICC business. Or, if the ICP determined an educational need, a proposal for a change in the infection control program to include an intensive educational program or a proposal to do a study of the transmission of organisms infecting wounds on the surgical floors would need review by the ICC.

## Review Functions

The ICC is charged by the JCAH with reviewing all data collected by the ICP, as well as policies, procedures, and protocols related to the risk of infections in the hospital. Specifically, the ICC reviews the following:

1. *Surveillance data.* Any data collected on nosocomial infections in patients or employees, environmental monitoring, and the results of outbreak investigations must be reviewed by the committee. Surveillance methods and data collected will be discussed in depth later.

2. *Policies and procedures.* All departments and areas must have infection control policies and procedures, which are reviewed by the ICC and approved or modified. In addition, certain policies are hospitalwide,

stemming from the overall hospital policy and procedure manual. For example, isolation policies and procedures are reviewed by the committee since all personnel directly or indirectly involved with patients must abide by these policies.

3. *Protocols.* Protocols for proposed studies as well as the infection control program itself are reviewed by the ICC. The infection control program structure (discussed later), including methods of surveillance, time allocations, and basic components of the program, are reviewed and approved by the committee.

### Recommendation Functions

After review of the results of infection control activities, policies, and procedures, and protocols related to infection control, the ICC makes recommendations to appropriate groups or areas in the hospital. This should be the major function of the committee, and its decisions should be on a high administrative level. The ongoing decisions in infection control practice are made by the ICP, with help as needed from appropriate committee members.

### FUTURE

In the past, the ICC has been the recognized basis for the institution's infection control program. Mallison has stated that "an effective infection control committee is the most important part of a program for control of nosocomial infections" (8). The JCAH standards can be interpreted in such a way that the committee actually develops and conducts the daily business of the infection control program. It is unreasonable to assume that the committee as a whole has the expertise or time to run the infection control program. The ICP, alone or in conjunction with the chairperson, should be responsible for this.

Many hospitals are beginning to examine the role and function of the ICC. These committees have for the most part been recommending rather than authoritative bodies. Hospitals must examine their purpose for the ICC—fulfilling regulatory agencies' requirements or a group committed to the prevention and control of nosocomial infections. More authority should be given to the ICC for implementation of its policies through the ICP, because a committee without this authority is an ineffectual group. The ICC should be a hospital committee whose authority is clearly supported and endorsed by the hospital board or executive committee. The ICC chairperson and the ICP should receive their direction and support from the hospital administration.

The ICC has an administrative and supervisory role in the infection control program, performing this function for other committees, departments, and areas of the institution as well. Through its review and approval functions, the committee sanctions and gives credibility to the daily activities and decisions of the ICP. The ICP develops the expertise needed to implement the program and, in turn, provides the committee with appropriate data, proposals for policy and procedure changes, and the clinical input to help in its decision-making process.

The JCAH has written its new accreditation manual in a style that allows it to be used as an assessment tool by the ICC and the ICP for evaluation of its program (9). In the future more attention may be focused on the ICC concerning the cost:benefit ratio of its infection control practices. As hospital revenues continue to be limited, the ICC will need to constantly modify its practices and assess its direction for reduction of nosocomial infections to their lowest possible level and demonstrate to administration the cost-effectiveness of their activities in achieving this goal (10,11). This will be discussed in Chapter 25.

Diagnosis-related groups (DRGs), as established in 1983 for the reimbursement of Medicare patient hospital costs, have presented the ICC and the ICP with an opportunity to interact directly with administration and demonstrate that nosocomial infections cost the institution in nonreimbursable expenditures (12–14). The ICC must show administration that a strong infection control program with adequate funding will reduce nosocomial infections and save money.

# REFERENCES


1. American Hospital Association: Bulletin 1, Chicago, American Hospital Association, May 21, 1958.
2. American Hospital Association: *Infection Control in the Hospital,* ed 4. Chicago, American Hospital Association, 1979, p 22.
3. *Accreditation Manual for Hospitals 1986: Infection Control.* Chicago, standards adopted by the Board of Commissioners of Joint Commission on Accreditation of Hospitals, 1985, p 71.
4. LaForce FM: The hospital infection control committee: A personal view. *Hosp Pract* 12(1):135, 1977.
5. Brachman PS: Nosocomial infection control: An overview. *Rev Infect Dis* 3(4):640–648 (1981).
6. Brachman PS, Haley HW: Nosocomial infection control: Role of the hospital administrator. *Rev Infect Dis* 3(4):783–784 (1981).
7. Himmelsbach CK: Role of hospital infection committee. Atlanta, Centers for Disease Control.
8. Mallison GF: A hospital program for control of nosocomial infections. *APIC Newsl* 2(1):1, 1974.

9. *Accreditation Manual for Hospitals 1986.* Chicago, standards adopted by the Board of Commissioners of Joint Commission on Accreditation of Hospitals, 1985, p ix.

10. Haley RW: *Managing Hospital Infection Control for Cost Effectiveness.* Chicago, American Hospital Association, 1986.

11. How to design a cost-effective infection control program. *Cost Containment Newsl,* August 13, 1985.

12. Beyt BE Jr, Roxler S, Cavaness J: Prospective payment and infection control. *Infect Control* 6(4):161, 1985.

13. Pinner RW, Haley RW, Blumenstein BA, et al: High cost nosocomial infections. *Infect Control* 3(2):143, 1982.

14. Haley RW, Schaberg DR, Von Allmen SD, et al: Estimating the extra charges and prolongation of hospitalization due to nosocomial infections: A comparison of methods. *J Infect Dis* 141(2):248,1980.

# 3

# The Infection Control Practitioner

**BACKGROUND OF THE INFECTION CONTROL PRACTITIONER**

The idea underlying the position of the ICP may have arisen when, during the Crimean War, Florence Nightingale said that the first requirement of hospitals is that they do no harm to the sick. In 1959, Torbay Hospital in England named the first "Infection Control Sister" as a liaison among all personnel and disciplines in the hospital with respect to asepsis. In the United States, Kathryn Wenzel was named to a similar position in 1963 at Stanford University Medical Center, following a U.S. Public Health Service conference (U.S. National Conference on Institutionally Acquired Infections), where the idea was suggested. Shirley J. Streeter entered a similar position at about the same time at the University of Illinois Research and Education Hospital (1).

The duties and responsibilities of ICPs have not changed much over the years but have become more specific as the field has been defined more clearly. The ICP has been, from the beginning, the central figure in the infection control program (2). The requirements for the position of ICP were varied and nonspecific; now, as more formal educational programs become available, the required preparation for employment in the field of infection control practice is also becoming more stringent. Wenzel's description in 1970 of the ICP's background includes experience in hospital nursing, and she stated that experience in communicable disease care and public health were helpful (2).

## CURRENT QUALIFICATIONS

Although it is not a requirement, the JCAH strongly recommends that an ICP be employed in every hospital. The standards do require an effective and active infection control program and specify many activities and functions that imply the need to designate a responsible person. The American Hospital Association manual states: "The establishment of such a position within a hospital administration represents an advance in infection control, and the position is one that hospitals should establish" (3).

There is no single program that qualifies a person to be an ICP; what is needed is a mixture of education, experience, personal qualifications, and formal and informal training programs that forms an appropriate background to infection control practice. In examining the field of infection control, Imperato added that "there is much variation in the quality of services provided by these nurses, because of tremendous variations in recruiting standards, training, and experience" (4). No single part of this mixture can stand alone, but the varied backgrounds supplement each other to provide the person with the knowledge necessary to practice in the field.

### Formal Education

A variety of backgrounds has led people into the position of ICP. At this time, most ICPs have a background in nursing through either a baccalaureate or a diploma nursing program. There are also ICPs with baccalaureate degrees in medical technology and master's degrees in public health, environmental sciences, nursing, microbiology, and other health care fields. With the exception of diploma-qualified nurses, the bachelor's degree is the minimal degree held by nearly all ICPs.

### Experience

Since at least 75% of the ICPs are nurses, their experience is mostly in nursing. The range of specialties is broad, however, including ICPs from medical, surgical, pediatric, obstetric, public health, and virtually all other areas of nursing. Many ICPs begin their work in infection control in the same hospital in which they acquired their nursing experience, and LaForce states that this is a definite advantage for a successful infection control program (5). Medical technologists usually have experience in the microbiology aspects of their field. Some practitioners additionally have administrative or supervisory experience in health care.

## Personal Qualifications

LaForce states that the ICP must be tactful, tough, well organized, energetic, and reliable (5). Imperato adds, as desirable qualities, punctuality, competence, and self-direction (4). The ICP functions within the hospital as an independent agent and therefore must have enough self-assurance and assertiveness to deal with people at all levels of the organization (6). Although the infection control program may be specifically outlined, the ICP has a lot of freedom in determining the priorities of day-to-day activities. Continuing education is also an area where the ICP needs self-discipline and motivation in order to supplement and to augment the background training and experience that that ICP brought to the position.

## KNOWLEDGE AND ABILITIES

Although some institutions require a nurse as their ICP, it is more important that the person in the position have a good knowledge of hospital skills and services. Mallison states that "the selection, support, training, ability, and effectiveness of the [practitioner] are prime factors in the adequacy of an overall hospital program for control of nosocomial infections" (7). The person selected must have the ability and be given the opportunity to expand and learn, in order to be able to know and deal with people and situations in the following areas. A combination of experience, education, on-the-job training, and formal and informal programs can be used to gain this knowledge.

### Nursing

The ICP must understand nursing procedures related to infection control, including isolation techniques; aseptic technique; proper use of all patient care equipment, such as Foley catheters, ventilators, intravenous catheters, as well as other equipment in the hospital environment; and adequate decontamination, disinfection, and sterilization techniques for the inanimate environment. The ICP should also understand the structure of the nursing department and the responsibilities of the levels of nursing personnel. Nursing is the department in which the ICP will probably spend the most time; therefore, ICPs with nursing backgrounds have a great deal of the required knowledge and expertise to deal with patient care situations.

### Microbiology

The ICP must have a good understanding of microbiology in general and specifically as it relates to patient and employee infections. In order to understand the agents that cause disease, a knowledge of normal human flora, natural pathogens, reservoirs, natural habitats, and characteristics of microorganisms is necessary. Knowledge of laboratory methods that identify microbes will be useful for the correct collection, handling, and interpretation of cultures from patients and the environment. An understanding of antimicrobial sensitivity patterns is essential in order to identify unusual organisms in the hospital. The practitioner who enters the field with a background in medical technology or microbiology will have a good knowledge base on which to build the clinical and other aspects of the infection control program.

### Infectious Diseases

The ICP must understand the most common nosocomial infections, as well as infectious diseases brought into the hospital from the community. The ICP also should know the etiology, course, and spectrum of a disease, its treatment and prevention, and the necessary precautions against infections, both in inpatients and in employees of the institution. A knowledge of immunology, host defense mechanisms, immune deficiency diseases, and other risk factors is also needed for a full understanding of the epidemiology of certain infections and the need for precautions to prevent transmission. A general understanding of antimicrobials is helpful, including action, spectrum, side effects, and the etiology of antimicrobial resistance among microorganisms.

### Epidemiology

A basic knowledge of epidemiology is necessary, and more advanced knowledge may be helpful in certain institutions. With an understanding of research methodologies, biostatistics, tests of significance, the appropriate selection of control groups, and other components of the epidemiologic method, the ICP will be able to make critical evaluations of research in the literature. Nearly all ICPs will be in a position to do some research in the field of infection control—to evaluate a procedure change, to measure changes before and after an educational program, or to do a prospective study of an infection control practice and measure its efficacy in preventing transmission of infection. All ICPs must be able to calculate infection rates and will need an understanding of basic biostatistics in order to interpret the literature as well as to work with the data collected on infections within their own institutions. A knowledge of epidemiologic principles also will be necessary to describe and deal with outbreaks of infections in the institution. The ICP whose educational background includes epidemiology, such as a master's degree in public health, will be well prepared in this area.

## Administration and Supervision

The ICP is the administrator of the infection control program and may be a department head in the hospital structure. As the manager of the infection control program, the ICP will need to know the JCAH and other regulations, including those of the state and local health departments, and how to interpret and implement them throughout the hospital.

Technically, the ICP supervises all hospital employees as their activities relate to infections. Since this is not a line supervision and the ICP does not directly influence job performance or evaluation of the employee, the ICP must have, or develop, effective interpersonal and management skills to motivate these employees to carry out the infection control practices of the institution.

The ICP will need to have administrative skills in areas such as budgeting, program planning, writing reports and keeping adequate records, and management. Skills in teaching, supervision, disciplinary actions, and coordinating different areas to accomplish an objective are necessary. The ICP must have good communication skills.

Infection Control Practitioners may enter the field with advanced educational preparation in administration or supervision, usually in the form of master's degrees in nursing administration, hospital administration, or public health administration. These people should be well qualified to interact with the various departments and levels of personnel in the practice of infection control.

## Environmental Sciences

Although closely related to epidemiology and microbiology, the environmental sciences are another area of expertise required in infection control practice. Infection Control Practitioners must help to formulate policies for departments such as Housekeeping, Maintenance, and Central Supply. The ICP must know the proper handling of biologic waste from clinical laboratories, the operating room, and the pathology laboratory. Ensuring that these areas are safe from an infection control standpoint requires a knowledge of handling systems, adequate disinfection techniques, and public health laws concerning disposal of different kinds of waste from the hospital environment. Certain ICPs enter the field as environmental sanitarians, sometimes with an advanced degree such as a master's degree in public health in environmental sciences, which provides an excellent background for dealing with infection control problems in these areas.

Regardless of the educational preparation a person brings to the field, the knowledge and abilities in infection control practice span several fields. Infection Control Practitioners should supplement their backgrounds with formal and informal education to acquire the necessary knowledge base. Some resources that are available to the beginning ICP are discussed below.

## RESOURCES

### Centers for Disease Control

The Centers for Disease Control (CDC) provide both formal and informal guidance to the ICP. Courses are offered that are specific to infection control practice, as well as training programs and seminars in advanced areas or topics related to infectious diseases. The beginning practitioner should become familiar with programs from the CDC by getting in touch with Centers for Disease Control, Center for Professional Development and Training, Atlanta, GA 30333.

The CDC also publishes several reports, including *Morbidity and Mortality Weekly Report* (8), which has valuable public health and epidemiologic notes. Additionally, CDC personnel have developed guidelines for the prevention of nosocomial infections that include the environment, employee health, and patient care practices. These guidelines are continually being updated as new data become available to support or reject current practices. These guidelines are available in manual form from National Technical Information Service, U.S. Department of Commerce, 5285 Port Royal Road, Springfield, VA 22161, telephone (703) 487-4650. Updated guidelines may be available on request to the ICP from Hospital Infection Program, Center for Infectious Diseases, Centers for Disease Control, Atlanta, GA 30333, and most have been published in the *American Journal of Infection Control.*

The CDC also has developed the *Guidelines for Isolation Precautions in Hospitals* (9), which includes a category-specific card system and a disease-specific system, either of which can be used for isolation. These are discussed in detail later.

### Association for Practitioners in Infection Control

In 1972 an organization was formed to respond to needs felt by a growing number of ICPs. The Association for Practitioners in Infection Control (APIC) has grown to over 7000 members and provides a resource for practitioners in a number of formal and informal ways.

Local chapters host educational programs for beginners, as well as continuing education for experienced practitioners. Affiliation with a chapter also provides ICPs with a peer group and the benefits of group problem solving and support. Membership provides subscription to the *American Journal of Infection Control*, which includes a calendar of training and continuing education programs available in the United States.

Information on APIC membership and benefits can be obtained by writing to: Membership Director, Association for Practitioners in Infection Control, 505 East Hawley Street, Mundelein, IL 60060.

## Other Training Programs and Associations

Hospitals, universities, and health departments throughout the United States are beginning to provide educational programs for ICPs. Certain universities have begun degree programs in infection control. The American Public Health Association, the American Society of Microbiology, and other health care organizations have added hospital epidemiology or infection control sections to their membership and include this topic in their publications and national meetings. The ICP should investigate these programs locally and nationally to obtain the desired training, experience, and continuing education.

## Other Books and References

The American Hospital Association manual *Infection Control in the Hospital* (3) is a valuable reference for infection control and should be studied in detail by every beginning practitioner. The JCAH standards are also helpful as a resource and can be used as an assessment tool by the ICP to determine the strengths and weaknesses of the infection control program (10). It can be obtained directly from the practitioner's hospital administrator. These and other suggested references are listed in Table 3-1 and should be evaluated carefully by the ICP for their usefulness.

## AUTHORITY OF THE INFECTION CONTROL PRACTITIONER

In 1974 the American Hospital Association estimated that an ICP should spend 10 hours in infection control practice for each 100 beds in the institution (3). In 1977, LaForce recommended a full-time ICP for every 200 beds, doubling the estimated need for infection control personnel (5). The need will vary from one hospital to another, depending on the complexity of care in the institution, the level and depth of infection control practice, and the involvement in and commitment to infection control of the hospital administration and medical staff.

**Table 3-1**
## REFERENCES FOR THE INFECTION CONTROL PRACTITIONER

---

**Books and Manuals**

American College of Surgeons: *Manual on Control of Infections in Surgical Patients,* ed 2. Philadelphia, Lippincott, 1984.

American Hospital Association: *Infection Control in the Hospital,* ed 4, Chicago (840 North Lake Shore Drive), 1979.

Axnick K, Yarbrough, M (eds): *Infection Control: An Integrated Approach.* St. Louis, Mosby, 1984.

Benenson Abram S (ed): *Control of Communicable Diseases in Man,* ed 14. Washington, DC, American Public Health Association (1015 Eighteenth Street, NW, Washington, DC 20036), 1985.

Haley RW: *Managing Hospital Infection Control for Cost Effectiveness.* Chicago, American Hospital Association, 1986.

Isolation Precautions for Hospitals, U.S. Department of Health and Human Services, Centers for Disease Control, Atlanta (Government Printing Office Public Documents Section, Superintendent of Documents, Washington, DC), 1983.

Kunin CM: *Detection, Prevention and Management of Urinary Tract Infections,* ed 2. Philadelphia, Lea & Febiger, 1979.

Roderick M (ed): *Infection Control in Critical Care.* Rockville, MD, Aspen Systems Corporation, 1983.

Smith PW: *Infection Control in Long-Term Care Facilities.* New York, Wiley, 1984.

Soule B (ed): *APIC Curriculum for Infection Control Practice,* vols I and II. Dubuque, Iowa, Kendall/Hunt Publishing Company, 1983.

Wenzel RP (ed): *CRC Handbook of Hospital Acquired Infections.* Boca Raton, FL, CRC Press, 1981.

**Periodicals**

*American Journal of Infection Control*
CV Mosby Company
11830 Westline Industrial Drive
St. Lewis, MO 63146
*Hospital Infection Control*
American Health Consultants
67 Peachtree Drive, NE
Atlanta, GA 30309
*Infection Control*
Charles B. Slack
6900 Grove Road
Thorofare, NJ 08086
*Infection Control Digest*
American Hospital Association
840 North Lake Shore Drive
*The Journal of Hospital Infections*
Academic Press
111 Fifth Avenue
New York, NY 10003
*Morbidity and Mortality Weekly Report*
Massachusetts Medical Society
CSPO Box 9120
Waltham, MA 02254-9120

---

The position of the ICP in the hospital administrative structure has been unclear. Since many ICPs are nurses, many are administratively in the Department of Nursing Service and report directly to the Director of Nursing. In 1970, Wenzel suggested that the ICP be under the jurisdiction of the Division of Infectious Diseases of the Department of Medicine and report to the division head, who would also be the chairperson of the Infection Control Committee (2). Other ICPs are directly responsible to the chief executive officer or one of the assistant or associate administrators of the hospital. Still others are based in the Microbiology, Pathology, Housekeeping, or Central Supply departments.

Infection Control Practitioners must be free agents in the hospital, unhindered by their administrative departments in investigating, implementing, recommending, and enforcing control measures. Infection Control Practitioners have successfully run infection control programs from all the above-mentioned departments, but many have expressed problems related to their administrative positions.

Infection Control Practitioners under Nursing Service, in particular, have found difficulties in some institutions in accomplishing their objectives; problems have arisen when a strong director of nursing has insisted on dictating the priorities of the infection control program without an adequate appreciation of the scope of infection control practice. Other problems have resulted from the ICP's inability to investigate freely and control problems related to Nursing Service, because of the ICP's position within that department.

Infection Control Practitioners in departments such as Microbiology, Housekeeping, or Central Supply have expressed problems in implementing control measures and in having an impact on patient-care practices in the hospital. An ICP in one of the many patient-care service departments may feel too removed from the main decision-making departments and people because of inadequate communication lines.

The ICP ideally should be under the highest administrative area or department within the hospital structure, in order to function freely in the system and to have direct communication lines to and from all hospital areas and departments. This area probably would be the hospital administration or the medical staff. The position itself should be on the level of a department head, such as Central Supply, Radiology, Housekeeping, and the like. A practitioner coming into a newly created position should examine the hospital structure carefully to ensure this freedom; a practitioner having communication problems or difficulties in recommending or implementing change or enforcing control measures should approach the appropriate people to discuss a restructuring of the position within the hospital hierarchy.

The ICP's salary has varied according to the level and location of the position and the background and qualifications of the person hired. These variations will continue until some regulated, uniform requirements, such as certification or licensure, are adopted by a regulating agency, such as the JCAH or APIC. In general, taking into consideration education and experience, the ICP should receive a salary comparable to that of the middle management department heads.

## FUTURE ROLE OF THE INFECTION CONTROL PRACTITIONER

At the present time, the training and experience in and the level of infection control practice are variables determined by the practitioner and the hospital. The practitioner brings a background to the position and, largely through self-direction and motivation, expands this background to fill in needed knowledge from formal and informal resources. The hospital structures the position administratively and has input into the position through employment requirements and its willingness to fund training and continuing education for the practitioner. Currently, these programs offer continuing education units in nursing, administration, or in whatever field the practitioner is experienced.

Organizations and agencies such as APIC and the American Nursing Association (ANA) have been actively involved in developing uniform requirements for infection control practice necessary for ICPs. APIC has been a leader in assessing the needs of the ICP. It has outlined eight standards of prerequisite knowledge, developed a two-volume curriculum for study (11) and initiated a certification examination to test the proficiency of the ICP. This, in addition to 2 years of infection control experience by the ICP, has led to a recognized certification process in infection control. Certification is a voluntary, nongovernmental process but has set a recognized standard of competency in infection control practices for a group that has diversified backgrounds, philosophies, and priorities. Competency on the examination entitles the practitioner to use the title, "Certified in Infection Control" (CIC).

The ICP must utilize management skills to make changes indicated by data assessment and must be attuned to the problems of fiscal restraint and continue to offer, with administrative support, effective infection control programs that monitor, analyze, and control nosocomial infections at minimal cost but without compromising patient care.

## REFERENCES


1. Garner JS: Nurse epidemiologist instrumental in infection control. *Assoc Operating Room Nurses J* 20(2):261, 1974.
2. Wenzel K: The role of the infection control nurse. *Nurs Clin North AM* 5(1):89, 1970.

3. American Hospital Association: *Infection Control in the Hospital,* ed 4. Chicago, American Hospital Association, 1979, p 29.

4. Imperato PJ, Drusin TM, Lewis M, et al: The New York City nurse–epidemiology program. *Bull NY Acad Med* 53(6):569, 1977.

5. LaForce FM: The hospital infection control committee: A personal view. *Hosp Pract* 12(1):135, 1977.

6. Cassem N: The infection control nurse—a nurse without a peer. Toronto, *Proceedings of the First Annual North American Eastern Conference on Infection Control,* 1973, p 4.

7. Mallison GF: A hospital program for control of nosocomial infections. *APIC Newsl* 2(1), 1974.

8. *Morbidity and Mortality Weekly Report,* Centers for Disease Control, Waltham, Massachusetts Medical Society.

9. *Guidelines for Isolation Precautions in Hospitals,* U.S. Department of Health and Human Services, Atlanta, Centers for Disease Control, 1983.

10. *Accreditation Manual for Hospitals 1986; Infection Control.* Chicago, standards adopted by the Board of Commissioners of Joint Commission on Accreditation of Hospitals, 1985.

11. Soule, BM (ed): *The APIC Curriculum for Infection Control Practice.* Association for Practitioners in Infection Control, vols 1 and 2, 1983.

# 4

# The Infection Control Program

The infection control program in an institution should be evaluated and revised annually by the ICC. Priorities of the program will need revision based on the results and analysis of surveillance data. Regardless of the size or type of institution or the level of patient care given, several general components of an infection control program will be present. These components fall into two general categories—surveillance and reporting, and control and prevention.

## COMPONENTS OF AN INFECTION CONTROL PROGRAM

### Surveillance and Reporting

Data collection, tabulation, and analysis have traditionally been the cornerstones of an infection control program. Within any institution, there are several sources and populations at risk that need monitoring.

#### *Patient Infections*

Data on patients with infections are collected in varying degrees of detail; in some institutions both nosocomial and community-associated infections are surveyed. The purposes of collecting these data are to establish baseline infection rates for different units or services, determine problem areas or areas where inservice education could lower infection rates, and identify outbreaks of infections rapidly.

EXAMPLE.   The ICP surveyed a surgical intensive care unit and collected data on all nosocomial infections for a 6-month period. The infection rate was highest for postoperative pneumonias, higher than the rate of urinary tract infections for the unit. Following observation of suctioning techniques, aseptic techniques in handling respiratory therapy equipment, and isolation procedures, the ICP gave a series of in-service education classes and informal discussions on these subjects for the intensive care staff. A 3-month follow-up of collected data revealed a lower infection rate for pneumonias, second to urinary tract infections, and follow-up observations showed greater awareness of aseptic techniques by nursing personnel.

### *Personnel Infections*

Infections among personnel must be monitored and these data analyzed. The ICP should be aware of employee exposure to communicable diseases, accidents related to contaminated equipment or material, and employees who come to Health Service exhibiting communicable diseases.

EXAMPLE. The ICP was called by the laboratory when the test result of a sputum culture from a patient on a medical floor was positive for *Mycobacterium tuberculosis*. From a review of the patient's chart and a discussion with medical and nursing personnel, the ICP determined that the patient had a productive cough, changes on x-ray films (the patient's admitting diagnosis was pneumonia), and had not been isolated. Working with the Health Service personnel, the ICP made a list of all the people exposed to the patient during his hospitalization. These people were notified, and Health Services provided purified protein derivative skin tests for tuberculosis (PPDs) within the week and again 8 weeks after exposure. No employees converted from negative to positive when the skin test results were read, and the ICP gave an in-service class to the medical unit personnel on the epidemiology of tuberculosis, stressing that tuberculosis should be suspected among certain groups of patients with the appropriate set of symptoms.

### *Environment*

Certain areas of the hospital environment must be monitored. All-steam autoclaves and ethylene oxide (EO) sterilizers must be routinely tested with live biologic indicators at the intervals required by the JCAH. The ICP may need to take microbiologic cultures of the environment during outbreaks of infection when environmental reservoirs are suspected. Environmental surveillance also includes continuous observation of the environment in patient care units and hospital departments for infection hazards.

EXAMPLE. While on rounds, an ICP noticed a stainless-steel covered pitcher labeled "for clean catches" in the clean utility room of a surgical unit. Inside were cotton balls in some solution. The ICP learned from one of the nurses that the pitcher contained sterile saline and soaked cotton balls; the nurses would take some out with their hands, put them into a paper cup, and give them to a patient with instructions to use the cotton balls for cleansing before obtaining a clean catch urine specimen. The ICP removed the pitcher and gave the nurses informal (and later a formal) in-service training on obtaining clean catches with soap, water, and fresh cotton balls, and explained the potential hazard of reservoirs of opened containers of "sterile" solutions. The ICP later found that the microbiology laboratory had received four clean catch specimens that grew 1000–10,000/ml of *Pseudomonas* sp. The pitcher contents were also positive for the same organism.

Because the urine specimens did not indicate clinical infection (>100,000 organisms/ml) the ICP would not have normally received the four reports. Through environmental surveillance, the ICP was able to find a potential hazard; although the patients did not have infections, all were potential kidney transplant recipients and may have preoperatively colonized their periurethral regions with this *Pseudomonas,* with the possibility of subsequent problems occurring after surgery.

### *Communicable Diseases*

The ICP is generally responsible for reporting all communicable diseases to the appropriate health authorities. Through close association with the microbiology laboratory, the practitioner can be notified of cultures or other tests positive for reportable organisms such as *Salmonella, Shigella,* or diseases such as tuberculosis, hepatitis, and others. Reportable diseases diagnosed without culture, such as measles, must be detected through routine surveillance or some other mechanism by which the ICP is notified.

All the data generated through surveillance activities must be reported. Specific methods of data collection and reporting will be discussed in Chapters 14–17. Nearly all the information is reported to the ICC for its evaluation. The evaluation should be used to restructure the infection control program on a continuing basis, improve patient care, and minimize infection risks to patients and hospital personnel.

## Control and Prevention

Of equal importance in the infection control program are control and prevention activities. Later discussion will show the relative emphasis that should be placed on surveillance and prevention activities in institutions of varying sizes and in infection control programs in varying stages of development. The following aspects of control and prevention activities should be components of any infection control program.

### *Teaching and Consulting*

All new employees must be taught infection control principles and the isolation policies and procedures in use at the institution. Continuing education in infection control for all departments and areas of the hospital is also required by the JCAH. This teaching should be based on surveillance data, observations of procedures and the environment, and requests from hospital personnel for in-service training. Depending on the size and affiliation of the institution, the ICP may teach nursing, medical, medical technologist, radiology, respiratory therapy, and other students.

Consultation, on a formal and informal basis, is probably the most important means of preventing and controlling infections. Some ICPs are responsible for supervising the placement of any patient into isolation, a policy that affords an opportunity for informal teaching and minimizes the chances of inappropriate isolation.

EXAMPLE.  The ICP was paged by a nurse on a medical floor because a patient was admitted whose test result for hepatitis B antigen ($HB_sAg$) was positive. The nurse asked whether this patient needed isolation, and if so, what kind. The ICP explained the hospital policy that $HB_sAg$-positive patients did not need a private room if their hygiene was good. Since the patient's liver function tests were normal, it indicated no active disease and a patient who was an asymptomatic carrier of $HB_sAg$. The ICP reminded the nursing personnel that even without active disease the patients blood and other body fluids were infectious and caution, such as the use of disposable gloves, should be used when handling needles or other articles contaminated with blood. She also pointed out that all laboratory and other procedure requisition forms should be marked "isolation—blood precautions" for alerting personnel involved in the processing and handling of these specimens and/or patients.

The ICP was able to teach the nursing personnel, on this informal basis, who the persons at risk would be, what procedures would expose them to the risk of acquiring or transmitting the virus, and what precautions were necessary because of the presumed level of infectiousness of this patient.

Consultation may also extend beyond the hospital itself, into the community, neighboring extended care facilities, or other institutions. Infection Control Practitioners frequently make use of each other's expertise.

EXAMPLE. A university medical center hired a play therapist for the pediatric areas of the hospital. The therapist used many pieces of hospital equipment as well as toys in interacting with children who were surgical patients, both before and after they underwent their operations, and with children who had various medical diseases. The ICP was consulted on the method of

decontamination and disinfection of this equipment. In addition to looking into the literature on the subject, the ICP consulted the ICP at a children's hospital in the same town, where a similar program had been in existence for several years.

### Administrative Activities

Another component of the infection control program includes all administrative activities necessary to implement the decisions of the ICC. The first of these activities is the generation of a hospitalwide infection control manual. This manual contains all hospital policies and procedures related to infection control. An example of a table of contents for an infection control manual can be seen in Table 4-1.

Second, the infection control program includes the development of infection control sections for every other hospital department's policy and procedure manual in addition to the hospitalwide manual that is available in each department.

EXAMPLE. A hospital infection control manual has a policy that states "patients with communicable diseases will be appropriately isolated". The procedures in the manual discuss proper gowning, gloving, and masking techniques, as well other procedures necessary for all people in the hospital who have contact with the patient.

The Radiology Department in the same hospital has a policy and procedure manual that is specific for that area. In the infection control section, one of their policies states "patients who require isolation can be seen in the Radiology Department, and appropriate precautions will be carried out in the department to minimize the risk of transmission of infections to others." Their procedures outline specific precautions to be taken, including handling of x-ray equipment, where the patient is to stay if waiting is necessary, and decontamination and disinfection procedures that are specific for the personnel, the area, and the equipment of that department.

The listing of specific policies and procedures for each hospital department is beyond the scope of this text. However, references are available, such as a manual that can be purchased and modified for use in any institution (1), as well as the American Hospital Association manual (2). The JCAH guidelines can be consulted, since they outline specific areas that must be covered for certain departments (3).

Third, a part of the infection control program is input into other administrative committees. The ICP is frequently a member not only of the ICC but of other standing committees of the medical staff such as Safety, Standardization or Product Evaluation, Pharmacy, and Medical Audit. The ICP serves as a representative of the infection control program and also is the hospital expert on infection control.

EXAMPLE. A state hospital began to take bids for Foley catheters. The policy was that unless there were specific reasons for refusing a product, the lowest bidder would get the year's contract. A standardization committee was formed of various persons in and outside patient care to evaluate products to insure that the product with the lowest bid would be acceptable by all concerned.

The Foley catheter that had the lowest bid did not have a specimen port and was made of silicone. The ICP recognized that needle aspiration for specimens could not be done because the silicone would not close over the needle hole; the only way to obtain specimens would be to break open the urinary drainage system. As a member of the Standardization Committee, the ICP brought up this objection and gave supporting data on the incidence and likelihood of urinary tract infections with open drainage systems. The committee agreed to sign a contract for a more expensive catheter that had a sampling port, so that specimens could be obtained without opening the drainage system.

The portion of time spent by ICPs in ICC activities is the greatest of all their administrative committee work. The ICP is responsible for communicating the findings, analysis, and results of all infection control program activities to the committee. The committee as a whole then can review and revise the program as needed.

### Special Studies

Regardless of the size of the institution, a portion of the infection control program should be devoted to the investigation of new products, old procedures, or other aspects of patient care that could lead to lower infection risks to patients and personnel.

EXAMPLE. In one hospital, the ICC approved the use of either an iodophor solution or chlorhexidine gluconate for handwashing in the newborn nursery. The ICP designed a simple study, using the geographic division of the nursery, to test the iodophor product against chlorhexidine gluconate for irritation of the hands. It was assumed that if a product was irritating, nurses would wash less frequently; this variable was explored, since both products were acceptable from an infection control standpoint if used properly.

## PRIORITIES OF AN INFECTION CONTROL PROGRAM

The components of the infection control program—surveillance, reporting, prevention, and control—are present in every institution but in varying

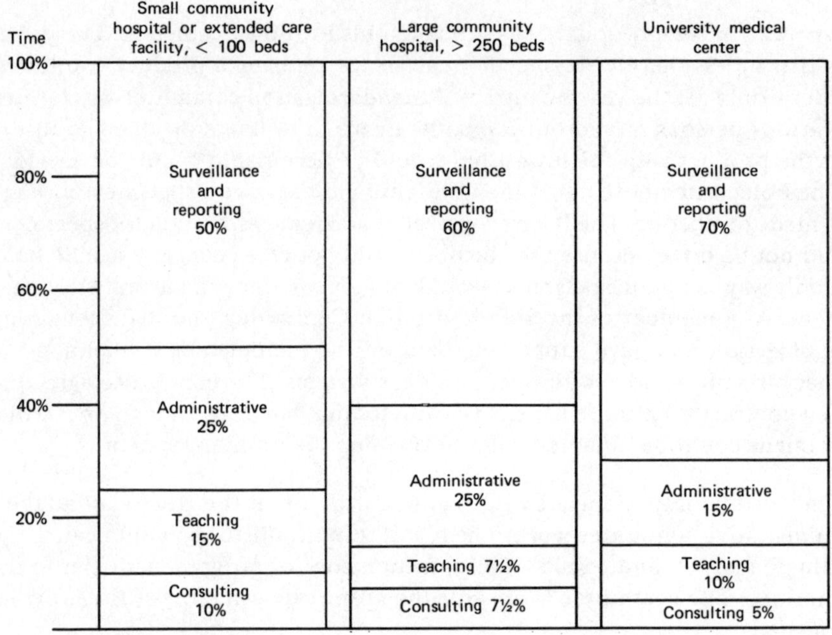


*Figure 4-1*

*Examples of time spent in setting up infection control programs, by size and type of institution. In setting up a program, much time is needed for surveillance and reporting infections to establish baseline infection rates. Smaller institutions will generally require less time to do total hospital data collection than will larger facilities because of the increased complexity of care. Little time is spent in teaching and consulting, partly because personnel do not know of the availability of the ICP. Administrative activities consume a great amount of time because of the need to develop infection control manuals, in both hospitalwide manuals and the infection control sections of departmental manuals.*

degrees. The priorities of an infection control program depend upon the size of the institution and level of care given, the ratio of ICPs to beds, and the stage of development of the program. If there are not enough ICPs to implement the program, not all components will be addressed adequately.

In the development of an infection control program, one of the first priorities is to determine baseline infection rates. Therefore, the ICP who is setting up a new program will spend proportionately more time in surveillance and reporting activities. In addition to becoming familiar with the hospital, the ICP will, through surveillance activities, be a highly "visible" person; other hospital personnel will learn that this person is available for answering

| Time | Small community hospital or extended care facility, < 100 beds | Large community hospital, > 250 beds | University medical center |
|---|---|---|---|
| 100% | Special studies 10% | Special studies 10% | Special studies 30% |
| 80% | Surveillance and reporting 20% | Surveillance and reporting 20% | |
| 60% | Administrative 10% | Administrative 20% | Surveillance and reporting 20% |
| | Teaching 45% | Teaching 15% | Administrative 10% |
| 40% | | | Teaching 20% |
| 20% | | Consulting 35% | |
| | Consulting 15% | | Consulting 20% |

**Figure 4-2**

*Examples of time spent in infection control activities in programs 1–2 years old, by size and type of institution. After a program has been well established, less time is needed for surveillance and reporting activities. Additionally, once infection control manuals (hospitalwide and departmental sections) have been completed, only annual review is necessary, so that administrative time can be decreased. More time is then allocated to teaching, consulting, or special studies.*

questions and for support in infection control decisions. This visibility is important for the success of an infection control program.

Figure 4-1 shows suggested time allotments for newly organized infection control programs in hospitals of varying sizes. Proportions of total time are used, regardless of the number of ICPs employed, assuming that the number is sufficient to implement a good program.

Priorities can and should change after the infection control program has been in operation for a time. The time needed for developing an infection control manual and helping department heads develop infection control sections in their manuals is much greater than the time needed to review this material annually. Likewise, the time that was used initially in surveillance activities to determine baseline infection rates should be allotted to prevention and control efforts after the program has been under way a year or more. Figure 4-2 shows suggested time allotments in the same three hospitals 1 or 2 years after implementation of an infection control program. In smaller hospitals, ICPs can more easily continue to collect data and may choose to do so in order to maintain high visibility. By contrast, in larger hospitals the ICP may have to spend more time for baseline data collection and would need to modify surveillance activities more drastically after these data have been collected, in order to accomplish other objectives.

## SUMMARY

The infection control program in any institution has the same basic components of surveillance, reporting, prevention, and control. Some of these aspects are covered in more detail in subsequent chapters. The beginning of an infection control program requires time commitment by the ICP, the ICC, and other hospital personnel to determine baseline infection rates and to establish policies and procedures to minimize infection risks. In McGuckin's opinion, however, continuous data collection activities are time-consuming and may be an inefficient way of conducting infection control (4). However, Haley states in the SENIC Report that establishment of intensive infection surveillance and control programs was strongly associated with reductions in rates of nosocomial infections (5). The ICC should revise the program in order to make it more active in terms of prevention and control of infections, and data collection activities should be continued in high-risk areas and limited in low-risk areas to those necessary for the detection of infection outbreaks and special studies.

## REFERENCES


1. Craig CP, Reifsnyder DN: Departmental Procedures for Infection Control Programs, New Jersey, Medical Economics Company, 1977.
2. American Hospital Association: *Infection Control in the Hospital*, ed 4. Chicago, American Hospital Association, 1979.
3. *Accreditation Manual for Hospitals 1986*. Chicago, standards adopted by the Board of Commissioners of Joint Commission on Accreditation of Hospitals, 1985.
4. McGuckin MA, Abrutyn E: Surveillance method for early detection of nosocomial outbreaks. *APIC J* 7(1):18, 1979.
5. Haley RW, Culver DH, White JW, et al: The efficacy of infection surveillance and control programs in preventing nosocomial infections in US hospitals. *Am J Epidemiol* 121(2):182, 1985.

# PART TWO

# EPIDEMIOLOGY OF NOSOCOMIAL INFECTIONS

# 5

# The Chain of Infection

In this chapter we will examine the epidemiology of nosocomial infections and specifically, how infections occur in the hospital setting. Three components are necessary for the development of an infection: a source of infectious organisms, a method of transmission, and a susceptible host. The mechanics and interaction of these three components are often referred to as the *chain of infection*. When all components are present under the right circumstances, an infection develops (Fig. 5-1).

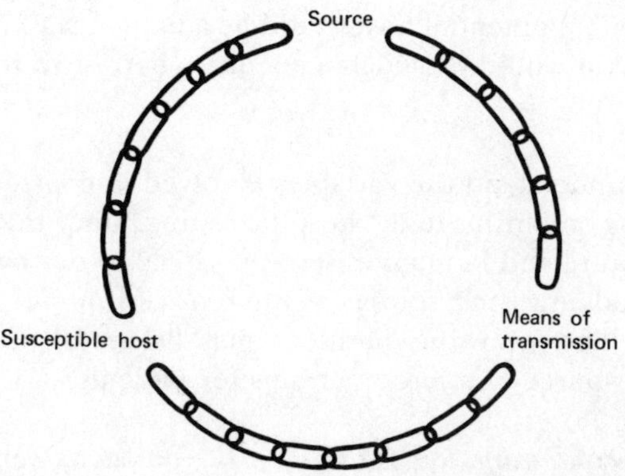


**Figure 5-1**

*For an infection to occur, all three parts of the infection chain must be present, and all criteria must be met.*

## SOURCES OF INFECTING ORGANISMS

Very few things in the world are sterile or remain sterile after contact with the environment. People are colonized with a multitude of microorganisms, as are other forms of life. Within hospitals, any person, including patients, personnel, or visitors, can be a source of infecting organisms. When one is a source of organisms to oneself, the resulting infection is called *endogenous*. An infection from a source outside the person's own body is called *exogenous*.

In addition to the animate environment, the inanimate environment in an institution provides possible sources of infecting organisms. It has been shown that the inanimate environment comprising walls, floors, sinks, drains, faucets, drapes, and countertops rarely is the cause of nosocomial infections (1,2). The most significant sources of infecting organisms in the inanimate environment are from objects that become contaminated with organisms from infected patients or organisms carried on the hands of personnel. They can then be transmitted to invasive devices such as intravenous or Foley catheters (3–5).

EXAMPLE. An intravenous fluid bottle that is cracked and has become contaminated should be considered a significant source of infecting organisms. The fluid is a good growth medium for the survival and proliferation of the organisms. The fluid is administered via tubing directly into the bloodstream, which is normally sterile, bypassing normal defense mechanisms, the skin in particular.

By contrast, a floor that has been contaminated by the feces of an incontinent patient presents a relatively lower infection risk under normal circumstances. The floor does not provide a good environment for the survival of microorganisms, since it is cold and dry. Furthermore, under normal circumstances contact with a potential host would be a patient walking over the floor barefoot. Intact skin would provide an adequate barrier to inoculation of the organisms.

The ICP must understand the variables involved in considering a potential source of infecting organisms in the hospital setting. Since microorganisms are widespread in nature and in many cases are critical to our own life functions, the ICP must evaluate each source of microorganisms for its potential for infecting others. The following questions may be useful in determining the relative risk of a source of microorganisms for patients and personnel.

1. *How much contamination is there on the object or person?* The object may have been grossly contaminated with microorganisms, such as a used, wet dressing from an infected wound, or the contamination may have been light, such as a dry blood pressure cuff. A person may have heavily contaminated

hands from helping a coworker change the sheets of an incontinent patient. By contrast, a nurse may have little exogenous contamination on the hands after adjusting the flow rate on a patient's IV setup.

2. *What is the virulence of the organism?* The patient with a *Pseudomonas* wound infection may be considered a source of infecting organisms to another patient who has a Foley catheter. These organisms, transmitted via the hands of personnel, may be considered more virulent because they are causing disease in the patient's wound. By contrast, the *Pseudomonas* that can be recovered from the sink may not cause disease when transmitted onto the second patient's Foley catheter. That is, a greater number of organisms may need to be directly inoculated into the bladder, for instance, for an infection to occur. The *Pseudomonas* causing the wound infection may be transmitted in fewer numbers, and infection may occur more readily because of their increased virulence, which is demonstrated by the fact that they are causing the disease in the first patient's wound. Additionally, certain organisms are naturally more virulent than others. Few *Shigella* organisms need to be ingested for infection to occur, whereas the normal adult needs to ingest a large number of *Salmonella* organisms in order to acquire a gastroenteritis due to this enteric pathogen. The following formula may express this better:

$$\text{Infection} = \frac{\text{number} \times \text{virulence}}{\text{resistance of host}}$$

The more virulent the organism, the fewer are needed to cause infection, and conversely, infection can still be caused by an organism of low virulence, provided enough of them are inoculated. The third factor is host resistance; the better the host's defense mechanisms, the less likely infection will occur, even by large numbers of virulent microorganisms. Conversely, relatively low numbers of avirulent organisms can cause infections in people with extremely low resistance, as evidenced by the infections and causative organisms in severely compromised patients.

3. *What does the object or person provide microorganisms in the way of a favorable environment for survival or growth?* An opened bottle of sterile saline used for irrigation of a patient's catheter is likely to become contaminated during use. The fluid provides a good medium for bacterial growth. If the fluid is allowed to stand at room temperature, some organisms may grow to large numbers that would subsequently be inoculated into the patient's bladder. Similarly, a carefully prepared hyperalimentation solution may also have been contaminated; therefore, these IV solutions are refrigerated, thus greatly slowing or stopping microbial growth. Additionally, both these solutions are dated and discarded, if not used within 24 hours, to minimize the risk of a time interval long enough for significant bacterial growth to occur. The

hands of personnel provide a moist, warm environment for bacterial survival. Therefore a nurse's hands can carry organisms from an infected patient to a potential host. By contrast, of less significance is the nurse's uniform, which can become contaminated with microorganisms as bed linens are changed, for example; however, if the uniform is dry, most bacteria soon die. Walls, floors, and other inanimate objects may become contaminated with potential pathogens, but many of the objects in a patient's environment do not provide the right conditions to permit bacterial survival over long periods of time.

4. *What kind of contact will the person or object (the source) have with a potential host?* A fiberoptic bronchoscope used on a patient who has bacterial pneumonia may become contaminated with microorganisms during this procedure. This instrument must be adequately decontaminated and disinfected before being used on another patient (3). This piece of equipment must be considered a significant potential source of infecting organisms, because during its use normal host defense mechanisms are bypassed and infectious organisms are inoculated directly into the lower respiratory tract (6). Other invasive equipment includes Foley catheters, intravenous equipment, and respiratory therapy equipment. By contrast, some equipment that becomes contaminated may not be used in invasive procedures. A blood pressure cuff or a tourniquet are patient-care devices that, although they can become grossly contaminated with microorganisms, generally come in contact with intact skin and therefore are considered less likely to transmit infections under normal circumstances. The hands of personnel, again, can become grossly contaminated, but the risk to patients from this source is also relative, depending on the invasiveness of the procedures done. A nurse with grossly contaminated hands (e.g., from a previous patient procedure) who turns a patient or helps the patient off a bedpan may not transmit organisms to that patient that will cause an infection. However, if the same nurse were to provide tracheostomy care or intravenous catheter care without handwashing, organisms from the nurse's hands could colonize and later infect that patient. The source should be considered with respect to the amount of contamination, the ability of organisms to survive or grow in the source, or the length of time from contamination to contact with a potential host, the virulence of the organism, and the relative invasiveness or intimacy of contact that the source will have with the potential host. The ICP must evaluate all these variables to determine and remove or control significant sources of infective organisms in the hospital environment.

## MEANS OF TRANSMISSION

The second necessary link in the chain of infection is the means of transmission, or the manner by which organisms get from the source to a potential host. Obviously, a source of potential pathogens can do no harm to a person unless that person has some contact with it, especially intimate or invasive contact. These methods of transmitting infectious agents have been divided into four general categories: contact, airborne, vehicle, and vector.

In addition to evaluating the relative significance of a source of microorganisms, the ICP must have a good understanding of the routes by which these organisms could spread to susceptible persons.

EXAMPLE.  A patient has active tuberculosis that has just been diagnosed and begins treatment with Isoniazid (INH) and Rifampin. The patient, who is in Respiratory Isolation, finishes dinner; the nurse wears a mask to enter the room and pick up the patient's tray. The tray is handled normally with the other patient trays by the Dietary Department personnel.

Although the patient's dietary utensils may be contaminated with the tubercle bacilli, the means of transmission of this organism is the airborne route; susceptible people need to inhale very small ($<10$ $\mu$m in diameter) particles containing the bacteria to become infected. Contaminated food or utensils, therefore, pose a minimal risk of transmission of tuberculosis and do not need special handling.

Knowledge of the routes by which infections are transmitted within hospitals will further aid the ICP in evaluating infection risks.

## SUSCEPTIBLE HOST

The last necessary link in the infection chain is the susceptible host. Without a person who is susceptible to infection, of whatever kind or in whatever site, an infection cannot occur.

EXAMPLE.  A child is admitted to a semiprivate room for diagnostic urologic tests; the child's roommate has nearly recovered from open-heart surgery to correct a congenital defect. They play together in their room, sharing toys; 48 hours later the urology patient develops clinical signs and symptoms of chickenpox. The roommate has a positive history of the disease during the previous year.

The urology patient could be considered the source of the infecting organism, the varicella-zoster virus. The means of transmission during the incubation period would be through contact on mucous membranes with droplets from the patient's upper respiratory tract (later, the contact route would also be possible from the open, draining lesions characteristic of the disease). The patient's roommate certainly was exposed to the virus by the appropriate means for transmission to occur, but he was not a susceptible host, since previous infection confers immunity. Therefore, the chain of infection was not completed, and an infection did not result in the roommate.

Certain events, especially those occurring during hospitalization, can alter host susceptibility and make patients as a group more susceptible to infections, as opposed to the population in the community.

EXAMPLE. Two patients are housed in the same room on a surgical floor; one has a *Pseudomonas* infection in a surgical wound, which is draining heavily. The other patient has a well-healed hernia repair wound and is nearly ready for discharge. Transmission of the *Pseudomonas* may occur via the hands of personnel or patient care equipment, but the roommate of the infected patient has essentially intact skin and no IV equipment, Foley catheter, or other invasive devices into which these organisms could be inoculated. The patient is nearly a normal host, on whom colonization with this organism would probably not lead to infection.

This patient's susceptibility would be increased, however, if the wound were open (break in normal barrier of the skin) or if a Foley catheter, an IV catheter, or a tracheostomy or endotracheal tube (invasive device) were inserted. Organisms transmitted to the patient's body could then invade and cause infection.

Another factor that increases host susceptibility is chronic underlying disease, such as diabetes, immune deficiency diseases, neoplasms, or leukemia. Therapeutic measures taken to deal with one medical problem may increase susceptibility to infections; for example, immunosuppression therapy, radiation therapy, antibiotic therapy, and insertion of medical equipment. Additionally, certain population groups have increased susceptibility to infections, such as the very young and the very old.

## BREAKING THE CHAIN OF INFECTION

The components of each part of the infection chain are summarized in Figure 5-2. Breaking the chain involves interrupting one or more event in the series, and this is the purpose of infection control practice (Fig. 5-3).

Because bacteria are ubiquitous in the hospital environment, infection control policies and procedures should be devised and enforced to limit and control these sources of potential pathogens, to prevent their transmission. Handwashing has been called the single most important measure in preventing the transmission of infections in hospitals (7,8). Specific handwashing

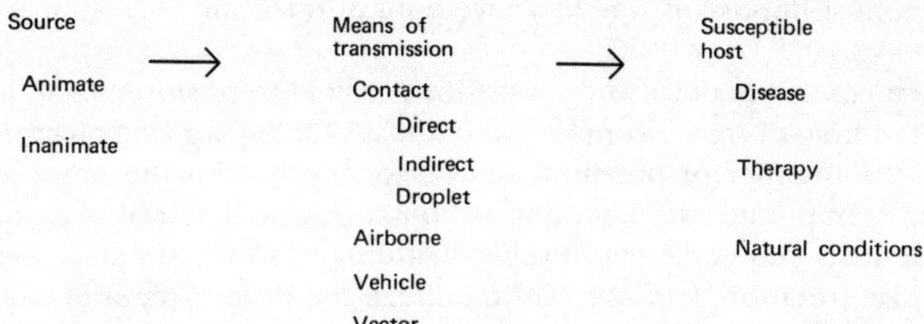


**Figure 5-2**

*A number of factors within each part of the infection chain are responsible for the many ways infections occur and can be spread within hospitals.*

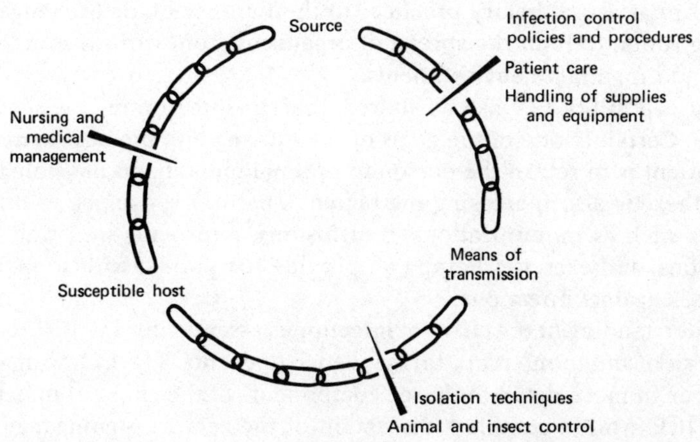


**Figure 5-3**

*Infection control activities focus mostly on breaking the infection chain by controlling the numbers and kinds of reservoirs of microorganisms in the hospital and limiting or preventing transmission of these organisms. Medical and nursing management are important in breaking the chain by making the patient less susceptible to infection and thus improving overall patient health.*

procedures are outlined in detail in Chapter 18, **Isolation Techniques**. Through adequate handwashing, the hands of personnel do not become sources of organisms that can be transmitted from one patient to another; this is the most important way that the chain of infection in hospitals can be broken.

Infection control policies and procedures related to trash removal, laundry service, handling of sterile supplies, and housekeeping are also measures that decrease the number of potential sources of bacteria in the hospital environment. Prompt and safe handling of contaminated material is required to protect patients and personnel. Proper handling of sterile supplies, including their storage, rotation, and use, will minimize the development of sources of infecting organisms.

The chain of infection can also be interrupted at the means of transmission stage. Isolation techniques, based on the method by which each infection is spread, are the most obvious ways of interrupting the sequence. The control of insects and rodents in the environment is another method that helps to control the spread of bacteria. The use of single-dose or single-use equipment, medications, and other supplies is an attempt to limit spread of infection by these items. The ICP has the overall responsibility for monitoring procedures in the hospital, from dietary practices to the number of air exchanges in the operating room, to limit the spread of organisms from various sources in the animate and inaminate environments.

Host susceptibility can also be altered, thereby interrupting the sequence at this stage. Certainly one of the goals of the nursing and medical management of the patient is to return the person to optimal mental and physiologic functioning. thereby also increasing the patient's natural resistance to infections. Measures such as immunizations, transfusions, improving nutritional status, medications, and exercise therapy all provide the patient with some increase in defenses against infections.

An understanding of the chain of infection is essential for the ICP in order to evaluate risks and to interrupt this sequence of events. The following chapters will outline in more detail the three components of the chain of infection and give the ICP a more complete discussion of the relative significance of each component.

## REFERENCES

1. Maki DG, Alvarado CJ, Hassemer CA, et al: Relationship of the inanimate hospital environment to endemic nosocomial infections. *N Eng J Med* 307 (25):1562, 1982.

2. McGowan JE, Jr: Environmental factors in nosocomial infections—a selected focus. *Rev Infect Dis* 3(4):760, 1981.

3. Kellerhals S: A pseudo-outbreak of *Serratia marcescens* from a contaminated fiber-bronchoscope. *APIC J* 6(4):5, 1978.

4. Maki DG, Hennekens CG, Phillips CW, et al: Nosocomial urinary tract infection with *Serratia marcescens:* An epidemiologic study. *J Infect Dis* 128(5):579, 1973.

5. Buxton AE, Anderson RL, Werdegar D: Nosocomial respiratory tract infection and colonization with *Acinetobacter calcoaceticus. Am J Med* 65 : 507, 1978.

6. Webb SF, Vall-Spinosa A: Outbreak of *Serratia marcescens* associated with the flexible fiberbronchoscope. *Chest* 68 : 703, 1975.

7. Steere AC, Mallison GH: Handwashing practices for the prevention of nosocomial infections. *Ann Intern Med* 83 : 683, 1975.

8. Garner JS, Favero MS: Guidelines for handwashing and hospital environmental control 1985. Hospital Infections Program, Atlanta, Centers for Disease Control, 1985.

# 6

# Sources of Infecting Organisms

In the course of running an infection control program, the ICP will have a close relationship with the microbiology laboratory of the hospital. Some ICPs enter the position with a background or specific education in microbiology, but most have not had much formal or even informal education in this area. The ICP must understand microbiology to be able to review and examine cases of infections intelligently and also to serve as a liaison between the laboratory and the rest of the hospital.

During surveillance activities, or special studies of infections, the ICP should be able to interpret results from the microbiology laboratory. In addition to the specific criteria for determining infections, the ICP should know normal body flora and what organisms are or can be pathogens in a certain body site, as well as the course of disease for the microorganism, treatment, and prognosis.

To make the best use of the microbiology laboratory, the ICP should know how to take specimens properly from the appropriate body site and how to handle them in order to obtain the best results for the money and time spent. The ICP will give classes on proper specimen collection techniques and therefore must have a good understanding of growth patterns of organisms, including the best methods of culture, how long to wait before results can be expected, and the different tests available to screen for particular organisms.

This chapter includes a discussion of microbiology for the ICP who has no background in this field. Although it is far from complete, it does cover the more common aspects of microbiology that the ICP should know during practice. Those ICPs who have not had any education or experience in microbiology should spend some time working in the microbiology laboratory; if this is not possible, the ICP should attend courses that are periodically offered on the subject. Because microbiology is the key to infection control practice, formal or informal education is essential to the ICP.

A discussion of microorganisms from the laboratory's standpoint follows, including some definitions, groupings and characteristics of microorganisms, and certain laboratory tests. The study of microbiology can be divided into four major groups: bacteriology, mycology, parasitology, and virology.

## BACTERIOLOGY

Various staining techniques are available for the identification of certain characteristics or groups of microbes. The Gram stain and the acid-fast stain techniques are probably the most important to the ICP.

The Gram stain is the most common technique; it rapidly identifies bacteria as gram-positive or gram-negative and shows the shape and size of the organisms when viewed under the microscope. There are variations in the Gram stain method; this is one example:

1. Heat-fix specimen to slide.
2. Pour crystal violet or gentian violet on slide for 10 seconds, then rinse with water.
3. Pour Gram's iodine on slide for 10 seconds, then rinse with water.
4. Carefully decolorize with 95% ethanol, then rinse with water.
5. Pour safranin on slide for 10 seconds, then rinse with water.
6. Air-dry or blot with paper towels.

Organisms that are gram-positive retain the crystal violet and iodine and resist decolorization; the organisms stain purple. Organisms that are gram-negative lose the crystal violet-iodine stain and pick up the counterstain (safranin) after decolorization; these organisms stain pink or red.

Organisms then can be viewed under the microscope and are described as gram-positive or gram-negative; organisms are further described by their size, shape, and grouping, such as rods, cocci, grouped in chains or in pairs, lancet-shaped, and so on. Certain organisms have characteristic shapes and groupings that, with the clinical picture, can lead the physician to an early presumptive diagnosis and prompt therapy.

The acid-fast stain is a technique using carbolfuchsin, acid alcohol, and methylene blue in succession.

**Table 6-1**
COMMONLY ISOLATED BACTERIA GROUPED BY STAIN
AND AEROBIC NEEDS

---

**Gram-Positive Cocci**

Aerobes
- *Staphylococcus aureus*
- *Staphylococcus epidermidis*
- *Streptococcus pneumoniae* (pneumococcus, diplococcus)
- *Streptococcus* sp. Groups A, B, D (including Enterococcus)

Anaerobes
- *Peptococcus* sp.
- *Peptostreptococcus* sp.

**Gram-Positive Rods**

Aerobes
- *Bacillus* sp.
- *Corynebacterium* sp.
- *Listeria* sp.

Anaerobes
- *Clostridium* sp.
- *Propionibacterium* sp.

**Gram-Negative Cocci**

Aerobes
- *Neisseria* sp.

**Gram-Negative Rods**

Aerobes
- Enterobacteriaceae
    - *Escherichia coli*
    - *Klebsiella* sp.
    - *Enterobacter* sp.
    - *Serratia* sp.
    - *Proteus* sp.
    - *Providencia* sp.
    - *Salmonella* sp.
    - *Shigella* sp.
- *Pseudomonas* sp.
- *Acinetobacter* sp.

**Small Gram-Negative Rods**

Aerobes
- *Hemophilus* sp.
- *Moraxella* sp. (diplobacilli)

Anaerobes
- *Bacteroides* sp.

**Acid-Fast Bacilli**
- *Mycobacterium tuberculosis*

---

**Table 6-2**

## BACTERIA COMMONLY ASSOCIATED WITH INFECTIONS OR DISEASES

| | *Characteristics on Staining* | *Infection or Disease* |
|---|---|---|
| **Gram-positive organisms** | | |
| Staphylococci | Clusters of cocci (grapelike) | Skin infections, endocarditis, bacteremia, pneumonia |
| Streptococci | Chains of cocci; pairs (*S. pneumoniae*) | Erysipelas, pharyngitis, scarlet fever, pneumonia, meningitis, endocarditis |
| Clostridia | Anaerobic rods usually containing spores (except *C. perfringens*) | Tetanus (*C. tetani*), botulism (*C. botulinum*), gas gangrene (*C. perfringens*), pseudomembranous colitis(*C. difficile*) |
| Corynebacterium diphtheriae | Club-shaped rods in palisade ("picket fence") | Diphtheria |
| Listeria | Small rods (pleomorphic) | Bacteremia, meningitis |
| **Gram-negative organisms** | | |
| *Klebsiella pneumoniae* | Rods | Pneumonia |
| *Escherichia coli* | Rods | Urinary tract infection |
| *Yersinia pestis* | Rods | Plague |
| *Bordetella pertussis* | Small rods or coccobacilli | Pertussis (whooping cough) |
| *Salmonella* sp. | Rods (nonlactose fermenting) | Diarrhea<br><br>Typhoid fever (*S. typhi*) |
| *Shigella* sp. | Rods | Diarrhea<br>Dysentery (*S. dysenteriae*) |
| *Neisseria meningitidis* | Cocci in pairs | Meningitis |
| *Neisseria gonorrhoeae* (gonococcus) | Cocci in pairs | Gonorrhea |
| *Vibrio cholerae* | Rods, comma-shaped | Cholera |
| *Pseudomonas aeruginosa* | Rods | Bacteremia, pneumonia, urinary tract infection |

**49**

1. Heat-fix specimen to slide.

2. Cover smear with filter paper and pour carbolfuchsin over slide.

3. Steam for 3–5 minutes; let stand for 5 minutes; then rinse with water (discard filter paper).

4. Pour acid alcohol onto slide until no more color appears, then rinse with water.

5. Pour counterstain (methylene blue) over slide for 20 seconds, then rinse with water.

6. Air-dry; examine with 100× oil-immersion lens.

Some mycobacteria are acid-fast; they retain the carbolfuchsin (red) and resist decolorization by the acid alcohol. Organisms that are nonacid-fast are decolorized and pick up the counterstain, methylene blue. The particular value of this technique is for the patient with suspected tuberculosis, since *M. tuberculosis* (and all other members of the genus *Mycobacterium*) is acid-fast. Since this organism can take weeks to grow in culture, a positive stain combined with clinical signs and symptoms is most helpful to the clinician and to the patient, whose therapy can then begin.

Organisms are also grouped by their need for and survival in oxygen. Anaerobes are organisms that in some way are harmed by oxygen, although there is much variability in the degree of toxicity of oxygen to different anaerobic organisms. Some simply grow better without oxygen present, but many bacteria categorized as anaerobes are obligate anaerobes, that is, they do not grow in cultures incubated aerobically. Facultative bacteria have a wider range: facultative anaerobes can grow in the presence of small amounts of oxygen (microaerophilic); facultative aerobes can grow in conditions of diminished oxygen. Another useful term in describing microorganism growth characteristics is *fastidious:* organisms that are fastidious are difficult to grow without specific and sometimes special nutrients or conditions set up for culture.

Table 6-1 is a listing of bacteria commonly isolated in patient infections (both nosocomial and community-associated), grouped by stain and aerobic needs. Table 6-2 outlines specific microorganisms or groups, laboratory characteristics, and diseases generally associated with invasion by each microorganism or group of microorganisms.

## MYCOLOGY

Fungi and yeasts are identified by techniques using potassium hydroxide (KOH), india ink, Giemsa stain, and acid-fast stain. Table 6-3 lists significant microorganisms and common infections or diseases; characteristics of stains or cultures can be found in bacteriology texts (1–3).

**Table 6-3**
FUNGI AND YEASTS COMMONLY ASSOCIATED WITH INFECTIONS
OR DISEASES

| Fungus Species | Infection or Disease |
| --- | --- |
| Candida albicans | Superficial infection (vaginitis, oral thrush), disseminated disease in compromised host |
| Nocardia sp. | Pulmonary infection, disseminated disease in compromised host |
| Cryptococcus neoformans | Meningitis, pulmonary disease in compromised host |
| Histoplasma capsulatum | Pulmonary, disseminated disease in compromised host |
| Aspergillus sp. | Pulmonary infection, opportunistic invader in the compromised host |
| Blastomyces dermatidis | Pulmonary infection |
| Coccidioides immitis | Pulmonary, usually subclinical |
| Phycomyces group<br>Mucor sp., Rhizopus sp. | Opportunistic invader in compromised host |

## PARASITOLOGY AND VIROLOGY

Parasites also are identified by stains, wet smears, or other laboratory techniques and are best reviewed by the ICP in a bacteriology or parasitology text. Parasites include *Entamoeba histolytica* and *Giardia lamblia*, as well as tapeworms, roundworms, and flukes. Although these pathogens are clinically significant, the laboratory methods for their identification are not as important for the ICP to understand.

Viruses are obligate intracellular parasites and can be divided into two groups: RNA viruses and DNA viruses. Table 6-4 shows some common infections and diseases associated with viruses.

Viruses are now recognized as potentially significant nosocomial pathogens. Some hospital laboratories, especially large teaching hospitals, are equipped to do viral cultures. Viral cultures must be grown in live tissue and therefore require additional skills and facilities in order to make the proper identifications. Many hospitals are, however, able to identify viral infections by serologic tests rather than culture. The descriptions of viral culture isolation and lab techniques are beyond the scope of this text.

**Table 6-4**
INFECTIONS AND DISEASES CAUSED BY VIRUSES

| *Infection or Disease* | *Virus* |
| --- | --- |
| Respiratory | Influenza |
| | Adenovirus |
| | Enterovirus |
| | Respiratory syncytial |
| | Parainfluenza |
| Central nervous system | Poliovirus |
| | ECHO virus |
| | Coxsackie virus |
| | Herpes simplex |
| | HIV |
| Rashes | Varicella zoster |
| | Herpesvirus |
| | Enterovirus |
| | Measles |
| Liver | Hepatitis A, B, NANB |
| | Cytomegalovirus |
| | Epstein–Barr virus (EBV) |
| AIDS | HIV |
| Infectious mononucleosis | EBV |

Other microorganisms are clinically significant, namely, spirochetes, chlamydiae, rickettsiae, mycoplasmas, and nematodes. The ICP is referred to bacteriology texts for further information on the isolation, serologic tests, or other means of identification of these pathogens.


## NORMAL FLORA, PATHOGENS, AND CULTURE TECHNIQUES

Normal flora are microorganisms that reside in many areas of the body without causing infection. These organisms vary from one geographic area to another, and also from one host to the next, based on such individual host factors as age, presence of chronic disease, temperature, and acidity (6). The microorganisms that normally reside on the body help to prevent colonization by pathogenic organisms and thus participate in the host's defense against invasion. When host factors are altered, however, or if these "normal" organisms are introduced into another body area, they can cause infection.

Transient organisms are picked up during patient care, for example, on a nurse's hands. These organisms can become part of the normal flora of the nurse's skin during care for that patient. After the nurse is no longer caring for the patient, these organisms usually are no longer found colonizing that nurse's hands. The acquisition of transient flora can be important during outbreak investigations, when an organism not normally carried on hands can become transient normal flora and thus be transmitted from patient to patient (7).

This section of the chapter is a discussion of the normal flora found in each body site, the possible pathogens, and appropriate culture techniques. Tables 6-5 and 6-6 summarize the normal flora and type of specimen for each body site.

**Table 6-5**
POSSIBLE NORMAL FLORA AND POSSIBLE PATHOGENS BY BODY SITE

| Body Site | Possible Normal Flora | Possible Pathogens |
|---|---|---|
| Respiratory tract | | |
| Nasopharynx | Alpha, beta, and nonhemolytic streptococci | *S. pyogenes* (Group A) |
| | *Neisseria* sp. | *Corynebacterium* |
| | Diphtheroids | *diphtheriae* |
| | Streptococci | *Bordetella pertussis* |
| | Gram-positive bacilli | |
| | | In large numbers or pure |
| | *Bacteroides* sp. | culture: |
| | *S. aureus* | *S. aureus* |
| | *S. pneumoniae* | *S. pneumoniae* |
| | *Hemophilus influenzae* | *Hemophilus influenzae* |
| | Gram-negative bacilli | Gram-negative bacilli |
| Trachea, bronchi, lungs, sinuses | Normally sterile | |
| Eye | Diphtheroids | *S. aureus* |
| | *S. epidermidis* | *N. gonorrhoeae* |
| | *Neisseria* sp. | Gram-negative bacilli |
| | Nonhemolytic or alpha streptococci | *M. lacunata* |
| | | *Hemophilus* sp. |
| | | *S. pneumoniae* |
| | | *P. aeruginosa* |

Table 6-5 (Continued)

## POSSIBLE NORMAL FLORA AND POSSIBLE PATHOGENS BY BODY SITE

| Body Site | Possible Normal Flora | Possible Pathogens |
|---|---|---|
| **Ear** | | |
| External | *S. epidermidis* | *P. aeruginosa* |
| | Diphtheroids | *S. pneumoniae* |
| | Alpha streptococci | Gram-negative bacilli |
| | *Bacillus* sp. | *H. influenzae* |
| Middle | Normally sterile | |
| Inner | Normally sterile | |
| **Gastrointestinal tract** | | |
| Mouth | Alpha, beta, and | *Salmonella* sp.[a] |
| | nonhemolytic streptococci | *Shigella* sp. |
| | Staphylococci | *Y. enterocoliticus* |
| | *Candida albicans* | *E. coli* (enteropathogenic) |
| | Diphtheroids | *V. cholerae* |
| | *Bacteroides* sp. | *Campylobacter* sp. |
| | *Fusobacterium* sp. | *G. lamblia* |
| | *Peptostreptococcus* sp. | *C. albicans* |
| | | (in large numbers) |
| | | *Arizona* sp. |
| Esophagus | Organisms found in the | Parasites |
| | mouth, pharynx, and food | *C. difficile* |
| Stomach | $10^3$–$10^5$ bacteria/g | |
| | (only transiently from food | |
| | and are rapidly killed by | |
| | high acidity) | |
| Duodenum | $10^3$–$10^5$ bacteria/g | |
| | (but is usually sterile) | |
| | Lactobacilli | |
| | Enterococci | |
| Lower ileum | $10^8$–$10^{10}$ bacteria/g | |
| | Lactobacilli | |
| | Staphylococci | |
| | *C. perfringens* | |
| | Streptococci | |
| Large intestine | $10^{11}$ bacteria/g | |
| | *Bacteroides* sp. | |
| | Lactobacilli | |
| | Enterococci | |
| | Staphylococci | |
| | *E. coli* | |
| | *Klebsiella* sp. | |
| | *Enterobacter* sp. | |
| | *Candida* sp. | |
| | *Proteus* sp. | |
| | *Pseudomonas* sp. | |

54

| Site | Normal flora | Pathogens[a] |
|---|---|---|
| Urinary tract | | |
|   Urethra | Organisms in anterior third only<br>*S. epidermidis*<br>Lactobacilli<br>Alpha streptococci<br>Diphtheroids<br>  (esp. *E. coli*) | In numbers<br>  >100,000 organisms/ml<br>Enterococci<br>Staphylococci<br>*C. albicans*<br>Gram-negative bacilli |
|   Bladder | Normally sterile | |
|   Ureters | Normally sterile | |
|   Kidneys | Normally sterile | |
| Body fluids: blood and cerebropsinal fluid | Normally sterile | Potentially any organism, including staphylococci, gram-negative bacilli, *C. albicans*, *N. meningitidis*, *H. influenzae*, streptococci, listeria, staphylococci, enteric gram-negative bacilli |
| Female genital tract | | |
|   Vagina | Anaerobic streptococci<br>Lactobacilli | *N. gonorrheae* |
|   Cervix | *S. epidermidis*<br>*E. coli*<br>Diphtheroids<br>*C. albicans*<br>Alpha, beta, and nonhemolytic streptococci | <br>*H. vaginalis*<br><br>*C. albicans* |
| Skin | Staphylococci<br>Diphtheroids<br>Alpha streptococci<br>*P. acnes*<br>Organisms same as those colonizing nearby body sites (bowel, mouth, nose, etc.) | *S. aureus*<br>*S. pyogenes* (Group A) |
| Wounds or abscesses | Normally sterile | *S. aureus*, beta hemolytic streptococci, gram-negative bacilli, anaerobic organisms |

[a] This list of pathogens applies to the entire gastrointestinal tract.

**Table 6-6**
TYPE OF SPECIMEN BY BODY SITE

| *Body Site* | *Specimen* |
| --- | --- |
| Respiratory Tract | |
| Nares | Sterile swab in transport media |
| Nasopharynx | Sterile swab in transport media |
| Throat | Sterile swab (dry for Group A Streptococci) in transport media |
| Lower respiratory tract | Sputum in sterile cup, suction trap, or syringe (transtracheal aspiration) |
| Eye | Sterile swab in transport media<br>Corneal scrapings directly inoculated |
| Ear | Sterile swab in transport media<br>Scrapings if fungi suspected |
| Gastrointestinal tract | Feces in clean cup<br>Rectal swab |
| Urinary tract | Urine in a sterile cup or syringe |
| Body fluids | |
| Blood | Two or three separate venipunctures, 10 ml each (adult) inoculated at the bedside |
| CSF | Sterile test tube (2 ml) |
| Female genital tract | Sterile swab in transport media<br>Needle aspiration (endometrial) |
| Skin | Sterile swab in transport media<br>Needle aspiration<br>Scrapings |
| Wounds or abscesses | Sterile swab in transport media<br>Needle aspiration |

## Respiratory Tract

The nasal passages are colonized predominantly with gram-positive organisms, including *Staphylococcus aureus* (20–80% of the population) and *S. epidermidis;* streptococci, including *Streptococcus pneumoniae* (5–15% of the population); *Neisseria* sp. (*N. meningitidis* in 0–4% of the population), *Hemophilus influenzae* (5–10% of population), and diphtheroids (6).

The nasopharynx can be colonized with some of the same microorganisms as the nose, such as streptococci (*S. pyogenes* [Group A], in 5–15% of the population), *Neisseria* sp. (*N. meningitidis* in 5–20% of the population), *H. influenzae,* and in fewer numbers, *S. aureus* and gram-negative bacilli such as *Escherichia coli, Proteus* sp., and *Pseudomonas aeruginosa.*

The trachea, bronchi, lungs, and sinuses are normally sterile. Possible pathogens include Group A streptococci, although, since these can be upper respiratory normal flora, clinical signs and symptoms are necessary to complete the diagnosis. *Corynebacterium diphtheriae* is the pathogen responsible for diphtheria, and *Bordetella pertussis* is the causative agent in whooping cough. Other microorganisms in pure culture or that occur in great numbers matched with the clinical picture can lead to a diagnosis of upper or lower respiratory tract infection.

Nose and nasopharyngeal cultures should not be taken to determine the etiology of acute or chronic sinusitis, but they may be taken to rule out a carrier of an organism implicated in an outbreak or to identify *C. diphtheriae.* Cultures of the nares are taken with a swab, extended as far back as possible in the nostril, and left in place long enough to obtain nasal secretions. Nasopharyngeal cultures are taken by using a nasal speculum. A special swab on a flexible wire is inserted through the speculum to the nasopharynx and is rotated and left in place for 30 seconds. It is important to transport these specimens immediately to the laboratory. The use of a transport medium will prevent the swab from drying out.

Throat cultures are taken in patients with acute tonsillitis or pharyngitis. The specimen is taken with a sterile swab; by depressing the tongue with an applicator, the posterior pharynx is swabbed, including any areas of purulence. The swab must not touch any other part of the oral cavity. Transport media are not needed in cultures for Group A beta hemolytic streptococci.

Sputum is cultured when a patient has clinical signs or symptoms of lower respiratory tract infection. A coughed specimen is best obtained in the early morning, since the patient's secretions have pooled overnight. After rinsing the mouth out with water, the patient is instructed to cough as deeply as possible. Induction by nebulizer is sometimes used to stimulate coughing and loosen secretions. Nasotracheal suctioning and transtracheal aspirates are better for sputum specimens, since there is likely to be little or no oropharyngeal contamination of the sputum. A culture may also be taken directly during bronchoscopy. Transtracheal aspiration and nasotracheal suctioning are discussed in more detail in Chapter 10, **Nosocomial Respiratory Tract Infections.**

Sputum is Gram-stained when it reaches the laboratory, to determine the quality of the specimen. Some labs, after examining the smear of the specimen, will reject sputum that has a predominance of epithelial cells, an indication of oral contamination. The presence of polymorphonuclear cells in the smear suggests that the specimen may be from the site of infection and therefore of good quality.

## Eye

The eye is normally colonized with organisms including diphtheroids, *S. epidermidis,* nonhemolytic streptococci, saprophytic fungi, and *Neisseria* sp. Pathogens can be *S. aureus, Moraxella lacunata, Neisseria gonorrhoeae, S. pneumoniae,* and certain gram-negative bacilli such as *Pseudomonas* sp.

Eye cultures are taken in patients with clinical evidence of purulent conjunctivitis or ulceration. Sterile swabs can be used for obtaining discharge, but there is frequently not enough material to collect. Direct scrapings of the cornea can be taken after application of a topical anesthetic. Transport media are necessary for swabs; scrapings can be directly inoculated into appropriate laboratory media.

## Ear

Normal flora of the outer ear includes common skin flora such as *S. epidermidis,* diphtheroids, and alpha hemolytic streptococci. The middle and inner ear are normally sterile. Pathogens include *P. aeruginosa,* pathogenic fungi (*Aspergillus* sp. in particular), *S. pneumoniae, H. influenzae,* and other gram-negative bacilli.

Ear cultures are taken or tympanocentesis is performed in patients with purulent otitis media. If the tympanic membrane has ruptured, cultures can be taken with a sterile swab after cleansing the external ear with an antiseptic. Purulent discharge is swabbed, and the specimen is placed in transport media.

## Gastrointestinal Tract

The mouth is colonized with a variety of aerobic organisms, with anaerobic organisms in the gums and tooth pockets. The organisms include alpha and nonhemolytic streptococci, staphylococci (usually *S. aureus*), diphtheroids, *Candida albicans* and other yeasts, *Bacteroides* sp., *Fusobacterium* sp., *Peptostreptococcus* sp., and others.

The stomach and duodenum contain minimal numbers of bacteria; if there is obstruction, more bacteria will be present in retained stomach contents, and gall bladder infection may result in more bacteria in the duodenum. The jejunum and upper ileum contain $10^5$–$10^8$ bacteria per gram. The lower ileum contains more microorganisms, including *Clostridium perfringens*, enterococci, staphylococci, and lactobacilli. The large intestine is heavily colonized with microorganisms, with anaerobic bacteria outnumbering facultative bacteria by a factor of 300 (8). Included in these anaerobes are *Bacteroides* sp., *Peptostreptococcus* sp., and *Clostridium* sp. The common aerobes in the large intestine, often called coliforms, include *E. coli, Enterobacter* sp., and *Klebsiella* sp.

Organisms that are pathogenic to the gastrointestinal tract include *Salmonella* sp., *Shigella* sp., *Arizona* sp., *Yersinia* sp., *Edwardsiella* sp., and *Campylobacter* sp. *Staphylococcus aureus* and *C. albicans,* which are normal flora, may be pathogens if found in pure culture or if they predominate (>50% of organisms). *Clostridium difficile,* an organism found in 2–4% of the population, is the major cause of pseudomembranous colitis and antibiotic-associated colitis. This organism has been implicated in nosocomial infections (9). Parasites are also included among gastrointestinal pathogens.

Stool cultures are indicated in patients with prolonged diarrhea or other clinical signs of enteric infections. Samples may also be taken in the investigation of an outbreak, where rectal carriage among patients or personnel is suspected. Feces or a rectal swab in transport media are acceptable; fecal material is better for the isolation of *Salmonella* sp.

## Urinary Tract

The anterior third of the urethra can be colonized with microorganisms such as *S. epidermidis,* diphtheroids, enterococci, alpha streptococci, and lactobacilli. The urinary tract above the anterior portion of the urethra is normally sterile, including the bladder, ureters, and kidneys.

Pathogens include the coliform bacteria and other gram-negative organisms, especially *E. coli.* Other possible pathogens, if found in numbers greater than 100,000/ml of urine, include *C. albicans,* enterococci, *S. aureus,* and, occasionally, *S. epidermidis.*

Urine specimen collection is described in more detail in Chapter 9, **Nosocomial Urinary Tract Infections.** Specimens of urine should be obtained in a sterile cup or syringe (suprapubic aspiration or aspiration from a Foley catheter) and transported promptly to the lab. If transport and inoculation onto media cannot occur within 2 hours, the specimen should be refrigerated or put into special transport media.

Urethral specimens are taken in patients with suspected gonorrhea, or, in males with nonspecific urethritis, a swab may be used to obtain urethral discharge after milking the urethra toward the orifice.

## Body Fluids

Blood and cerebrospinal fluid are normally sterile. Nearly all common microorganisms already mentioned can primarily or secondarily infect these sites. Additionally, specimens may become contaminated by skin flora during collection. The more common organisms found in blood cultures include staphylococci; gram-negative organisms such as *E. coli, Klebsiella* sp., and *Pseudomonas* sp.; streptococci; and *Bacteroides* sp. Subacute bacterial endocarditis (SBE) can be caused by alpha hemolytic streptococci (*S. viridans*), enterococci, staphylococci, gram-negative organisms, fungi, yeasts, or anaerobes. Specimen collection techniques are outlined in more detail in Chapter 12, **Nosocomial Bacteremia**.

Cultures of the cerebrospinal fluid are taken by the physician, after handwashing, gloving, draping, and a good skin prep. These specimens should be transported immediately to the laboratory. Since the pathogens are often fastidious, they may not survive refrigeration.

## Female Genital Tract

The lower female genital tract is colonized with a variety of microorganisms, including anaerobic and aerobic streptococci, *E. coli, S. epidermidis,* and *C. albicans.* A definite pathogen is *N. gonorrhoeae,* and possible pathogens include *Hemophilus vaginalis* and *C. albicans.* Indications for culture are purulent vaginitis and postpartum endometritis, as well as investigation of contacts of people who have venereal diseases. A swab of vaginal secretions or needle aspiration for endometrial cultures is taken with the patient in lithotomy position, after insertion of the speculum. Specimens should be delivered as soon as possible to the lab, or inoculated immediately, if *N. gonorrhoeae* is suspected.

## Skin

The skin is colonized with microorganisms such as *S. epidermidis,* diptheroids, alpha streptococci, and *Propionibacterium acnes.* Additionally, areas of skin near colonized body sites, such as the nose, mouth, and rectum, will be colonized with some of the normal flora from those sites. The common skin pathogens are *S. aureus* and *S. pyogenes* (Group A). Other microorganisms can cause superficial skin infections; subcutaneous infections can be caused by anaerobic organisms such as *Clostridium* sp.

Cultures should be taken of the skin when the patient has boils, furuncles, carbuncles, or other eruptions. In addition, skin cultures may be taken in an outbreak investigation, such as before and after handwashing to detect skin colonization with the responsible pathogen. The best culture method is aspiration of vesicles with a needle and syringe. After a gentle skin prep, taking care not to rupture the lesion, as much material as possible is aspirated. If lesions are open and draining, a sterile swab can be used to obtain a specimen. If fungal infection is suspected, dry skin scrapings are an adequate specimen.

## Wounds or Abscesses

Normal postoperative wounds are sterile, although they may be superficially contaminated by surrounding skin flora. Many organisms can become pathogens in a wound; most commonly isolated are *S. aureus, S. pyogenes* (Group A), *Pseudomonas* sp. and other gram-negative bacilli, and anaerobes such as *Clostridium* sp. and *Bacteroides* sp. Abscesses are frequently caused by anaerobes or a combination of aerobic and anaerobic organisms.

Specimens are indicated if the patient develops purulence in a wound or signs and symptoms of an abscess. The best method is needle aspiration after a skin prep or after cleansing an open wound with saline. Fresh pus from an open wound will give the best indication of the responsible pathogens. A more detailed description of wound culturing is given in Chapter 11, **Nosocomial Wound Infections**.

Other body sites may be cultured, and there are specific protocols for culturing certain suspected pathogens. The microbiology laboratory personnel should be consulted for any unusual specimen or particular technique needed.

## MICROBIOLOGY OF NOSOCOMIAL INFECTIONS

### Changing Trends

In the 1950s, one-third or more of all bacteremic patients were infected with *S. aureus;* by 1965 this proportion declined to about one-fifth. Concurrent with the decline in *S. aureus* bacteremias was a marked increase in bacteremias caused by enteric bacteria, from one-eighth in 1935, steadily rising to one-third to one-half or more currently (10,11). There is now a predominance of gram-negative microorganisms causing nosocomial disease as opposed to the staphylococcal and streptococcal infections of the 1950s and 1960s (12).

The longer survival of critically ill patients as well as selective antibiotic pressures are resulting in reports of nosocomial infections by organisms previously thought to be nonpathogenic (13–15) and reports of increased antimicrobial resistance in isolates (16–18). The genetic and biochemical bases and clinical implications of antimicrobial resistance are beyond the scope of this text. The ICP may attend seminars or search the literature for information on this subject.

## Special Tests for Epidemiologic Use

Antibiotic sensitivity tests provide useful information for the clinician in the consideration of appropriate antimicrobial therapy. Results of susceptibility testing should be monitored and discussed by the ICC. Additional tests useful in the investigation of outbreaks are phage typing for staphylococci and M and T typing for streptococci. Most of these tests are not done in hospital laboratories; they are performed when appropriate by reference laboratories such as the Centers for Disease Control. When such tests are needed, the hospital should work through the state health department to get the tests done. There are other procedures that the microbiology laboratory can perform to link a cluster of cases or isolates more closely to the same epidemiologic strain.

## ROLE OF THE INFECTION CONTROL PRACTITIONER

The ICP can be a liaison between the microbiology laboratory and the other hospital personnel. Hospital personnel need to obtain specimens properly and to mark laboratory slips appropriately. The ICP may be able to offer instruction in both areas. The laboratory, on the other hand, must report appropriate information to hospital personnel.

The laboratory slip is an often neglected part of the culture process. The ICP can offer in-service courses that discuss the importance of including the following information: accurate date and time of collection, patient and unit identification, patient diagnosis, and/or suspected infection. If the personnel are screening for a specific organism, direct consultation with the microbiology personnel, before the specimen is taken, will save time and money for the hospital and the patient. The ICP can provide useful information to clinicians and can encourage frequent communication with the laboratory.

The microbiology laboratory should report clinically significant results. The personnel should not have to do sensitivity testing on inappropriate organisms or organisms felt to be contaminants, or perform tests on specimens that are contaminated, or isolate and identify organisms that are normal flora. In certain circumstances, these studies may need to be done; if this is the case, again the laboratory slip should be clearly marked with unusual requests. The ICP may have a role in supporting the decision of laboratory personnel to reject contaminated specimens or to limit the identification or further testing of certain cultures. The ICP can again serve as a liaison, consultant, and teacher in this area and help to improve communication between the microbiologist and the clinician (19).

# REFERENCES


1. Lennette EH, Balows A, Housler WJ, Jr.: *Manual of Clinical Microbiology,* ed 3. Washington, DC, American Society for Microbiology, 1984.

2. Moffett HL (ed): *Clinical Microbiology.* Philadelphia, Lippincott, 1975.

3. Finegold SM, Martin WJ: *Diagnostic Microbiology,* ed 6. St Louis, Mosby, 1982.

4. Valenti WM, Betts RF, Hall CB, et al: Nosocomial viral infections: II. Guidelines for prevention and control of respiratory viruses, herpes-viruses, and hepatitis viruses. *Infect Control* 1(3):165, 1980.

5. Wenzel RP, Deal EC, Hendley JA: Hospital-acquired viral respiratory illness on a pediatric word. *Pediatrics* 60:367, 1977.

6. Mikat DM, Mikat KW: *A Clinician's Dictionary Guide to Bacteria,* ed 4. Eli Lilly Company, Indianapolis, IN, 1981.

7. Knittle MA, Eitzman DV, Baer H: Role of hand contamination of personnel in the epidemiology of gram-negative nosocomial infections. *Pediatrics* 86(3):433, 1975.

8. Youmans GP, Paterson PY, Somers HM: *The Biologic and Clinical Basis of Infectious Diseases.* Philadelphia, Saunders, 1975.

9. Heard SR, O'Farrell D, Holland D, et al: The epidemiology of *Clostridium difficile* with use of a typing scheme: Nosocomial acquisition and cross-infection among immunosuppressed patients. *J Infect Dis* 153(1):159, 1986.

10. Finland M: Changing ecology of bacterial infections as related to antibacterial therapy. *J Infect Dis* 122(5):419, 1970.

11. Centers for Disease Control: Nosocomial infection surveillance, 1983. *CDC Surveillance Summaries* 33(2SS):9SS, 1984.

12. Eickhoff TC: New antibacterial treatment of nosocomial infections. *Bull NY Acad Med* 51(9):1056, 1975.

13. Young VM, Myers WF, Moody MR, et al: The emergence of coryneforme bacteria as a cause of nosocomial infections in compromised hosts. *Am J Med* 70:646, 1981.

14. Thomas FE, Jackson RT, Melly MA, et al: Sequential hospitalwide outbreaks of resistant *Serratia* and *Klebsiella* infections. *Arch Intern Med* 137:581, 1977.

15. Brown A, Davis L, Yee RB, et al: Endemic *Serratia marcescens* in the Veterans Administration Hospital in Pittsburgh, PA, 1971–1976. *Health Lab Sci* 15(3):159, 1978.

16. Schaberg DR, Alford RH, Anderson R, et al: An outbreak of nosocomial infection due to multiply resistant *Serratia marcescens:* Evidence of interhospital spread. *J Infect Dis* 134(2):181, 1976.

17. Weinstein RA, Nathan C, Gruensfelder R, et al: Endemic aminoglycoside resistance in gram-negative bacilli: Epidemiology and mechanisms. *J Infect Dis* 141:338, 1980.

18. Harris AA, Levin S, Trenholme GM: Selected aspects of nosocomial infections in the 1980s. *Am J Med* 78 : 3, 1984.

19. Lee A, Mclean S: The laboratory report: A problem in communication between clinician and microbiologist? *Med J Aust* 2 : 858, 1977.

# 7

# Means of Transmission of Infections

The ICP spends a lot of time investigating the means of transmission of various diseases or microorganisms and working to prevent or minimize the transmission within the hospital. Certain diseases may have known means of transmission (Table 7-1), and precautions to prevent this from occurring are clear-cut. The transmission of certain microorganisms, however, may be less clear, as well as the mechanism of patient colonization or disease during an outbreak. The ICP must be concerned about both the transmission of communicable diseases and the mechanism by which patients within the hospital are colonized by a common organism that later results in endogenous infections.

**Table 7-1**
COMMON DISEASES OR INFECTIONS AND THEIR
MEANS OF TRANSMISSION

| Disease | Means of Transmission |
|---|---|
| Chickenpox | Contact: direct, indirect, droplet |
| Diarrhea | Contact: direct, indirect |
| Rubella | Contact: droplet |
| Hepatitis | Contact: direct, indirect |
| Rubeola | Contact: droplet |
| Wound infection | Contact: direct, indirect |
| Tuberculosis | Airborne |
| Urinary tract infection | Contact: direct, indirect |

Transmission can be broken into four main categories: contact, airborne, vehicle, and vector (1). Some diseases or microorganisms can be spread by more than one route, and preventive or control measures can differ for each route.

## TRANSMISSION BY CONTACT

Contact is the most common way infectious agents are transmitted from one person to another. There are different ways within the contact route that infections are spread, and each is controlled somewhat differently.

### Direct Contact

Direct contact occurs whenever one person touches another. During this contact, organisms colonizing each person can be transmitted, or active infectious material (such as secretions from draining lesions) can be spread from one to the other. Within the hospital, direct contact is an ongoing process: daily care is done by nursing personnel directly touching patients; in pediatric units, outpatient areas, and psychiatric units there may be direct contact between patients; employees have direct contact with each other as they share duties and interact with each other. In an intensive care unit, a nurse may have prolonged, close contact with more than one patient in a short period of time. There is a great potential for transmitting organisms—those causing infections as well as normal flora—from one patient to another via the hands. Since hands can provide adequate survival and even growth requirements for microorganisms, nurses can become colonized with those organisms that have colonized or infected the patient with whom the nurse has direct contact. This "transient flora" can persist as long as the nurse comes into contact with the patient, as long as the patient remains under that nurse's direct care.

The best means of preventing transmission by direct contact is through handwashing, since the hands have the most contact with patients. Gowning and gloving are more strict precautions to prevent transmission, either to the patient, from the patient, or the health care giver through the use of a protective covering that is discarded after use. The use of antiseptic soaps with residual action against microorganisms has been suggested for intensive care areas. This is intended to prevent transient colonization of employees' hands with potential pathogens when handwashing cannot be accomplished after each and every contact. Antiseptic soaps have also been suggested for use before invasive procedures, such as surgery or before intravenous or Foley catheter insertion (2–3).

Cohorting of nursing personnel is another means of limiting spread through direct contact. Certainly if there were one nurse for each and every patient, spread from patient to patient via the hands would not occur (although spread of disease from the patient to the nurse or vice versa would still be possible by the contact route). The idea of grouping patients with similar organisms or diseases, consistently cared for by the same nurse or nurses, has merit during an outbreak. These nurses would not have direct contact with noncolonized or noninfected patients; therefore, if the infectious material were picked up and carried by personnel, it could not be transmitted to patients who were not already positive for the organism or disease.

## Indirect Contact

Indirect contact occurs when a person touches an inanimate object that has been contaminated by another person. In the hospital environment there is a multitude of objects shared by patients: common toys in a pediatric outpatient department; a stethoscope and sphygmomanometer, beds, and other pieces of equipment used for one patient after another. As stated in Chapter 5, the importance of the inanimate environment in the spread of disease-causing agents should be evaluated.

Preventive measures include isolation techniques: double bagging of contaminated laundry and dressings to ensure that they do not contact other patients or susceptible personnel, gowning and gloving of personnel while handling linen and equipment in an isolation room, and special disposal of needles; the list covers the entire range of cleaning, disinfection, and sterilization techniques and the handling of infectious waste in the hospital environment (3). It is important that certain pieces of equipment, such as instruments and devices that break the skin, always be handled with care before or after patient use. It is also important, however, that other parts of the inanimate environment be examined carefully during outbreaks when the indirect contact route of spread is suspected; for example, the common use of a playroom and toys should be restricted during a suspected outbreak of chickenpox in a pediatric unit.

## Droplet Spread

The droplet route of spread involves contact with infectious upper respiratory secretions. Infections spread in this manner require proximity between the infected and the noninfected persons. When a person coughs, talks, or sneezes, relatively large ($>5$ $\mu$m in size) droplets are disseminated from the upper respiratory tract. Because of their size, most travel about 3 ft before settling to a horizontal surface such as furniture or the floor. Infections spread via the upper respiratory tract, although these large droplets require that the noninfected person come in contact with the particles within this 3-ft range, before they fall. Infections occur when the susceptible host inhales the particles and that person's mucous membranes come in contact with the infectious particles.

Masks may help to prevent contact with infectious droplets from a person who is communicable through this route. Physical distance may also be a control, for example, by placing the person alone in a room. Additionally, infected people may wear masks to decrease the number of droplets that they disseminate.

## AIRBORNE TRANSMISSION

Some particles from a person's upper respiratory tract are smaller than the droplets, that is, less than 5 $\mu$m in diameter. In addition, the moisture in some droplets evaporates before they fall, and these particles, called *droplet nuclei,* are small enough to get into air currents in an environment and remain suspended. Although many organisms cannot survive in this nearly dry state, some do, in particular the tubercle bacillus, staphylococci, and streptococci. In this situation, organisms can be spread from one patient to the next without direct or indirect (via inanimate objects) contact between the patients or even without the actual presence of the disseminating person. An example of this is seen in the report of an outbreak of postoperative wound infections by *S. pyogenes* (Group A), during which the carrier–disseminator had just left the operating room and the subsequent patient became infected. These organisms survived long enough in the environment to infect the next surgical case via the airborne route (4).

Additionally, organisms can become aerosolized from contaminated inanimate objects and will then be transmitted via the air. Procedures such as sweeping, using dry dust mops or cloths, and shaking out linen can aerosolize particles that may contain, for example, the tubercle bacillus. *Legionella pneumophila,* the organism responsible for legionnellosis (Legionnaires' disease; Pontiac fever), has been isolated from water in air-conditioning cooling towers. The mode of transmission of this organism appears to be airborne, during evaporation of water droplets from the cooling tower, which are then drawn into air intakes (5).

Preventive measures include good ventilation systems; ideally, air is supplied from outside and is exhausted directly to the outside. If air is recirculated in high-risk areas such as the operating room, it should be filtered with a 90% efficiency filter. The operating room should be under positive pressure relative to the surrounding area (6). Control of patients with tuberculosis and other diseases where the airborne route is of concern includes a private room with negative pressure, the door kept shut, and the use of masks when entering the room.

## TRANSMISSION BY VEHICLES

Specific infections can be spread through contaminated blood, drugs, food, or water. Blood is routinely tested for $HB_s Ag$ and HIV in an attempt to prevent transmission of these diseases through the vehicle of blood. Accurate donor histories and the reduction of use of blood from paid-donor centers can reduce the risk of infection transmission via this route.

Periodically drugs and intravenous solutions are recalled by the Food and Drug Administration (FDA) because of contamination. A large outbreak related to contaminated intravenous solutions is an example of spread of infection via this vehicle (7). Prevention and control of transmission from contaminated drugs or other commercial products mainly include a high level of awareness and prompt action if a product is suspect (8). Withdrawing the product from patient use, saving the product for investigation, and notifying the proper authorities are essential activities. Time will be wasted if the hospital attempts to culture suspected material; the responsibility for investigating, including culturing, commercially prepared items in hospitals rests with the FDA. The ICP's responsibility is to investigate up to the point of determining the likelihood that a product is contaminated, withdrawing and saving the product, and notifying the proper authorities.

Drugs and solutions can become contaminated after being opened in the hospital and can then serve as a vehicle in the transmission of infection. This is a problem within the hospital, and the ICP should investigate to determine the source of the problem. A review of the procedures used in the handling of drugs, IV and irrigating solutions, and blood may be helpful in preventing or controlling transmission.

Food and water can also be vehicles in the transmission of infecting organisms. Although not common in the hospital setting, there is potential for foodborne outbreaks resulting from improper handling or storage techniques in the Dietary Department (9). The ICP's role in reviewing policies and procedures and in teaching personnel in this department will serve to minimize the risk of transmission by this route.

## TRANSMISSION BY VECTORS

Infections spread by the vector route have an animal or insect as an intermediate host between two persons. Although this type of infection transmission is generally not significant within the hospital, patients with plague or rabies, for instance, can become directly communicable to other persons. Isolation precautions and a high level of suspicion in geographic areas where these infections are more common will help to minimize the risk to other patients and personnel.

Infections and potentially pathogenic microorganisms are spread within the hospital by a variety of routes. The ICP must determine the route of spread in each case and recommend procedures or precautions to break the chain of infection by stopping its transmission. The range of precautions, from handwashing, to housing of patients, to disinfection and sterilization, to isolation precautions, all contribute in different ways to stop transmission of organisms. The ICP must evaluate the source's degree of infectivity, determine the means of transmission, and institute appropriate steps to prevent transmission of a sufficient number of organisms to a susceptible host.

## REFERENCES


1. *CDC Guideline for Isolation Precautions in Hospitals*. U.S. Department of Health and Human Services, Atlanta, Centers for Disease Control, 1983.

2. Steere AC, Mallison GF: Handwashing practices for the prevention of nosocomial infections. *Ann Intern Med* 83 : 683, 1975.

3. Garner JS, Favero MS: Guidelines for handwashing and hospital environmental control 1985. Hospital Infection Program, Atlanta, Centers for Disease Control, 1985.

4. Schaffner W. Lefkowitz LB, Goodman JS, et al: Hospital outbreak of infections with group A streptococci traced to an asymptomatic anal carrier. *N Engl J Med* 280(22) : 1224, 1969.

5. Garbe PL, Davis BJ, Weisfeld JS, et al: Nosocomial Legionnaires' disease: Epidemiologic demonstration of cooling towers as a source. *JAMA* 254(4) : 521, 1985.

6. Garner JS: Guidelines for prevention of surgical wound infections, 1985. Hospital Infections Program, Atlanta, Centers for Disease Control, 1985.

7. Centers for Disease Control: Follow-up on septicemia associated with contaminated intravenous fluid from Abbott Laboratories. *Morbidity and Mortality Weekly Rep* 20(12) : 110, 1971.

8. Centers for Disease Control: Contaminated povidone—iodine solution—northeastern United States. *Morbidity and Mortality Weekly Rep* 29(46) : 553, 1980.

9. Centers for Disease Control: Shigellosis in a children's hospital—Pennsylvania. *Morbidity and Mortality Weekly Rep* 28(42) : 498, 1979.

# 8

# Host Susceptibility

Healthy people have several mechanisms for fighting infection: (1) mechanical barriers such as intact skin and mucosal lining of body cavities, (2) appropriately functioning white blood cells, (3) cellular immunity, and (4) cells capable of manufacturing antibodies (humoral immunity). As stated earlier (Chapters 5–7), an infection or disease occurs when a microorganism of significant virulence or colony size is able to circumvent, inactivate, or overwhelm the normal host defenses. Organisms that are capable of doing this in a healthy person are known as *pathogens*. Organisms that are part of a healthy person's normal flora rarely cause infection but can cause infection when the host's defenses break down. These organisms are called *opportunistic*.

Many hospitalized patients have one or more broken or deficient defense mechanisms, thus predisposing them to acquiring an infection. Additionally, people with active infections may be hospitalized, so that severely compromised hosts may be housed in the same area, perhaps, as severely infected persons.

The ICP must have an understanding of normal host defenses, deficiencies or breaks in the normal defenses, and how each defense (or lack of it) affects a person's risk of acquiring an infection. In this chapter some of these issues are discussed, as well as certain measures that will decrease host susceptibility within the hospital.

## IMMUNOLOGIC FACTORS IN HOST DEFENSE

Three types of cells are involved in the host immunologic defense system that prevent infection: cells capable of phagocytosis, cell-mediated immunity

(CMI), and humoral immunity (HI). Additionally, complement is involved in antigen–antibody reactions that inactivate and destroy the microorganisms. All of these cells originate in the bone marrow as basic stem cells and when subjected to microchemical stimuli maturate and perform specific immunologic functions. These cells acting singly and together provide the host with a competent immunologic system. References are available for a complete review of immunology (1–3).

## Phagocytosis

Phagocytosis is the capture and killing of microorganisms. There are two overlapping categories of phagocytic cells: the circulating granulocytes known as *neutrophils* or *polymorphonucleocytes* (*polys*) and the macrophage, which is a highly specialized monocytic cell. The first type, the polys, are capable of traversing intact capillary walls, moving in response to a chemical stimulus (chemotaxis), attaching and engulfing the microorganism, and releasing toxic substances that kill the organism (4). Only mature polys, which are released from the bone marrow, are capable of phagocytosis. The immature forms are called bands. An increase in polys and bands in the peripheral blood is an indication of infection.

By contrast, macrophages emerge from the bone marrow and circulate as immature or relatively undifferentiated cells (monocytes) capable of clearing particulate matter and invading microbes from the blood. Differentiated, these cells become fixed and wandering phagocytic cells. Macrophages have greater phagocytic capacity, engulfing particles, debris, and dead polys (5).

Another important function of the macrophage is its ability to process antigens and secrete interleuken 1 (formally known as *lymphocyte-activating factor*), which activates T and B lymphocytes (6).

Polys are short-lived and usually succumb within a few hours after a phagocytic event, while macrophages are long-lived and can sustain a chronic long-term relationship with pathogens. Macrophages are capable of selfproliferation in a local lesion, whereas polys are dependent on the bone marrow and circulating blood for a fresh supply to the lesion. Macrophages have greater phagocytic capacity for engulfing particles, debris, and damaged cells than polys—an important activity in wound healing.

## Cell-Mediated Immunity

T lymphocytes are the immunologic cells responsible for CMI. They originate in the bone marrow and maturate and differentiate in the thymus gland. These thymus-derived lymphocytes are helper, effector, and suppressor cells.

Helper T cells stimulate B lymphocytes to produce antibody and help to differentiate effector T cells into two distinct cell types. One type of effector T cell can gather macrophages and produce delayed hypersensitivity reaction at an intradermal infection site. A PPD skin test for tuberculosis is a delayed hypersensitivity reaction. Other effector T lymphocytes produce lymphokines, which are chemical substances that kill certain viruses, fungi, parasites, and tumor cells. Interferon is a lymphokine. Both types of effector cells can attack and destroy tissue grafts that they perceive as foreign substances.

Suppressor T cells act as immunologic regulators and turn off hypersensitivity reaction and the inflammatory response before an unacceptable level of healthy tissue is destroyed. These regulator cells also stop antibody production when an adequate supply has been produced to eradicate the bacteria. T Lymphocytes are preprogrammed to recognize only one antigen. Cell-mediated immunity occurs when T lymphocytes are sensitized by contact with bacterial antigens at the site of infection or in the lymph nodes. These sensitized T cells have immunologic memory and are capable of self-proliferation to increase their numbers to destroy that particular microbial antigen when it is again presented to the host. The T cells also release lymphokines that are macrophage inhibitory factors (MIF). This causes immobilization and accumulation of the macrophages to kill more quickly or at least to contain the pathogen, giving rise to such defenses as the granuloma that forms around tubercle bacilli (7).

## Humoral Immunity

The third part of the immunologic defense system is antibody production and complement activity. The B lymphocyte is the cell responsible for antibody production. When a macrophage takes up a foreign antigen, it produces interleukin 1, which stimulates helper T cells to produce interleukin 2, which, in turn, activates B lymphocytes to produce plasma cells to secrete immunoglobulins (antibodies). Figure 8-1 is a simple diagram of the process. There are five classes of immunoglobulins: IgG, IgM, IgA, IgD, and IgE. These antibodies have three main functions: opsonization, agglutination, and neutralization. IgA and IgM are involved in opsonization and complement fixation. Opsonization occurs when the antibody coats a bacterium, making it more attractive to the poly and facilitating phagocytosis. Polys have receptor sites on their surfaces. The binding of complement and antibody to the surface of microorganisms allows the poly to attach its receptor sites, especially to heavily encapsulated organisms such as *S. pneumoniae* and *H. influenzae,* which are particularly resistant to binding to polys and macrophages. IgA is the predominate immunoglobulin in mucosal secretions of the gut and respiratory tract. The primary function of IgA is to bind to viruses and protozoa.

This interferes with their ability to adhere to membrane surfaces and thus reduces their capacity to invade underlying tissue. The immunoglobulin E initiates allergic responses with release of histamine and other vasoreactive substances.

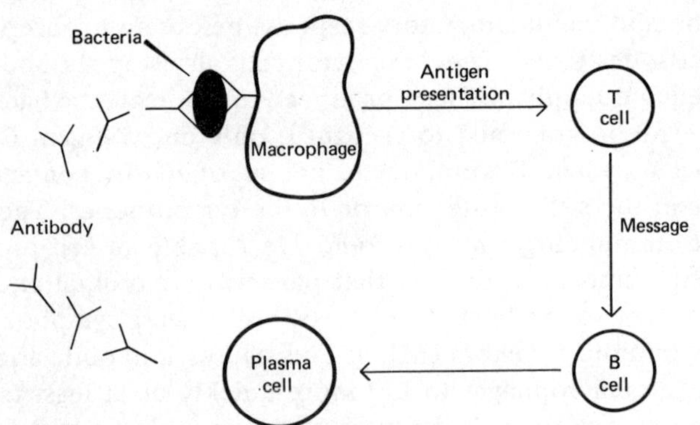


*Figure 8-1*

*One of the actions of the macrophage is to present the bacterial antigen to the T lymphocyte; the T cell then sends a message to the B lymphocyte. The B cell differentiates into a plasma cell and produces antibody specific for that antigen.*

Agglutination occurs because antibodies have more than one combining site and agglutinate bacteria by combining and branching. This makes a complex that is more easily phagocytized and more easily filtered in the lymph system. Neutralization occurs when the antibody coats the membrane of a host cell and prevents virus from attaching, therefore preventing invasion of the cell by the virus.

At birth, infants have antibodies from the mother; within the first month, the child begins to make its own antibody; the adult level of antibody is reached at about 12 years of age.

The complement system is the other part of humoral defense. It involves nine proteins and some enzymes, which act on one another in a cascade, often activated by the presence of antibody (8). Activation of the complement pathway results in opsonization, immune adherence, chemotaxis, and lysis of the bacterium.

# OTHER GENERAL HOST DEFENSES

Other host defenses include the skin, lung, and gastrointestinal anatomy. The integrity of the skin is an important bacterial barrier for the host. Skin secretions also provide a barrier, as do normal flora. The host defenses of the lungs are outlined in more detail in Chapter 10, **Nosocomial Respiratory Tract Infections**. Respiratory tract defenses include the cough and sneeze reflex, mucociliary escalator, and alveolar macrophages.

The gastrointestinal tract provides defenses against bacterial and viral invasion by its normal motility, immunoglobulins in the gut, and gastric acid.


# DEFECTS OR DEFICIENCIES IN HOST DEFENSE MECHANISMS

There are diseases and conditions, both natural and iatrogenic (physician-caused), that result in immunologic deficiencies or alterations in the other general host defense mechanisms. Impaired host resistance results from any of four basic defects: reduced functional phagocytes, diminished CMI, faulty antibody production, or damage to mechanical barriers (9).

Table 8-1 summarizes the more common diseases that affect the humoral immune response and lists the common pathogens associated with this defect. Table 8-2 shows diseases and pathogens associated with a deficiency in cellular immune response, and Table 8-3 shows diseases and pathogens present in people with depressed polymorphonuclear leukocyte bactericidal functions (10,11).

**Table 8-1**

DISEASES OR CONDITIONS AND COMMON PATHOGENS
ASSOCIATED WITH DEPRESSED HUMORAL (CIRCULATING
ANTIBODIES AND COMPLEMENT) IMMUNE RESPONSE

| *Diseases or Conditions* | *Common Pathogens* |
|---|---|
| Nephrotic syndrome | *S. pneumoniae* |
| Antimetabolite or cycotoxic drug therapy | Streptococci |
| Multiple myeloma | *P. aeruginosa* |
| Lymphatic leukemia | *P. carinii* |
| Lymphosarcoma | *H. influenzae* |
| Congenital hypogammaglobulinemia | |
| Splenectomy | |
| Complement defects | |

**Table 8-2**

### DISEASES OR CONDITIONS AND COMMON PATHOGENS ASSOCIATED WITH DEPRESSED CELLULAR (T-CELL) IMMUNE RESPONSE

| *Diseases or Conditions* | *Common Pathogens* |
| --- | --- |
| Hodgkin's disease | *M. tuberculosis* |
| Cancer | *Candida* sp. |
| Uremia | *Listeria* |
| Corticosteroid therapy | Herpesvirus |
| Sarcoidosis | Toxoplasma |
| Antimetabolite or cytotoxic drug therapy | *P. carinii* |
| AIDS | *P. carinii* |

**Table 8-3**

### DISEASES OR CONDITIONS AND COMMON PATHOGENS ASSOCIATED WITH DEPRESSED LEUKOCYTE BACTERICIDAL FUNCTION

| *Diseases or Conditions* | *Common Pathogens* |
| --- | --- |
| Myelocytic leukemias | Staphylococci |
| Chronic granulomatous disease | *Serratia* sp. |
| Burns | *Pseudomonas* sp. |
| Acidosis | *Candida* sp. |
| Corticosteroid therapy | *Aspergillus* sp. |
| Drug-induced granulocytopenia | *Nocardia* sp. |

Patients with lymphatic leukemia, lymphosarcoma, or multiple myeloma have reduced immunologlobulin or antibody levels; patients with granulocytic leukemia, as well as patients receiving certain corticosteroid therapy, have fewer polymorphonuclear leukocytes or impairment of their functioning. Patients with Hodgkin's disease have deficiencies in cell-mediated immunity (10). Immunodeficiency diseases can sometimes result in impairment of more than one defense system.

The organisms that commonly infect immunocompromised patients differ, based on the type of immune deficiency; patients with low amounts of circulating (humoral) antibodies tend to become infected by staphylococci, streptococci, and gram-negative bacilli. Patients with deficiencies in T-cell functioning (cell-mediated) tend to become infected with mycobacteria, fungi, viruses, and intracellular parasites.

Other diseases or conditions affecting host susceptibility include diabetes, which makes a person more susceptible to infections of the skin and soft tissues and the urinary tract (8). This increased susceptibility is due largely to vascular disease, making tissue avascular and therefore at risk. Additionally, ketoacidosis affects phagocytic functioning.

Anesthesia has been shown to decrease activity of alveolar macrophages in the lungs; also, endotracheal intubation, alteration of normal flora, and the delivery of dessicated gas alter lung defense mechanisms. Chapter 10 outlines these mechanisms and impairments in more detail. Colonization of the posterior nasopharynx with gram-negative microorganisms, which is associated with subsequent pneumonia, is increased among alcoholics and diabetics (12).

Age affects the immune response; the very young and the very old are more susceptible to infections. Immunologic immaturity renders neonates susceptible to a variety of microorganisms, which may result in overwhelming infections, including opportunistic pathogens such as herpes virus, *Listeria monocytogenes,* and *Candida* sp. (13). In the elderly, the increase in chronic debilitating diseases, malignancies, and waning immunologic responses results in reactivation of old diseases such as tuberculosis (14) and herpes zoster (15), as well as infections by staphylococci, streptococci, and gram-negative bacilli.

Nutritional status affects host susceptibility. Nonspecific factors include the integrity of the mechanical barriers, such as the skin and mucous membranes, to infection. Antibody production and leukocyte functions may also be impaired by malnutrition, as is cellular (T-cell) immunity (16).

Patients often come to hospitals with one or more chronic diseases or impairments in defense mechanisms. Once the patient is hospitalized, therapeutic measures, such as antimicrobial drugs, corticosteroids, radiation therapy, antineoplastic drugs, and insertion of foreign material may further predispose that patient to infection. These measures are discussed in more detail elsewhere (11) and in the chapters specifically dealing with nosocomial infections.


## MEASURES TO INCREASE HOST RESISTANCE IN THE HOSPITAL

Although there have been many advances in the understanding of immunologic defense systems, the prevention or control of infections among immunocompromised hosts remains difficult, and morbidity and mortality from infections remain high.

The use of protective isolation was for many years one way of decreasing the contact of the immunocompromised host with potential pathogens. Recent studies indicate that protected environments with filtered air or simple protective isolation requiring single room, gown, mask, and gloves are costly, cumbersome, and do not appear to be any more effective in reducing infections in the immunocompromised host than frequent and effective hand-washing (17,18).

A second approach to the problem would be to remove as many host defense impairments as possible. Defects in general defenses, such as intrusive devices (Foley catheters, IVs, endotracheal tubes) should be removed as soon as possible. Immunotherapy, immunization, and other methods of reconstituting the patient's residual immune response have been attempted. The use of transfer factor, levamisole, interferon, and thymus gland transplants are examples of experimental therapies undertaken in an attempt to restore a patient's immunocompetence (19). Vaccines against gram-negative rods have also been tried among critical care patients, in order to minimize colonization and subsequent infection (20).

The third approach to protecting these patients is the early recognition and prompt treatment of infections. Identification of those patients at high risk may enable the clinician to identify latent or occult infections, such as old tuberculosis. Screening studies may indicate immunocompromised patients at risk, because of their history, of diseases such as varicella; screening also identifies patients in need of protection from influenza or candidates for pneumococcal vaccine (21).

The ICP may elect to do surveillance of nosocomial infections based on host susceptibility; the severity of underlying diseases and the number and kind of medical and surgical procedures performed are related to infection risks. An outline of a surveillance system based on underlying disease as a predictor of nosocomial infection has been described elsewhere (22) (Chapter 14).

The ICP has the responsibility of understanding host defense mechanisms and susceptibility factors. The impairment of complex systems of immune defense results in varying levels of host susceptibility and subsequent infections. The ICP should know not only what factors increase and decrease susceptibility but also what preventive and control measures are effective for each type of immunologic disorder.


# REFERENCES


1. Lachman PJ, Peters DK: *Clinical Aspects of Immunology,* ed 4, vol 1. Boston, Blackwell Scientific Publications, 1982.

2. Stites DP, Stobo, JD, Fudenberg HH: *Basic and Clinical Immunology,* ed 5. Los Altos, CA, Lange Medical Publications, 1984.

3. Bach JF: *Immunology,* ed 2. New York, Wiley Publications, 1982.

4. Wade BH, Mandell GL: Polymorphonuclear leukocytes: Dedicated professional phagocytes. *Am J Med* 74(4): 686, 1983.

5. Werb Z: Granulocytes and macrophages. In Stites DP, Stobo JD, Fundenberg HH, *Basic and Clinical Immunology,* ed 5. Los Altos, CA, Lange Medical Publications, 1984.

6. Dinarello CA: Interleukin 1 and the acute-phase response. *N Engl J Med* 311(22) : 1413, 1984.

7. Fineberg R: T cells and B cells: Their role in infectious disease. *Infect Dis Pract* 7(2) : 1, 1983.

8. Hammond WP, Dale DC: Infections in the compromised host. *Hosp Med* 14 : 87, 1978.

9. Young LS: Nosocomial infections in the immunocompromised adult. *Am J Med* 70 : 398, 1981.

10. Eickhoff TC: Infections in immunosuppressed patients. *Drug Therapy* November: 19, 1972.

11. American Hospital Association: *Infection Control in the Hospital,* ed 4. Chicago, American Hospital Association, 1979, p. 12.

12. Mackowiak PA, Martin RM, Jones SR, et al: Pharyngeal colonization by gram negative bacilli in aspiration prone persons. *Arch Intern Med* 138 : 1224, 1978.

13. Weston, WL, Carson BS, Barkin RM, et al: Monocyte–macrophage function in the newborn. *Am J Dis Child* 131 : 1241, 1977.

14. Kasik JE, Schuldt S: Why tuberculosis is still a health problem in the aged. *Geriatrics* 77, March 1977.

15. Myers M: Varicella and herpes zoster: Comparisons in the old and young. *Geriatrics* 77, March 1977.

16. Neumann CG: Interaction of malnutrition and infection. *Arch Intern Med* 137 : 1364, 1977.

17. Armstrong D: Protected environments are discomforting. *Am J Med* 78 : 685, 1984.

18. Nauseff WM, Maki DG: A study of the value of simple protective isolation. *N Engl J Med* 304(8) : 488, 1981.

19. Wing EJ, Remington JS: Cell mediated immunity and its role in resistance to infection. *West J Med* 126(1) : 14, 1977.

20. Jones RJ, Roe EA: Low mortality in burned patients in a Pseudomonas vaccine trial. *Lancet* 2(1) : 401, 1978.

21. Ahronheim GA: Preventing infection in the immunocompromised patient. *Can Med Assoc J* 118 : 1479, 1978.

22. Britt MR, Schleupner CJ, Matsumiya S: Severity of underlying disease as a predictor of nosocomial infection. *JAMA* 239 : 1047, 1978.

# 9

# Nosocomial Urinary Tract Infections

The urinary tract is the most common site for a nosocomial infection. One-third to one-half of all nosocomial infections occur in the urinary tract. Approximately 1% of all patients hospitalized in the United States each year acquire a urinary tract infection (UTI), of which there may be as many as 800,000 cases or more per year. Urinary tract infections are most prevalent among geriatric and critically ill patients and occur more commonly after urinary catheterization (1,2). The infection can lead to pyelonephritis, septicemia, and other serious sequelae that have significant morbidity and mortality (3,4).

There are many host and environmental factors that result in urinary tract disease, as well as many forms of infection. This chapter deals primarily with nosocomial lower UTIs, those factors that contribute to the acquisition of this infection associated with hospitalization, and the role of the ICP in prevention and control.

## ANATOMY AND PHYSIOLOGY OF THE URINARY TRACT

It is well beyond the scope of this text to cover the complete anatomy and physiology of the urinary tract. The gross anatomic features of this system are shown in Figure 9-1; differences in the lower urinary tract between the male and female are shown in Figures 9-2 and 9-3. Urine is produced by the kidneys at a rate of 1 ml per minute and is moved by peristaltic action to the bladder through the ureters, which are about 25–30 cm long. The bladder is a storage organ that varies in capacity. When the bladder holds 100–150 ml of urine, a normal adult will feel the urge to urinate; when it reaches 350–400 ml, this causes discomfort.

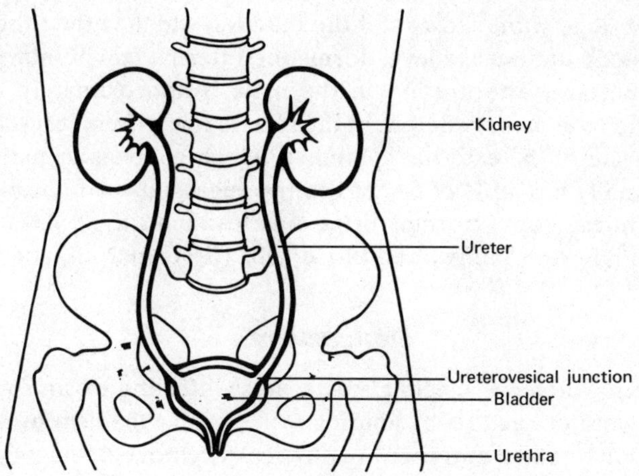



**Figure 9-1**
*Gross anatomy of the urinary tract.*

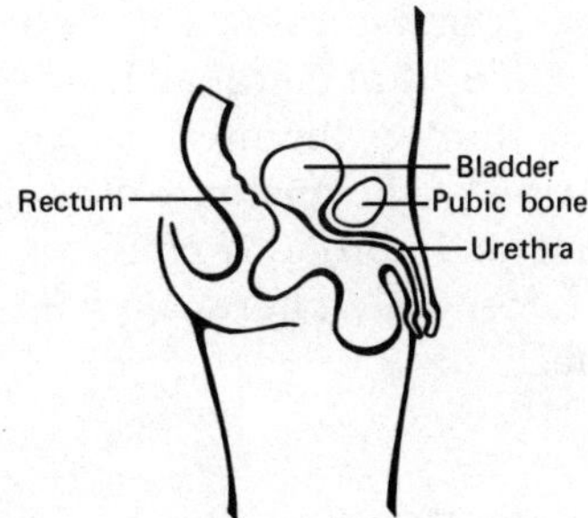



**Figure 9-2**
*The lower urinary tract in the male.*

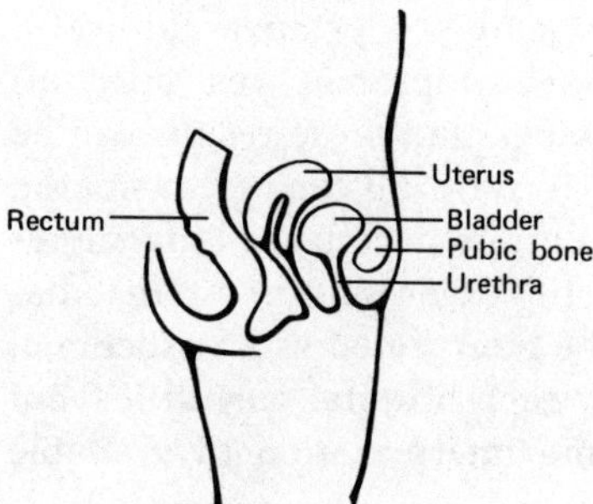



**Figure 9-3**
*The lower urinary tract in the female.*

The bladder wall has four layers: the fascia, which envelopes the bladder; the muscular layer; the submucosa; and the mucosa, which is the inner lining. At the bladder neck the muscle layer forms the internal (involuntary) sphincter around the urethra. The urethra in the male is approximately 20 cm long, passing through the penis, whereas in the female it is 3–5 cm long. The urethral orifice is the site of the external sphincter, which controls urination.

Urine normally has a pH of 5–7.5, with no sugar, albumin, or blood. Under high-power microscopy, normal urine has less than five white blood cells (WBC) per ml, fewer than two red blood cells (RBC) per ml, and no bacteria.

## Host Defenses

The bladder has defense mechanisms against infecting organisms. The constant washing out of bacteria by voiding urine is a mechanism by which bacteria that may have gained entrance are physically removed. Phagocytic function within the bladder wall has been suggested as another defense (5), as is the antibacterial character of the urine itself.

## Normal Flora

The anterior urethra in both males and females can be colonized with microorganisms, including *Staphylococcus epidermidis,* diphtheroids, lactobacilli, and alpha streptococci. Above the anterior third of the urethra, the urinary tract in the normal person is sterile. Because of the anatomy of the genitourinary tract and the proximity of the rectum, an improperly collected specimen can easily become contaminated with resident microflora and lead the clinician to a misdiagnosis of urinary tract infection.

## NOSOCOMIAL URINARY TRACT INFECTION

Nosocomial urinary tract infection, for the purposes of data collection, has been defined as the development of symptoms and/or a positive culture in a patient who was admitted without urinary tract symptoms. Most hospitals require urinalysis from patients on their admission, and these results can be used as a baseline. A urinalysis with fewer than 10 WBC/ml can be considered infection-free for the asymptomatic patient. Twenty-four hours or longer after admission, any specimen taken that grows $>10^5$ organisms/ml or that has $>10$ WBC/ml with or without symptoms may be interpreted as a nosocomial urinary tract infection. The specific criteria for each hospital may differ, but ICPs must be consistent in their collection and interpretation of available data.

Data for finding UTIs among hospitalized patients are available from the microbiology laboratory. The ICP may develop a method for retrieving information (such as patient name and nursing unit) for all patients with positive urine cultures. Locating patients with positive urinalysis (>10 WBC) and symptoms without a urine culture will be more difficult; this information will probably come from discussions with nursing personnel or a review of nursing Kardexes for antibiotic orders. It is important to teach nursing personnel to take urine cultures when patients become symptomatic, to rule out other problems and to identify the infecting organism. The microbiology laboratory remains, however, the primary data source for UTIs, since most true urinary tract infections will be cultured.

## Specimen Collection

Because of the anatomy of the urinary tract and the proximity of the urethral orifice in females to the vagina and rectum, the proper collection of urine for examination and culture is crucial for an accurate diagnosis. The ICP must understand and teach good specimen collection techniques and should understand the interpretation of various results that may indicate faulty technique. Specimens are acceptable if they are fresh, that is, if they have been examined within 30 minutes of collection or refrigerated immediately after collection and kept for no longer than 4 hours before examination. Methods of specimen collection include midstream clean catch, catheterization, and suprapubic aspiration.

### Clean Catch Specimen Collection

Because the urine can easily become contaminated by bacteria or white or red blood cells as it passes through the urethral orifice, a clean catch urine can be falsely positive. Important steps in the procedure include cleansing before urination to remove discharge that may pass into the specimen, collection of a midstream specimen, and care that the specimen is not contaminated in handling.

Mechanical cleansing with soap and water is adequate preparation for obtaining a urine specimen from both males and females. Whether cotton balls, washcloth, or towelettes are used, the mechanical removal of exudate is essential. The uncircumcised male should hold the foreskin retracted throughout the cleansing, rinsing, and throughout the specimen collection. The female should keep the labia separated throughout the specimen collection procedure.

Some institutions use antiseptics for cleansing the periurethral area before collecting urine specimens. Certain antiseptics, such as benzalkonium chloride, may become contaminated (6) and may deposit microorganisms that then may be carried by the urine into the specimen cup, giving a false-positive result. The author (M. C.) is familiar with one institution that used saline-soaked cotton balls stored in a container and replenished as needed for clean catch procedures, and these cotton balls became contaminated with *Pseudomonas* sp., which grew in the urine specimens obtained in this manner. The best method for cleansing involves the use of single-item cleansing towelettes or fresh soap and water to prevent this contamination from occurring. An additional problem with the use of antiseptics for meatal cleansing is the possibility that antiseptic in small amounts will get into the specimen and prevent the growth in culture of those microorganisms that are actually causing disease in the patient. Soap and water, with good rinsing, may be the easiest and least expensive method of cleansing before midstream urine collection.

To allow any remaining periurethral bacteria, bacteria that may be inside the anterior urethra, white or red blood cells, or cleansing solution to be washed away, the patient should begin to void in the commode. The specimen is then collected in the midstream; this represents the most accurate sample of bladder contents collected by this method. A first-voided specimen in the morning will give the best indication of infection, since organisms will have been allowed to multiply in pooled urine.

Care in handling the specimen includes the use of a sterile specimen cup, avoiding contamination while capping, and immediate transport to the microbiology laboratory. When patients are instructed to obtain the specimens, good instruction is essential, since most laypeople do not believe that urine is sterile and are not trained in aseptic technique.

### *Catheter Specimen*

When, because of weakness, obesity, or other medical problems, a patient is unable to give or cooperate in the procedure to obtain a midstream clean catch specimen, catheterization may be necessary. The procedure should be the same as that for indwelling catheterization, in terms of aseptic technique, and has been outlined in other references (7,8). The smallest catheter that can be used to drain the bladder is best, since there will be minimal trauma during the procedure.

If the patient has an indwelling Foley catheter, a specimen can be obtained without breaking the system open. Latex catheters can be aspirated, as shown in Figure 9-4, using a 21- or 25-gauge needle and 3-ml syringe. The catheter or drainage port can be cleansed with an antiseptic before aspiration of the specimen. For urinalysis or culture, 2–3 ml of urine is adequate. Silicone catheters cannot reseal over needle holes, but most catheters now have ports designed specifically for specimen aspiration (Fig. 9-5). The ICP should be actively involved in the selection of Foley catheters in order to assure that the urinary drainage system does not need to be broken to obtain specimens.

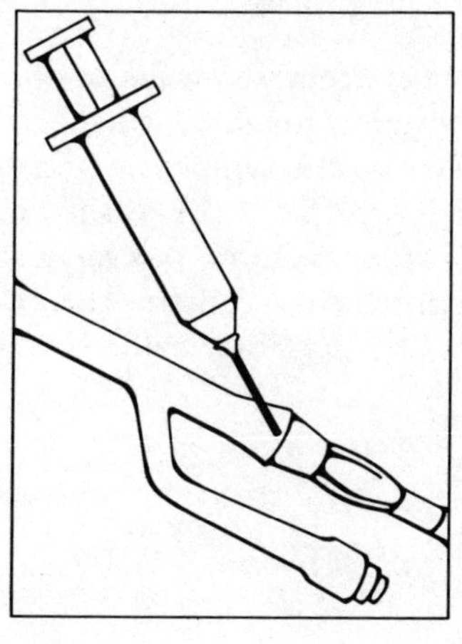

Figure 9-4
A needle is inserted at an angle into the
catheter, between the junction of the drainage
tubing and the tubing from the balloon. Urine
is aspirated into the syringe for culture or other
tests.

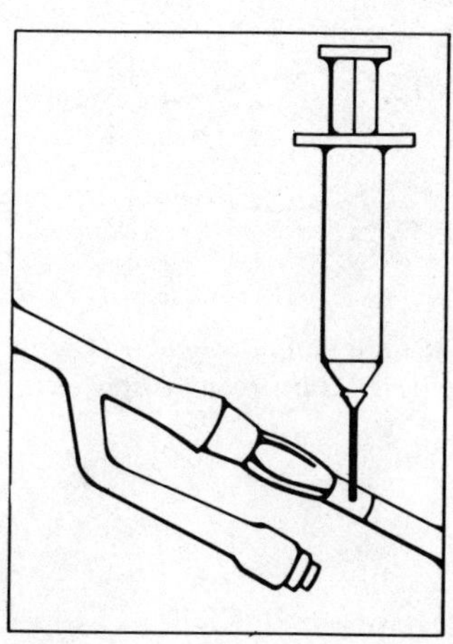

Figure 9-5
A needle can be inserted into the drainage port
of urinary catheters designed for specimen aspiration.

Foley catheter tips are not acceptable for culture, since they give no indication of the colony count in the urine and therefore cannot be interpreted. Additionally, it is likely that the tips will become contaminated when withdrawn through the urethra (9).

### Suprapubic Aspiration

Suprapubic aspiration of bladder contents is the most accurate means of obtaining urine for culture. A 20-gauge needle is inserted through anesthetized skin into the full bladder. The insertion site is between the symphysis pubis and the imbilicus, over the bladder when it is full and palpable (8), as shown in Figure 9-6. Patients who must have long-term catheterization may have a suprapubic catheter for urinary drainage. Specimens from the catheter can be obtained by needle aspiration in the same manner as from Foley catheters.

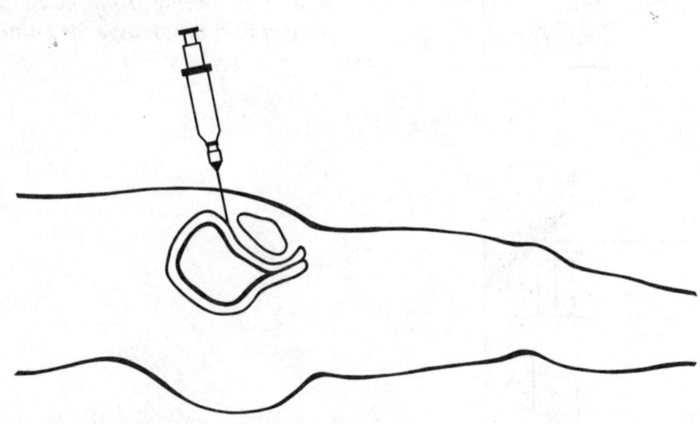

*Figure 9-6*

*Suprapubic bladder tap is performed, using sterile technique after an adequate skin prep; specimens of urine obtained in this manner give more accurate results than do specimens collected any other way.*

## Interpretation of Culture Results

A colony count of greater than 100,000 organisms/ml is considered an infection, based on studies correlating counts this high from voided specimens with positive suprapubic taps. Any specimen that has more than two different organisms in numbers greater than 100,000, or organisms that are nonpathogenic, should be considered possibly contaminated, and the specimen should be repeated (10). These organisms include diphtheroids and non-hemolytic streptococci, as well as small numbers of other normal flora of the perineal area.

## Mechanism of Infection

Since most nosocomial UTIs occur after Foley catheterization or some other form of urinary instrumentation, most infection control practices are aimed at the handling of this equipment and the patients undergoing these procedures.

Bacteria can enter the bladder of a catheterized patient at four places, as shown in Figure 9-7 (11).

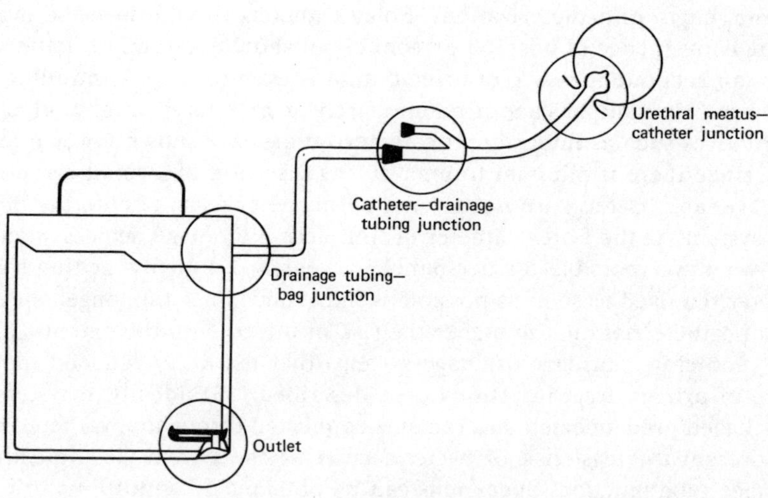


*Figure 9-7*

*Bacteria can enter the urinary drainage system at four different places: the urethral meatus–catheter junction, the catheter–drainage tubing junction, the drainage tubing–bag junction, and the outlet that drains urine from the bag.*

1. *The meatus-catheter junction.* It is thought that bacteria can enter the bladder at the time of catheter insertion in adequately prepped patients whose anterior urethras are heavily colonized with microorganisms. In addition, in the patient with an indwelling catheter in place, bacteria

can enter the bladder through the thin space between the catheter and the mucosal surface lining the urinary tract.

2. *The junction of the catheter and the drainage tubing.* Breaking the system open in an unsterile manner to obtain specimens or to irrigate has been shown to allow contamination and subsequent infection.

3. *The junction of the drainage tubing and catheter bag.* Reflux of urine from the bag into the tubing may occur, allowing bacteria to migrate into the bladder.

4. *The drainage port on the urine bag.* Contamination of the drainage outlet has been associated with the presumed migration of bacteria into the bladder (8).

## PREVENTION AND CONTROL OF URINARY TRACT INFECTIONS

The most obvious way to reduce catheter-associated UTIs is to limit the number and length of catheterizations. Foley catheters should never be inserted for the convenience of hospital personnel but should be used for patients for whom an accurate measure of urine output is essential on a continuing basis or where urine output cannot be measured or monitored in any other way. Alternatives such as intermittent catheterization have shown lower infection risks, since there is minimal trauma during insertion of a small catheter for drainage, and bacteria are not given a permanent means of entering the urinary system via the Foley catheter (12). External drainage devices should be used whenever possible for personnel convenience. Equally, getting a Foley catheter removed as soon as possible is important, since the longer the duration of catheterization, the higher the risk of infection to the patient (11).

In 1966 closed urinary drainage systems that markedly reduced the incidence of urinary tract infections were described (13). Ideally, a system that is packaged preconnected and remains connected throughout catheterization will present the least risk of bacteria entering the system via the catheter–drainage tube junction. Specimens can be obtained for culture or urinalysis by using a needle and syringe as previously described. Specimens for other tests can be obtained from the port on the drainage bag.

Catheters should be inserted by adequately trained personnel. Since the periurethral area is heavily colonized with microorganisms, careful cleansing is essential to minimize the number of organisms pushed into the bladder at the time of insertion. Additionally, knowledge of and skill in the insertion technique will prevent unnecessary trauma during cleansing or insertion; such trauma could increase the risk of infection. After insertion, the catheter must be secured to prevent more trauma during patient movement.

Recent studies have indicated that daily meatal care with either an antiseptic preparation or soap and water are not effective in reducing meatal colonization and, in fact, may increase rates of bacteriuria in patients with indwelling catheters. Manipulation of the catheter during meatal care increases the incidence of urethral colonization and precludes any benefit of antiseptic activity (12,14). Cleaning of the buttocks and thighs, especially after a bowel movement or fecal incontinence, may help to reduce microbial contamination of this area.

Irrigation of the catheter may be necessary to wash out plugs or clots after urinary surgery, for example. If these problems are anticipated, a three-way catheter, as shown in Figure 9-8, will obviate the need for opening the catheter system. If, however, the catheter becomes plugged and irrigation is needed, strict sterile technique using sterile equipment and gloves is essential. Fresh sterile irrigation solution and irrigation setup must be used each time the catheter is irrigated. Acetic acid or neomycin–polymyxin solutions have been shown to reduce the incidence of UTIs among long-term catheterization patients (8), although sterile saline will accomplish mechanical flushing. A recent study comparing neomycin–polymyxin irrigation via a three-way closed catheter system to no irrigation in a closed catheter system showed no difference in the incidence of catheter-associated UTIs (15). The patients undergoing irrigation had more resistant organisms isolated in their infections and also had evidence of more breaks in the catheter drainage system.

The catheter system must be maintained in such a way that the urine flows away from the bladder by gravity. The bag must always be below the level of the bladder, but it must never rest on the floor. Reflux valves may be helpful, but the maintenance of gravity flow at all times is the best assurance. Observation for kinks is important to prevent blocking of the catheter and pooling of urine.

Any accidental opening of the catheter with subsequent contamination warrants replacement of the system. Otherwise, the catheter system should not be changed routinely, since this may increase trauma and the risk of infection. Rolling the catheter between the fingers is a good way to detect potential plugs; if the catheter feels sandy when rolled, the system should be replaced before it becomes plugged. Care must be taken in emptying the urine from the bag so that the drainage outlet is not contaminated by hands, the collection pitcher, or the floor, thus becoming a source of infection. Each catheter bag should have an individually labeled urine container to prevent cross-contamination (11).

Prophylactic antibiotics should generally not be used for asymptomatic bacteriuria because of the risk of colonization and infection with more resistant nosocomial organisms(8).

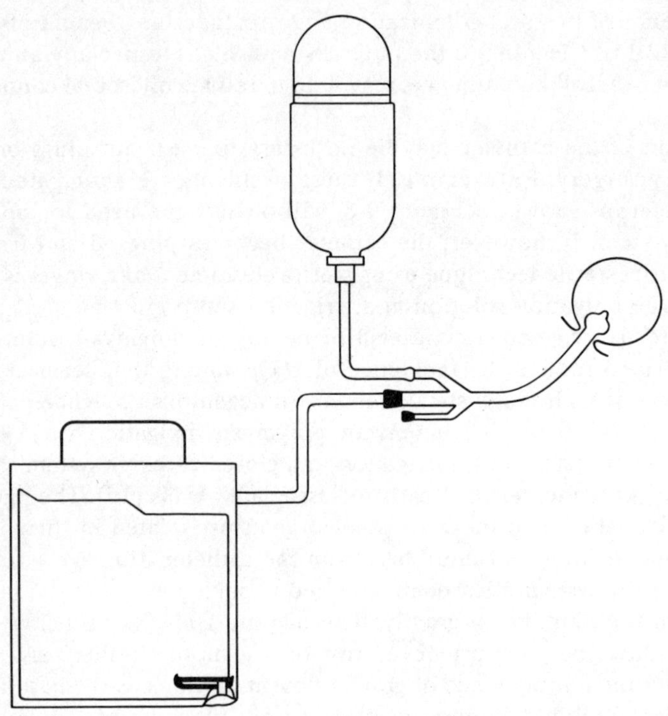

*Figure 9-8*

*A three-way catheter has three lumens: one for irrigation fluid to enter the bladder, one for irrigation fluid and urine to drain from the bladder, and one leading to the balloon that keeps the catheter in the bladder.*

Many mechanisms that reduce the risk of infection associated with Foley catheterization are related to the prevention of resident perineal flora from entering the system. Transmission from patient to patient can also occur via the hands of nursing personnel. Outbreaks of UTIs caused by organisms not generally found in the perineal flora have shown that this cross-infection can occur. Additionally, as with other procedures, nonsterile equipment, solutions, or commercial prepackaged products can result in infection. The CDC recommends that patients with indwelling Foley catheters be separated geographically whenever possible to minimize the risk of transmission via the hands of hospital personnel (11,16).

Because of the high incidence of catheter-related infections, emphasis has focused on preventive measures discussed in this chapter. Attention to proper catheter insertion and maintenance has reduced incidence of urinary tract infections by 31% (17).


## Role of the Infection Control Practitioner

The ICP has the responsibility of monitoring UTIs as well as other nosocomial infections in the health care facility. More useful than an ongoing surveillance system would be special studies to review technique, solutions, duration of catheterization, and other factors to determine where intervention might result in lower incidence rates.

In accordance with JCAH standards, there must be policies and procedures covering the insertion and care of urinary catheters. The ICP can make sure that these are in accordance with the latest set of guidelines from the CDC. These guidelines must be reviewed and updated as needed, at least annually, by the ICC.

The ICP also has the responsibility for teaching appropriate techniques to nursing and other health care personnel handling catheters. The ICP can have perhaps the greatest impact on the incidence of urinary tract infections by teaching and monitoring proper insertion and care techniques.

Last, the ICP has input into the selection of catheters and catheter-care products. The ICP should be aware of the mechanisms thought to be effective in reducing infection risks and should choose a product based on the maintenance of these practices (18). For example, the length of the tubing and the construction of the tubing-drainage bag junction should be examined with the practical problems of kinking and subsequent obstruction in mind; the type of sampling port or other provision for obtaining specimens is another aspect the ICP should consider in selecting a urinary catheter. The ICP must match the desired practices for good catheter insertion and care techniques with the product specifications to minimize risk from a poorly constructed product.


## SUGGESTED PROCEDURES

The following are suggested procedures for proper specimen collection and catheter insertion. Expansion is needed for each procedure to incorporate each facility's specific nursing service format for procedures. Only the basic points are included in the procedures presented below, and the procedures may vary slightly based on products or methods used.

## Midstream Urine Collection

### *Female*

1. Wash hands.
2. Position patient with legs spread or in stirrups.
3. Spread labia and continue to hold labia throughout specimen collection.
4. Cleanse the periurethral area gently with soap, warm water, and cotton balls. Each cotton ball is used once, from front to back, and discarded.
5. Rinse, using cotton balls and water, again front to back, once only for each.
6. Have the patient begin to void.
7. Collect the specimen midway in the voiding and do not touch the inside of the sterile cup during interception of the stream of urine.
8. Send the specimen to the laboratory immediately or refrigerate.

### *Male*

1. Wash hands.
2. Retract the foreskin if present and hold throughout entire procedure.
3. Cleanse the urethral meatus gently with soap, warm water, and cotton balls.
4. Rinse, using cotton balls and water.
5. Have the patient begin to void.
6. Collect the specimen midway in the voiding and do not touch the inside of the sterile cup during interception of the stream of urine.
7. Send the specimen to the laboratory immediately or refrigerate.

## Foley Catheter Insertion

### *Female*

1. Wash hands.
2. Position patient with legs spread or in stirrups. Make sure that there is good lighting in the work area.
3. Inspect perineum and wash with soap and water and rinse, if secretions are visible. Wash hands.

4. Set up sterile field, put on sterile gloves, test balloon, and lubricate catheter.

5. Wearing sterile gloves, spread labia and continue to hold labia throughout catheter insertion procedure.

6. Using forceps, cleanse periurethral area gently with antiseptic and cotton balls. Each cotton ball is used once, from front to back, and discarded. Do not contaminate sterile gloved (free) hand.

7. With sterile gloved hand, insert lubricated preconnected catheter.

8. After inflating balloon, secure catheter with tape to the patient's leg.

### *Male*

1. Wash hands.

2. Make sure there is good lighting in the work area.

3. Wash penis with soap and water and rinse, if secretions are present. Wash hands.

4. Set up sterile field, put on sterile gloves, test balloon, and lubricate catheter.

5. Wearing sterile gloves, retract foreskin if present and continue to hold in this position throughout catheter insertion procedure.

6. Using forceps, clean the periurethral area gently with antiseptic and cotton balls. Do not contaminate sterile gloved (free) hand.

7. With sterile gloved hand, insert lubricated preconnected catheter.

8. After inflating balloon, secure catheter with tape to the patient's leg.

## Needle Aspiration of Specimen from Catheter

Follow manufacturer's direction when obtaining specimens from catheters with special drainage ports.

1. Wipe latex catheter with antiseptic between the catheter–drainage tube junction and the balloon port.

2. Insert a 25-gauge needle and 3-ml syringe into the catheter at a 45° angle.

3. Aspirate specimen.

4. Send specimen to the laboratory immediately or refrigerate.

*Note:* Latex catheters will close over the needle hole, whereas silicone will not; therefore, a drainage port is needed for silicone catheters.

## Foley Catheter Irrigation

1. Use fresh sterile irrigation solution and sterile irrigation setup each time procedure is done. Solution must be labeled and discarded after 24 hours if not used. Irrigation syringe should be sterile for each procedure.

2. Set up sterile field: sterile drape, towel, Asepto or large (50-ml) syringe, and sterile basin with irrigation solution.

3. Wipe junction of catheter and drainage tubing with antiseptic.

4. Wearing sterile gloves, disconnect catheter from drainage tubing and place on sterile towel.

5. Instill irrigation fluid into catheter according to physician's orders. Do not put Asepto syringe directly into irrigation bottle; use prepoured solution only.

6. Reconnect catheter to drainage tubing securely.

## REFERENCES


1. Turck M, Stamm W: Nosocomial infections of the urinary tract. *Am J Med* 70 : 651, 1981.
2. Centers for Disease Control: Nosocomial infection surveillance, 1980–1982. *CDC Surveillance Summaries* 32(455) : 155, 1983.
3. Gross PA, Neu HC, VanAntwerpen C, et al: Deaths from nosocomial infections: Experience in a university hospital and a community hospital. *Am J Med* 68 : 219, 1980.
4. Platt R, Polk FB, Murdock B, et al: Mortality associated with nosocomial urinary-tract infection. *N Engl J Med* 307(11) : 637, 1982.
5. Kaye D: Host defense mechanisms in the urinary tract. *Urol Clin North Am* 2 : 407, 1975.
6. Centers for Disease Control: Hazards of infection associated with the use of aqueous benzalkonium chloride. Atlanta, Centers for Disease Control, 1974.
7. De Groot J: Basic principles of infection control and urethral catheterization. *Infect Control Urol Care* 3(1) : 5, 1978.
8. Kunin CM: *Detection, Prevention and Management of Urinary Tract Infections,* ed 3. Philadelphia, Lea & Febiger, 1979.
9. Gross PA, Harkavy LM, Barden GE, et al: Positive foley catheter tip cultures—fact of fancy? *JAMA* 228(1) : 72, 1974.
10. Nicolle LE: Urine cultures and long-term indwelling catheters. *Arch Intern Med* 145 : 1794, 1985.

11. Wong ES, Hooton TM: *Guidelines for Prevention of Catheter-Associated Urinary Tract Infections*. Hospital Infections Program, Atlanta, Centers for Disease Control, 1982.

12. Garibaldi RA, Burke JP, Britt MR, et al: Meatal colonization and catheter-associated bacteriuria. *N Engl J Med* 303 : 316, 1980.

13. Kunin VM, McCormack RC: Prevention of catheter-induced urinary-tract infections by sterile closed drainage *N Engl J. Med* 274(21) : 1155, 1966.

14. Burke JP, Garibaldi RA, Britt MR, et al: Prevention of catheter-associated urinary tract infections: Efficacy of daily meatal care regimens. *Am J Med* 70 : 655, 1981.

15. Warren JW, Platt R, Thomas RJ, et al: Antibiotic irrigation and catheter-associated urinary-tract infections. *N Engl J Med* 299 : 570, 1978.

16. Okuda T, Endo N, Osada Y, et al: Outbreak of nosocomial urinary tract infections caused by Serratia marcescens. *J Clin Microbiol* 20(4) : 691, 1984.

17. Haley, RW, Culver DH, White JW, et al: The efficacy of infection surveillance and control programs in preventing nosocomial infections in U.S. Hospitals. *Am J Epidemiol* 121(2) : 182, 1985.

18. Gurevich I: Selection criteria for closed urinary drainage systems. *Supervisor Nurse* 10(Feb) : 39, 1979.

# 10

# Nosocomial Respiratory Tract Infections

Respiratory tract infections account for about 15–20% of all nosocomial infections among hospitalized patients. *Hemophilus influenzae, Streptococcus pneumoniae,* beta hemolytic streptococci, and *Staphylococcus aureus* were described as common infecting organisms in pneumonias in the late 1940s. In subsequent years, following the advent of antibiotic drugs, the agents responsible for pneumonias have changed (1). Gram-negative rods are becoming increasingly important as agents that cause pneumonia in general hospitals as well as in referral hospitals dealing with severely compromised patients.

Nosocomial respiratory tract infections occur in 0.5–5% of all hospital admissions; of these cases, gram-negative bacterial pneumonias account for over one-half and have an associated high mortality rate, especially among patients with malignancies (2,3). Other nosocomial respiratory tract infections are caused by anaerobes, staphylococci, and fungi.

Although viral upper respiratory infections are easily spread within hospitals (4,5) and may present problems to ICPs, this discussion will focus on lower respiratory infections, in particular, gram-negative rod pneumonia. Host defenses, the epidemiology of this kind of infection, and methods for prevention and control will be discussed.

## ANATOMY AND PHYSIOLOGY

The respiratory system is equipped with complex protective mechanisms to prevent injury or infection. General anatomic and physiologic descriptions of the respiratory system can be found in medical and nursing texts. A more detailed discussion of host defense mechanisms, shown in Figure 10-1, may be

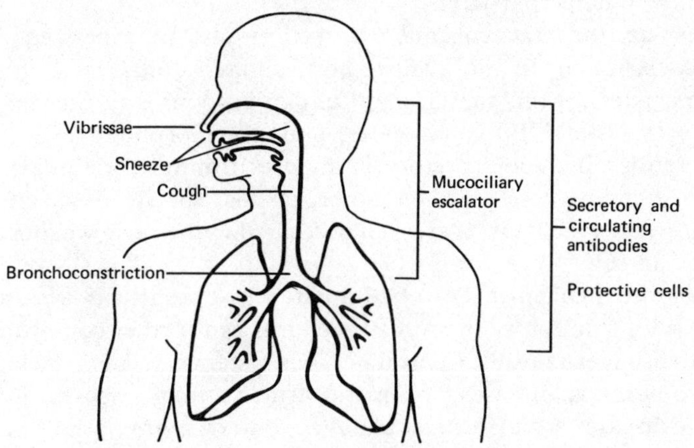


*Figure 10-1*

*The respiratory defense mechanisms in the normal person. These mechanisms are designed to trap and expel foreign material, including microorganisms.*

useful, however, for the understanding of nosocomial lower respiratory tract infections.

## Host Defenses

### *Nose and Nasopharynx*

The nose is structured in such a way that large inhaled particles are trapped by nasal hairs (vibrissae) and the mucus layer. This mucus blanket then moves particles toward the nasopharynx, where they are swallowed or expectorated. Additionally, the nasal passages have receptors that stimulate a sneeze or cough when irritated.

Organisms that become trapped in the nasal passages can stimulate an immune response by mobilizing lymphocytes, polymorphonuclear leukocytes, macrophages, and antibodies. Inflammation is an immune defense because of increased blood flow to the nose, delivering cellular defenses. Particles 10–20 $\mu$m in size bypass the nose and are trapped in the nasopharynx, where some of the same defenses are stimulated.

### *Trachea, Bronchi, and Lungs*

Particles less than 5 $\mu$m in diameter can bypass upper respiratory defenses and be deposited in the lungs. Not all particles that enter lower respiratory air spaces are deposited; most are washed back out with subsequent breaths. Additionally, lung clearance mechanisms are efficient in removing most inhaled particles.

Irritation in the tracheobronchial tree results in reflex coughing and bronchoconstriction. In the healthy host, ciliated epithelial cells move deposited particles toward the larynx. Cellular responses in the lungs include macrophages, T and B lymphocytes, and polymorphonuclear leukocytes. Lung secretions include secretory antibodies (immune globulins IgA, IgG, IgM) that help macrophages to engulf organisms. Specific descriptions of respiratory defense mechanisms are well described in the review paper by Dowell and Freeman (6).

Host defense mechanisms can be impaired by chronic diseases, and hospitalization with respiratory therapy procedures can further compromise respiratory defense mechanisms. Central nervous system disorders, including coma and neuromuscular diseases, chronic obstructive lung diseases, and immune deficiency diseases are disorders that affect one or more of the host defenses. Hospitalization, including the use of endotracheal tubes or tracheostomies, can impair the host further. The patient most at risk of a nosocomial lower respiratory infection is the one with a combination of chronic disease and iatrogenic factors that result in infection (2).

## Normal Flora

The upper respiratory tract, including the nose, nasopharynx and throat, is colonized with organisms such as alpha streptococci, diphtheroids, *S. epidermidis*, *S. aureus*, and *S. pneumoniae*. *Neisseria* sp. also colonize this area, a small number of people are colonized with *N. meningitidis*, and some are colonized with *H. influenzae*.

# NOSOCOMIAL RESPIRATORY TRACT INFECTION

Nosocomial lower respiratory tract infection has been defined as the development of a new infiltrate as seen on x-ray films or a combination of signs and symptoms, including an increase in cough with purulent sputum, fever, and leukocytosis. Such infections occur in up to 5% of patients admitted to the hospital, particularly among critically ill patients. Colonization of the upper respiratory tract of hospitalized patients by gram-negative bacilli seems to play a major role in the subsequent development of nosocomial pneumonia. In a study of critical care unit patients, 45% became colonized in the posterior pharynx with gram-negative bacilli (7). Up to a quarter of these patients develop nosocomial infections (8,9).

## Impairment of Host Defenses

Colonization and subsequent infection are based on the impairment of host defenses by clinical conditions or by external factors related to hospitalization. These conditions include chronic disease and severity of current illness, such as chronic obstructive lung disease, cystic fibrosis, leukemia, CNS depression (coma), and electrolyte imbalance (6). These disorders affect the sneeze and cough reflexes, mucociliary clearance activity, and other defenses. Dehydration leads to dry mucous membrane surfaces and thickens secretions, making it difficult to expel this material. In the hospital, host defenses may be impaired by the use of cytotoxic and corticosteroid drugs and anesthesia (10), which can affect lung macrophage activity. The use of some respiratory therapy equipment, such as endotracheal tubes, bypasses upper respiratory mechanisms altogether.

## Mechanism of Infection

The mechanism by which a colonized patient becomes infected is thought to be through the aspiration of upper respiratory secretions. Figure 10-2 is a

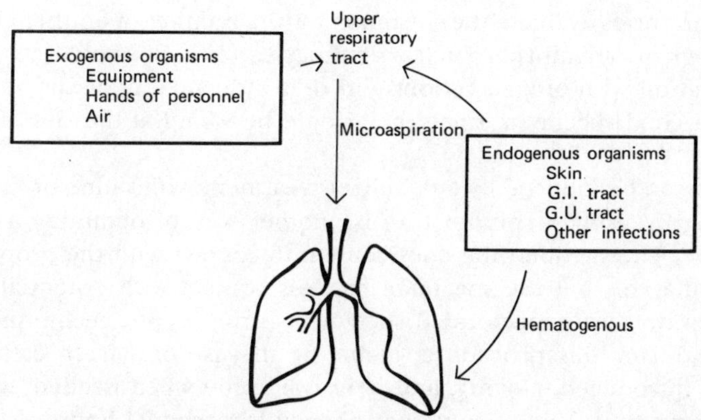


*Figure 10-2*

*Organisms responsible for nosocomial lower respiratory tract infections can be acquired by the host from exogenous sources, especially in a critical care unit. Infectious organisms from endogenous sources, including normal flora from other body sites or infections elsewhere, can seed the lungs via the bloodstream and can colonize the upper respiratory tract as well.*

diagram of the different ways by which nosocomial respiratory tract infection occurs (11,12). The upper respiratory tract of patients with impaired host defenses becomes colonized with gram-negative bacilli such as *Klebsiella* sp., *P. aeruginosa, Enterobacter* sp., *E. coli,* or *Proteus* sp. The additional pressure of antibiotics, frequently used in intensive care, may encourage the colonization of the upper respiratory tract with nonsusceptible or highly resistant organisms (13). These organisms can come from the patient's own gut or genitourinary flora, through direct contact. Exogenous colonization occurs from the hands of personnel, contaminated respiratory therapy equipment, droplets, or even food. Infection occurs when the patient aspirates minute quantities of upper respiratory secretions, because of the decreased cough and sneeze reflex, impaired mucociliary transport, or intubation that allows secretions to enter the lungs around the tube or from condensation inside the tube.

## Specimen Collection

The diagnosis of nosocomial pneumonia is made on clinical grounds rather than on the basis of a culture result. Expectorated sputum specimens can easily become colonized with oropharyngeal organisms; interpretation, therefore, is difficult. An early morning specimen is best, since secretions will have pooled overnight. The patient should be instructed to rinse his or her mouth with water and to cough deeply and expectorate into a sterile specimen cup without touching the inside. A careful explanation to the patient is essential to obtain a true sputum specimen rather than saliva. As stated in Chapter 6, some laboratories evaluate the specimen for the number of epithelial cells and the number of polymorphonuclear leukocytes (14). Epithelial cells indicate contamination with oral secretions and thus indicate a poor specimen; polys indicate a good specimen, since they would be found at the site of infection (15).

Sputum can be induced by a nebulizer treatment with saline or medication. Suctioning by using a sputum trap is another way of obtaining a specimen for culture. The suction tube does come into contact with the oropharynx or the nasopharynx, but the specimen has less contact with potential contaminants than does an expectorated specimen. Strict aseptic technique must be observed during this procedure, including the use of a fresh catheter each time it is introduced, gloving, and irrigation, only when needed, with sterile saline from a unit dose or container opened less than 24 hours earlier.

Fiberoptic bronchoscopy has also been used to obtain specimens for culture, but this method has the same limitations as expectorated and suctioned specimens, namely, contamination with upper respiratory flora (16,17). Contamination occurs in part when the bronchoscope is inserted, in the same way that nasopharyngeal suction catheters become contaminated.

Translaryngeal aspiration and transtracheal aspiration are useful procedures when performed by a well-trained person. It is especially useful in the isolation and identification of anaerobes (18), since oral contamination by other specimen collection means can mislead the clinician. Figure 10-3 shows the method by which this procedure is done. There have been complications associated with this procedure, including hemorrhage (19), pneumomediastinum (20), and infection (21). This procedure, however, is the most valid in providing the clinician with a specimen indicative of the organisms causing disease in the lungs. Positive blood cultures in a patient with signs and symptoms of lower respiratory infection will be the best indication of the pathogens involved.

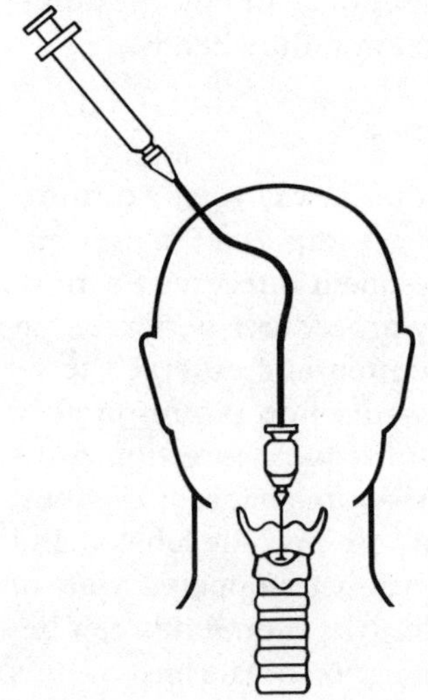

*Figure 10-3*
*Translaryngeal aspiration is accomplished by a percutaneous puncture through the cricothyroid membrane. Transtracheal aspiration is performed at a site below the larynx (subcricoid). (Redrawn with permission from The Upjohn Company,* <u>Anaerobic Bacteria and Disease</u>, *Kalamazoo, MI, The Upjohn Company, 1975, p 22).*

## PREVENTION AND CONTROL

Prevention of nosocomial respiratory tract infections is based on minimizing transmission and colonization of patients' upper respiratory tracts with gram-negative rods, and good respiratory hygiene so that the colonized patient has a lower risk of developing pneumonia. Measures to accomplish this include nursing care techniques, hospital isolation policy, and care of respiratory equipment (22).

## Handwashing

Handwashing is essential, especially in a critical care unit. Outbreaks of respiratory infections by such opportunistic pathogens as *Acinetobacter calcoaceticus* have occurred among severely compromised patients in critical care units. One mode of transmission suggested in this setting was via the hands of personnel, from one patient to the next in an open care unit (23,24). A thorough discussion of the proper handwashing technique can be found in Chapter 18, **Isolation Techniques.**

The transmission of *P. aeruginosa* from sinks to patients has been known to occur (25), but is probably not a common occurrence. Hands should be washed in a sink and splashing should be avoided. In intensive care units where cross-colonization or cross-infection is a problem, or handwashing facilities are not easily accessible, the ICP should consider the use of an antiseptic handwashing solution. Ideally, the unit should be remodeled to allow for safer patient care, but this is obviously not always possible. If nurses are not able to wash as often as needed, the use of an iodophor or chlorhexidine gluconate may help by the residual antibacterial action on the hands.

## Respiratory Care Techniques

General respiratory techniques such as keeping the airway open; turning, coughing, and deep breathing; and early ambulation are important in preventing pooling of lower respiratory secretions and subsequent infection. Suctioning is probably one of the most common pulmonary procedures performed in critical care settings. The ICP should review the written and observed technique used for suctioning. Catheters should be inserted into the respiratory tract once only and a fresh one obtained for each subsequent insertion. Sterile gloves should be worn. Irrigation is done to loosen tenacious secretions; any container of irrigation fluid opened for this purpose must be labeled and discarded at 24-hour (maximum) intervals; small, rubber-stoppered vials of saline or single-use irrigation ampules are available. Irrigation fluids can become contaminated and can inoculate huge numbers of organisms via this procedure (23). Complete guidelines on suctioning technique are available from the CDC (22).

Care of endotracheal tubes and tracheostomies is important, since the accumulation of secretions at a tracheostomy site or within an endotracheal tube can lead to aspiration. There should be policies and procedures written for the routine cleaning of tracheostomy tubes and sites. Additionally, the provision of humidified air is important to prevent drying of respiratory mucosa, with the resulting impairment of ciliary function (22).

Use of special equipment such as Wright respirometers and Ambu bags should be monitored; the common use of any respiratory therapy equipment from one patient to the next without adequate disinfection can result in the transfer of microorganisms (26).

## Respiratory Therapy Equipment

The risks of nosocomial respiratory infections associated with the use of inhalation therapy equipment is well documented in the literature. In particular, outbreaks have been related to nebulizers (27), and colonization of the respiratory tract has been related to nearly all respiratory equipment used. A review and recommendations for the care of this equipment is available from the CDC (22).

Many patients receiving respiratory therapy treatment are intubated; therefore, the oxygen or gas mixture delivered to the patient is humidified. Additionally, nebulizers can give the patient medication or can loosen secretions via very small particles of the solution. Nebulizers have been implicated more strongly in the transmission and acquisition of nosocomial infections. Figures 10-4, 10-5, 10-6, and 10-7 show the difference between humidified air (or gas) and nebulized solution. A humidifier bubbles the gas through the water so that the gas picks up water molecules (Fig. 10-4). Humidifier reservoirs with large numbers of bacteria may produce a contaminated aerosol (28). A nebulizer results in a gas that actually contains small water (or other solution) droplets, large enough to contain bacteria. There are three ways nebulization occurs:

1. The venturi jet nebulizer passes gas rapidly over a tube immersed in solution. The solution is drawn up the tube, and small droplets are pulled into the gas (Fig. 10-5).
2. The spinning disk method involves solution poured onto a disc, which is spinning rapidly. The solution is broken up into large and small droplets (Fig. 10-6).
3. The use of ultrasonic energy nebulizes solution by vibration, breaking it into small droplets (Fig. 10-7).

Because nebulizers deliver particles of solution small enough to bypass normal respiratory defense mechanisms, they can be a significant source of infecting organisms. The ICP should make sure that policies and procedures are in effect to minimize the risk from this equipment. Nebulizer and humidifier reservoirs should be rinsed with sterile water and refilled, rather than sterile solution simply added to a reservoir that is nearly empty. The numbers of microorganisms in the remaining solution could grow to large numbers if allowed to remain by refilling without rinsing.

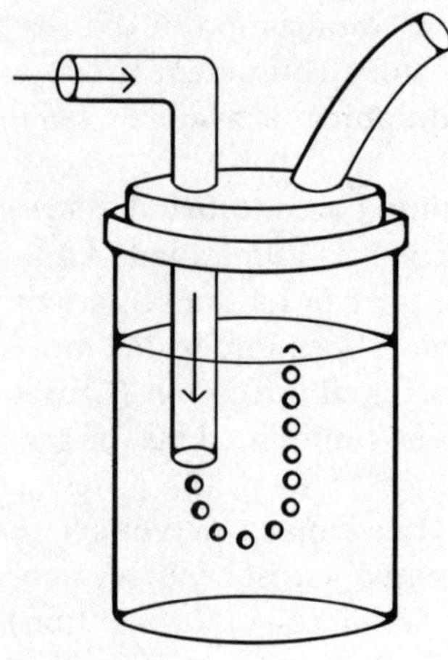



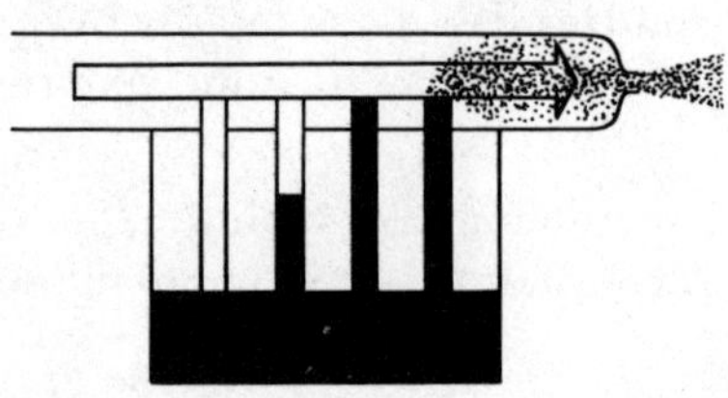

**Figure 10-5**
The Venturi jet nebulizer draws solution into the stream of gas that passes rapidly over the tube immersed in the reservoir. (Redrawn with permission, Malecka-Griggs B, Reinhardt DJ, Georgia State University, Atlanta, Ga.)

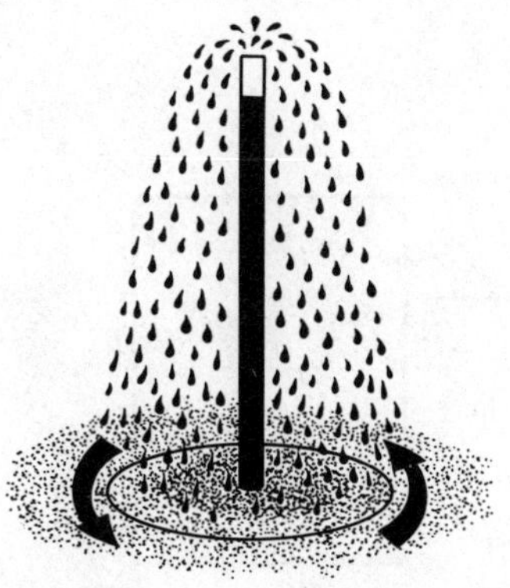



In this nebulizer, the rapidly spinning disk produces an aerosol when the solution is poured onto it, creating large and small droplets. (Redrawn with permission, Malecka-Griggs B, Reinhardt DJ, Georgia State University, Atlanta, Ga.)

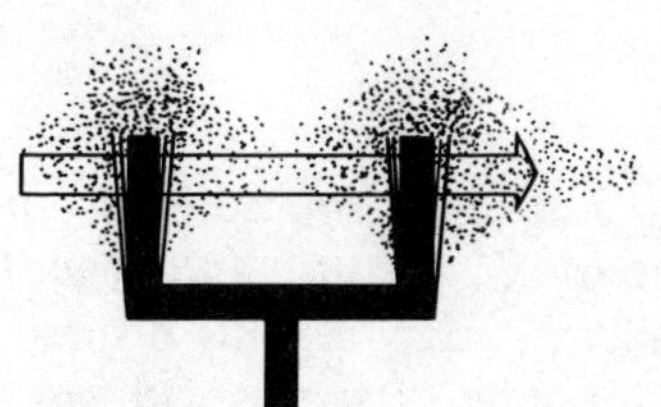



In this nebulizer, the solution is vibrated by ultrasonic energy, thereby breaking up the solution into small droplets. (Redrawn with permission, Malecka-Griggs B, Reinhardt DJ, Georgia State University, Atlanta, Ga.)

Continuous volume ventilation circuits (Fig. 10-8) should be changed at least every 48 hours (22) and disinfected or sterilized between patient uses by steam autoclaving, ethylene oxide, pasteurization, or activated glutaraldehyde. The use of disposable circuits eliminates cleaning and disinfection problems; each hospital should examine cost-effectiveness and other considerations in the selection of materials and procedures. Other recommendations are available (22) and are based on attempts to keep the level of bacterial contamination low enough so that pulmonary infection does not occur.

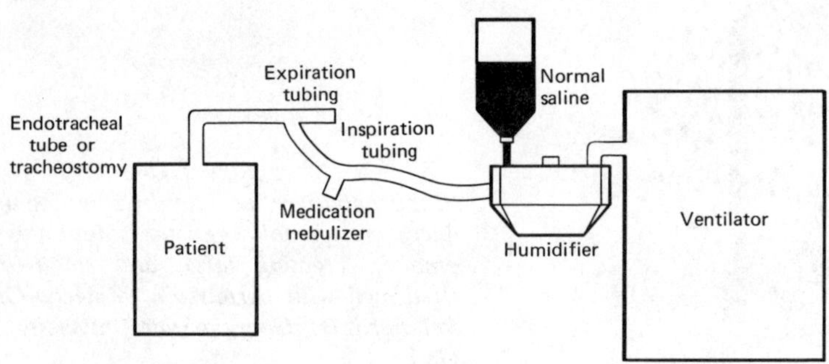


*Figure 10-8*
*Continuous-volume ventilator.*

## Isolation

Patients with bacterial pneumonias generally do not need isolation, except those infected with *S. aureus* or *S. pyogenes* (Group A). A true staphylococcal or streptococcal (Group A) pneumonia is an extremely serious disease, which can be shown by a pure culture of one or the other. Patients with sputum cultures growing mixed organisms, including *S. aureus* or Group A *S. pyogenes,* may not have had a true staphylococcal or streptococcal pneumonia, since these organisms can be normal flora in the upper respiratory tract. Respiratory isolation, or at least geographic separation, may be warranted for the patient who has pneumonia caused by a highly resistant, gram-negative microorganism, particularly if the patient is in an intensive care unit. The ICP should develop policies and procedures for such situations if the transmission of resistant gram-negative rods has been a problem in the institution.

Nosocomial respiratory tract infection is a serious consequence of hospitalization and usually follows respiratory therapy (30). The ICP should monitor these infections, especially in critical care areas, and be alert for possible breaks in technique that may lead to cross-infection, especially by opportunistic organisms.

# REFERENCES


1. Lepper MH: Opportunistic gram negative rod pulmonary infections. *Dis Chest* 44(1): 18, 1963.

2. Gross PA, Van Antwerpen C: Nosocomial infections and hospital deaths. *Am J Med* 75: 658, 1983.

3. Rhame FS, Striefel AJ, Kersey JH: Extrinsic risk factors for pneumonia in the patient at high risk of infection. *Am J Med* 78: 42, 1984.

4. Wenzel RP, Deal EC, Hendley JO: Hospital-acquired viral respiratory illness on a pediatric ward. *Pediatrics* 60: 367, 1977.

5. Hoke CH: Control of nosocomial influenza: Recommendations based on a review of the recent literature. *APIC J* 6(4): 14, 1978.

6. Dowell AR, Freeman ER: Lung defense mechanisms: their importance in respiratory care. *Respir Care* 22(1): 50, 1977.

7. Johanson WG Jr., Pierce AK, Sanford JP, et al: Nosocomial respiratory infections with gram-negative bacilli: The significance of colonization of the respiratory tract. *Ann Intern Med* 77: 701, 1972.

8. Tillotson JR, Finland M: Bacterial colonization and clinical superinfection of the respiratory tract complicating antibiotic treatment of pneumonia. *J Infect Dis* 119: 597, 1969.

9. Penn RG, Sanders WE, Sanders C: Colonization of the oropharynx with gram-negative bacilli: A major antecedent to nosocomial pneumonia. *Am J Infect Control* 9(2): 25, 1981.

10. Manawadu BR, LaForce FM: Impairment of pulmonary antibacterial defense mechanisms by halothane anesthesia. *Chest* 75S: 242S, 1979.

11. Teres D: Management of respiratory infections in the intensive care unit. *Int Anesthesiol Clin* 14(1): 163, 1976.

12. Dixon RE: Nosocomial respiratory infections. *Infect Control* 4(5): 376, 1983.

13. Goodpasture HC, Romig DA, Voth DW, et al: A prospective study of tracheobronchial bacterial flora in acutely brain-injured patients with and without antibiotic prophylaxis. *J Neurosurg* 47: 228, 1977.

14. Murray PR, Washington JA Jr.: Microscopic and bacteriologic analysis of expectorated sputum. *Mayo Clin Proc* 50: 339, 1975.

15. Van Scoy RE: Bacterial sputum cultures: A clinician's viewpoint. *Mayo Clin Proc* 52: 39, 1977.

16. Bartlett JG, Mahew JW, Alexander JM, et al: Should bronchofiberoscopy aspirates be cultured? *Am Rev Respir Dis* 114: 73, 1976.

17. Fossieck BE Jr., Parker RH, Cohen MH, et al: Fiberoptic bronchoscopy and culture of bacteria from the lower respiratory tract. *Chest* 72(1): 5, 1977.

18. Bartlett JG, Rosenblatt JE, Finegold SM: Percutaneous transtracheal aspiration in the diagnosis of anaerobic pulmonary infection. *Ann Intern Med* 79 : 535, 1973.

19. Schillaci RF, Jacovoni VE, Conte RS: Transtracheal aspiration complicated by fatal endotracheal hemorrhage. *N Engl J Med* 295 : 488, 1976.

20. Kalinski RW, Parker RH, Brandt DA, et al: Diagnostic usefulness and safety of transtracheal aspiration. *N Engl J Med* 276 : 604, 1967.

21. Lourie B, McKinnon B, Kibler L: Transtracheal aspiration and anaerobic abscess. *Ann Intern Med* 80 : 417, 1974.

22. Simmons BP, Wong ES: Guidelines for prevention of nosocomial pneumonia. Hospital Infections Program, Atlanta, Centers for Disease Control, 1982.

23. Castle M, Tenney JH, Weinstein MP, et al: Outbreak of a multiply resistant Acinetobacter in a surgical intensive care unit: Epidemiology and control. *Heart Lung* 7(4) : 641, 1978.

24. Buxton AE, Anderson RL, Werdeger D: Nosocomial respiratory tract infection and colonization with Acinetobacter calcoaceticus. *Am J Med* 65 : 507, 1978.

25. Teres D, Schweers P, Bushnell LS, et al: Sources of Pseudomonas aeruginosa infection in a respiratory/surgical intensive therapy unit. *Lancet* 1 : 415, 1973.

26. Cunha BA, Klimek JJ, Gracewski J, et al: A common source outbreak of Acinetobacter pulmonary infections traced to Wright respirometers. *Postgrad Med J* 56 : 169, 1980.

27. Ringrose RE, McKowan B, Felton FG, et al: A hospital outbreak of Serratia marcescens associated with ultrasonic nebulizers. *Ann Intern Med* 69 : 719, 1968.

28. Gervich DH, Grout CS: An outbreak of Acinetobacter infections from humidifiers. *Am J Infect Control* 13(3) : 210, 1985.

29. Craven DE, Connolly MG Jr., Lichtenberg DA, et al: Contamination of mechanical ventilators with tubing changes every 24 or 48 hours. *N Engl J Med* 306 : 1505, 1982.

30. Boslego JW: Nosocomial pneumonia. *J Nosocomial Infect* 1(1) : 17, 1985.

# 11

# Nosocomial Wound Infections

About a quarter of all nosocomial infections are surgical wound infections, and surgery itself is a contributing factor in 75% of all nosocomial infections (1). This chapter discusses the multitude of factors affecting wound healing and the occurrence of infections following surgery. The ICP may, in an ongoing manner or periodically, investigate and gather data on wound infections. An understanding of the known factors involved in wound infection prevention and control is essential in order to interpret data on wound infections and intervene appropriately in this aspect of infection control practice.

## WOUND HEALING

A wound is a break in the continuity of the skin, subcutaneous layers, and any other anatomic structure that is disrupted during a surgical procedure or a traumatic event. Any organs involved in the original wounding will have partial or complete loss of function. Other events that occur include a sympathetic stress response on the part of the host, as well as bleeding and clotting. Additionally, wounds are contaminated with bacteria in virtually all surgical procedures. The numbers of microorganisms, handling of the wound, and host defenses balance to determine whether or not infection results. The body's defense mechanisms are usually adequate to control a bacterial inoculum of $10^5$ organisms per cubic millimeter or less (2); for any greater number of bacteria, as can result from a contaminated traumatic injury (3), the infection risks are higher, unless wound management techniques remove the bacteria. There is also contamination from foreign material as well as dead cells that are present in the wound. Factors important in the prevention of wound infection will be discussed in depth later; nearly all are designed to prevent bacterial contamination from occurring or to minimize their number, to remove the bacteria or make the area the least favorable for bacterial proliferation, or to improve host defense mechanisms to handle effectively the contamination that does occur.

After a wound has been inflicted or after surgery, capillary permeability is increased at the wound site, allowing the leaking of water, complement, electrolytes, plasma proteins, and other blood components into the wounded area. Polymorphonuclear leukocytes, which are essential for the control of infection, also migrate to the site, as do macrophages. During this inflammatory stage, the bacteria that have gained entrance into the wound begin to proliferate. Depending on the ability of the cells that have migrated to the area to control this proliferation, wound infection may occur in the next days or weeks.

Proliferation of epithelial and endothelial cells occurs next in the medium of fluid and material that has been deposited in the wound. Granulation tissue covers and fills the space in the wound and serves as a bacterial barrier.

Remodeling is the final stage of wound healing (3) and can take place over a long period of time. During this phase the final repairs are made, with realignment and organization of cellular material, resulting in the healed wound.

## NORMAL FLORA

The microorganisms that can infect a surgical wound are dependent on the site of the wound with respect to the surrounding skin, the handling of the wound itself, and the internal organ systems crossed during the procedure. In general, the skin above the waist will be colonized with the predominant organisms of the upper respiratory tract; the skin below the waist will be colonized with the same organisms generally found in the bowel. Organisms residing in other organ systems have been discussed in Chapter 6.

There is no normal flora for a surgical wound, although there can be surface contamination of a wound with any number of different flora from the surrounding skin or the flora of drained body systems.

## NOSOCOMIAL WOUND INFECTION

A wound is described as infected based on its clinical signs, particularly an increase or change in the drainage. Purulence is the best guide to the presence of wound infection. A cholecystectomy wound normally drains after surgery; a marked increase in drainage, or a change from serous to purulent drainage, indicates infection. Other signs of a possible infection include temperature and redness, induration, or increased pain at the wound site. Two types of postoperative infections can occur: infections of the incision site and infections of structures adjacent to the incision. Of the two types, incision site infections account for 60–80% (4).

For data collection and comparative purposes, wound infections should be grouped according to the type of operation and the likelihood of contamination during surgery. The risk of a wound becoming infected following surgery of the bowel, for example, would be expected to be higher than that following surgery in a joint, where no contaminated body system was crossed. The most widely used classification for wounds are clean, clean–contaminated, contaminated, and dirty, as defined by the National Research Council (5).

- *Clean:* Clean wounds are those in which neither the gastrointestinal, respiratory, genitourinary tract, nor the pharyngeal cavity is entered and, during surgery, no inflammation is found. Also, these are cases where no breaks in aseptic technique occur.

- *Clean–contaminated:* Clean operations in which the gastrointestinal tract, respiratory or genitourinary tract is entered, but no significant spillage occurs during the procedure.

- *Contaminated:* Wounds in this category include surgical procedures where there is a major break in aseptic technique, gross spillage from a contaminated system, or acute inflammation without pus or fresh traumatic wounds.

- *Dirty:* Dirty wounds include old traumatic wounds and wounds with pus or where a perforated viscus is found.

Incidence rates of wound infections can be calculated, using the number of infections in each group as the numerator and the number of operations performed in each category as the denominator. Although there is much variability among reports, rates for each group in a large study of 62,939 postoperative wounds were clean, 1.5%; clean–contaminated, 7.7%; contaminated, 15.2%; dirty, 40% (6).

Several studies have shown the added expense of a postoperative wound infection in terms of cost and increased length of hospital stay. A study of six common operations (appendectomy, cholecystectomy, bowel resection, total abdominal hysterectomy, cesarean section, and coronary artery bypass graft) was conducted, using the presence of pus as the criterion for wound infection. Using controls matched for age, sex, operation, and underlying disease process, the results generally showed double postoperative stays and significant increases in cost of hospitalization for patients who acquired a nosocomial wound infection (7).

The ICP has several means of finding cases of wound infections for data collection purposes. The microbiology laboratory will be a source; a cultured wound does not indicate the presence of infection but does indicate suspicion of infection. Nursing care plans and nurses' notes may be another means of screening for special wound care precautions or procedures. Discussions with nursing personnel with explanations of criteria (purulence in particular) may be most useful, since wound care is a major activity on a surgical floor.

### Specimen Collection

Whenever possible, specimens from an infected wound should be fresh pus. Drainage on an occlusive dressing that has been on a wound for a period of time can be misleading; organisms from surrounding skin may be recovered, especially if a surface culture is taken, and may be mistaken for the pathogens. After removing the old dressing, old drainage should be wiped away, with sterile wipe, either dry or moistened with sterile saline. A specimen should be taken from deep in the wound, to obtain fresh pus. A specimen obtained in a syringe (with the needle removed) is best to preserve any anaerobes present; expel air from the end of the syringe, recap or insert the needle into a rubber plug, and transport the specimen immediately to the laboratory. Sterile swabs should be placed in transport media and should not be allowed to dry. Concurrent blood cultures, taken at the time of a febrile episode when the wound is suspected as the primary site, are most useful in determining the pathogen.

## PREVENTION AND CONTROL

Prevention of wound infections lies mainly in the area of preoperative and intraoperative procedures and technique. Historical advances in surgical technique include: the introduction of the cap and gown by Neuber in 1883; Halsted's use of rubber gloves; and, in 1897, the first use of the mask by Fluegge and Mikulicz-Radecki. In 1913, Halsted recommended the use of skin towels. Shoe covers were introduced in 1940, and in 1942 Ecker and DeBakey reported on the use of an impermeable adhesive coating on the skin as a bacterial barrier around the surgical site (8).

Much research has been done with respect to clean surgery, to determine factors that affect the subsequent occurrence of infection. Halsted's principles are still true in the handling of the wound during the operative procedure: gentleness, hemostasis, adequate blood supply, asepsis, no tension, careful approximation, and obliteration of dead space. It is important that adequate attention be given any wound during the preoperative, intraoperative, and postoperative phases, since the possibility for infection is great during each phase.

## Preoperative Concerns

Significant areas of concern in the preoperative period include the general health of the patient and the presence of underlying diseases or conditions such as obesity, diabetes, malnutrition, or increased age. It has been found that patients who showed these traits exhibited higher wound infection rates (2). Preoperative showering with an antiseptic soap was found to be of value, as was a surgical prep with an antiseptic solution. The patients who were shaved preoperatively had higher infection rates when the shave was done a number of hours before surgery; small nicks in the skin were thus given time to be colonized and became minute infection sites. Shaving immediately before surgery, no shave at all, or the use of a depilatory cream resulted in lower infection rates. The longer the patient was hospitalized before surgery, the higher the infection rate, according to the same large prospective study (6).

The value of topical and systemic antibiotics in the immediate preoperative, operative, and short postoperative period remains controversial (9). Those reports indicating a positive effect of antimicrobial agents on wound infection rates advocate their use on patients who are at high risk of acquiring infection, based on host or wound factors. Systemic antibiotics may be of value in certain operative procedures when given to high risk patients in the immediate operative period to provide an adequate drug level before and during the surgical procedure itself (10).

## Operative Concerns

Long operative procedures have been associated with increased infection rates; also, operations performed between midnight and 8:00 AM showed higher rates. Certainly, the amount of contamination at surgery has an effect on the resulting wound infection rate; other operative areas of concern include the use of cautery, which increases infection risks, and drained wounds, which show infection rates higher than undrained wounds; wounds with separate punctures for drains have lower rates than those in which the drain is brought out through the primary incision site. Closed wound suction drains have proved valuable in reducing infections from hematomas (2). The practice of delayed primary wound closure reduces infection rates in contaminated wounds (11).

The use of unidirectional or laminar airflow in operating rooms may lower the microbial load in the air of the surgical suite.

A 5-year prospective, randomized study using ultraclean air in joint replacement revealed a reduction in joint infections. The same survey also showed that prophylactic antibiotics had a greater affect on infection than clean air and were more cost-effective (12,13). Ultraclean air systems are costly for a hospital to install and are currently not recommended for use in U.S. hospital operating suites. Emphasis is placed on surgical hand scrub, impervious surgical attire, adequate air exchanges, and reducing patient endogenous flora prior to surgery (14,15). Ultraviolet light also reduces airborne contamination; results of a large study showed that it was useful only during very clean surgical procedures (4). Recently investigators have shown lower infection rates with the use of paper and tightly woven fabrics instead of the traditional loose woven muslin surgical scrub suits (16,17).

Adequate sterilization of surgical instruments is essential, and regular monitoring of sterilizers with live biologic indicators is necessary. This topic is discussed further in Chapter 17. Education of personnel in the proper techniques for sterilization will insure proper use of sterilizing machinery. Proper aseptic technique during the surgical procedure is also an obvious factor in the lowering of postoperative wound infections.

## Postoperative Concerns

The prevention of infection in clean, primarily closed wounds in the immediate postoperative period involves preventing direct contamination of the wound, although bacteremic spread from another infected site can occur. Care in maintaining a dry dressing is important for 8–12 hours after surgery; clean, closed wounds can be exposed after that time. Cruse states in his study of postoperative wounds that the clean wound infection rate is determined in the operating room, and events in the postoperative period are not significant (6). Care in maintaining intravenous lines and respiratory therapy apparatus may be important, however, in preventing the seeding of an implanted device with microorganisms from an infection at a remote site.

### *Dressings*

Wound care in the patient with an open or drained wound can be important in preventing infection or to aid the body in healing (18). Dressings are used for different reasons in different settings, and the need for a certain kind of dressing may change as the wound itself changes.

- *Protection:* A dressing protects the wound from contamination by the airborne and contact routes of spread. A dressing that is changed at adequate intervals can protect the wound from drainage by wicking exudate away from the incision; drainage in the warm, moist environment of an occlusive dressing can provide a good growth medium for microorganisms. By absorbing drainage away from the wound, a fresh dressing makes this medium less favorable. Reinforcement of a dressing is not recommended; if there is drainage, it should be changed.

- *Topical medication:* A dressing can provide a means for the application of antiseptics or antimicrobials to the wound site. Packing a wound can deliver solution deep into an open area and can also debride the wound when removed; the mesh of the dressing will entrap necrotic material that will be removed with the packing.

- *Support and immobilization:* A dressing can provide support to and immobilize an area that needs rest to heal. Pressure can be applied, as well as elevation, to minimize the transudation of fluid into the area. Other uses of a dressing include esthetic considerations (for a disfiguring wound), patient comfort, and, as a source of information to the medical and nursing personnel, the dressing can be a record of exudate from the wound in a given period of time.

### Isolation

When a wound becomes infected, isolation may be warranted to prevent transmission of virulent microorganisms to another patient. Precautions should be taken for all wounds, including bagging dirty dressings in a plastic bag, sterile technique, and proper handwashing before and after wound care.

A wound that drains enough to require a change of dressing twice in a 4-hour period, or one where the drainage cannot be contained by a dressing, requires wound and skin precautions. The specific techniques are outlined in Chapter 18, **Isolation Techniques.** It may be the ICP's responsibility to monitor wound infections, and make decisions about moving patients in and out of isolation.

The ICP has a role in monitoring wound care techniques as well as infection rates that suggest breaks in technique. Each hospital must have policies and procedures with respect to wound care and isolation; these policies must be reviewed and approved annually by the ICC. The ICP and the ICC also interact with operating room personnel to formulate policies regarding preoperative and intraoperative practices in the institution.

The ICP should calculate infection rates for each class of surgery: clean, clean–contaminated, contaminated, and dirty. Many hospitals also monitor the surgical wound infection rate for each surgeon. This information should be reported at regular intervals to the ICC and to all surgeons through the chief of the surgery service. This practice of active surveillance, monitoring wound care techniques and frequent reporting of infections rates to surgeons has reduced surgical wound infections by 35% (19).

Additionally, the ICP will be involved in the selection of scrub and prepping solutions and wound care products, and should be aware of the important factors in minimizing wound infections.

## SUGGESTED PROCEDURES

### Wound Care

1. Wash hands.
2. Set up and open sterile supplies.
3. Put on clean disposable gloves and remove soiled dressing.
   a. Observe drainage for later recording in nursing notes.
   b. Discard dressing in plastic bag.
   c. Remove gloves.
4. Wash hands if soiled during above procedure.
5. Put on sterile gloves.
6. Cleanse wound, using aseptic technique.
   a. Remove debris and necrotic material gently, using antiseptic solution and gauze pads.
   b. Observe wound carefully for changes.
   c. Cleanse wound from the center outward, cleaning only a small area with each pad before discarding. If the wound has one area or a separate wound that has purulent drainage, make sure that different cleansing materials are used in that area; any irrigation should flow from the clean to the dirty area.
7. Redress the wound, based on the amount of drainage and type of dressing needed.
8. Discard gloves in plastic bag.
9. Seal the plastic bag and discard.
10. Wash hands.

## REFERENCES


1. Centers for Disease Control: Nosocomial infection surveillance, 1980–1982. *CDC Surveillance Summaries* 32(4SS): 1SS, 1983.
2. Cruse PJ: Infection surveillance: Identifying the problems and the high-risk patient. *South Med J* 70(Suppl 1): 4, 1977.
3. Schilling JA: Wound healing. *Surg Clin North Am* 56(4): 859, 1976.

4. Centers for Disease Control: Trends in surgical wound infection rates—U.S. *Morbidity and Mortality Weekly Rep* 29 : 47, 1980.

5. National Academy of Science, National Research Council, Division of Medical Sciences, Ad Hoc Committee of the Committee on Trauma: Post-operative wound infections: The influence of ultraviolet irradiation of the operating room and of various other factors. *Ann Surg* 160(Suppl) : 1, 1964.

6. Cruse PJ, Foord R: The epidemiology of wound infection. *Surg Clin N Am* 60 : 27, 1980.

7. Green JW, Wenzel RP: Postoperative wound infection: A controlled study of the increased duration of hospital stay and direct cost of hospitalization. *Ann Surg* 85(3) : 264, 1977.

8. Schilling JA: Mechical means of isolating the surgical wound. The hazards of surgical infection: A symposium. *Hosp Topics,* March 1962.

9. Chodak GW, Plaut ME: Use of systemic antibiotics for prophylaxis in surgery: A critical review. *Arch Surg* 112 : 326, 1977.

10. Veterans Administration Ad Hoc Interdisciplinary Advisory Committee on Antimicrobial Drug use. Kunin CM (chairman): Prophylaxis in surgery. *JAMA* 237(10) : 1003, 1977.

11. Brown SE, Allen HH, Robins RN: The use of delayed primary wound closure in preventing wound infections. *Am J Obstet Gynecol* 127 : 713, 1977.

12. Lidwell OM: Effects of ultraclean air on operating rooms in deep sepsis in the joint after total hip or knee replacement: A randomized study. *Br Med J* 285 : 10, 1982.

13. Lidwell OM: The cost implications of clean air systems and antibiotic prophylaxis in operations for total joint replacement. *Infect Control* 5(1) : 36, 1984.

14. Garner JS: Guidelines for Prevention of surgical wound infections, 1985. Hospital Infections Program, Centers for Disease Control, Atlanta, 1985.

15. American College of Surgeons: *Control of Infections in Surgical Patients,* ed 2. Philadelphia, Lippincott, 1984.

16. Maylan JA, Kennedy BV: The importance of gown and drape barriers in the prevention of wound infection. *Surg Gynecol and Obstet* 151 : 465, 1980.

17. Belkin NA: Evaluating surgical gowning, draping fabrics. *Assoc Operating Room Nurses J* 34(3) : 499, 1981.

18. Castle M: Wound care. *Nursing 75* 5(8) : 40, 1975.

19. Haley RW, Culver DH, White JW, et al: The efficacy of infection surveillance and control programs in preventing nosocomial infections in U.S. hospitals. *Am J Epidemiol* 121 : 182, 1985.

# 12

# Nosocomial Bacteremia

Bacteremia can be a primary infection or a secondary complication of an infection at another site. The incidence of bacteremia in hospitals varies from reports of 20 cases per 10,000 hospital admissions (1) to over 200 cases per 10,000 admissions (2).

Nosocomial bacteremia is defined as the isolation of any organisms from a properly obtained blood culture specimen in a patient with clinical signs of sepsis who was admitted with no signs or symptoms of infection nor a positive blood culture. Nosocomial primary bacteremia develops in 6 of every 1000 hospital admissions, producing infection in approximately 120,000 patients per year (3). These infections can add 7–14 days to the hospital stay and cost more than $1.5 billion annually (4–5).

Two-thirds of all nosocomial bacteremias are caused by aerobic gram negative bacilli (3), and in the last decade deaths attributed to gram-negative bacilli bacteremia have increased at a faster rate than all other causes (6).

Bacteremia occurs more frequently in patients with severe underlying diseases, and mortality varies from 20 to 80% depending on whether shock is present (7). Outbreaks of infection with associated nosocomial bacteremias can be detected quickly when bacteremias are used as sentinel indicators of the problem.

Intravenous cannulas, arterial monitoring devices, and Swan-Ganz catheters are the most frequent causes of primary nosocomial bacteremias; cardiovascular, arterial, intraabdominal, central nervous system, and burn infections cause approximately one-third of all secondary nosocomial bacteremias. Dissemination of bacteria from other nosocomial sites such as surgical wounds, pneumonias, and urinary tract infections cause the remainder (3).

This chapter discusses primary nosocomial bacteremias that are associated with intravascular devices such as IVs and intraarterial monitors. Secondary bacteremias can be reduced by attention to prevention and control of the nosocomial primary sites as discussed in Chapters 9–11. Such a focus has been chosen rather than a general discussion of all bacteremias, because of the ICP's responsibility for monitoring practices related to intravenous catheter insertion and management and also because of the potential for a reduction in the incidence of this infection by adherence to infection control policies and procedures.

## INTRAVENOUS CATHETERIZATION

The plastic catheter for intravenous infusion was introduced in 1945, and the first reports showed no complications from its use. Shortly after the more widespread use of these catheters, however, more reports appeared citing serious complications, especially thrombophlebitis and septicemia.

Maki and his colleagues, Goldmann, and Rhame (8,9) provide an excellent review of the history of intravenous cannulation, showing a report as early as 1957 associating the length of time of catheterization and the occurrence of infection (10). The authors indicate, however, that intravenous catheterization was not considered a significant source of nosocomial infection until much later, and prospective studies did not begin to appear until 1973.

Problems associated with intravenous catheterization have been identified and continue to be significant in terms of patient morbidity and mortality. The use of catheterization for the total nutritional support of a patient has been associated with a high frequency of complications; this problem will be discussed later.

### Sites, Kinds, and Uses of Intravenous Cannulation

Intravenous catheters can be inserted into a number of body sites. Originally the site of choice was the femoral vein; however, now peripheral placement in upper extremities, surgical placement (cutdown) of subclavian catheters, and catheters inserted into the umbilical vein of newborns are common IV catheterization areas and techniques.

Materials used for IV infusion include plastic and steel. The steel needle (scalp vein needle) has been used extensively in pediatrics; because of problems with infiltration, these needles need frequent replacement. Plastic catheters provide a more secure route for administration of fluids.

Intravenous infusion serves several purposes in the care of the hospitalized patient. First, fluids and electrolytes can be restored quickly; moreover, total nutrition can be provided for patients who cannot otherwise be fed or who need supplemental nutrition. An IV catheter provides a route for the continuous or emergency delivery of medications. Last, a catheter provides a means of monitoring central venous pressure or other changes in the vascular status in the critically ill patient. The benefits of intravenous cannulation are clear; the problems are based on a break in the integrity of the skin and in the direct access to the sterile bloodstream via a foreign body, the catheter. The risks must be weighed against the benefits in determining the need for IV catheterization.

# PRIMARY NOSOCOMIAL BACTEREMIA

Intravascular devices carry an inherent risk of infection. The increased use of these devices for hemodynamic monitoring, parenteral nutrition, chemotherapy, and venous access has increased the potential for primary bacteremia. Since catheter-associated infections are the most common types of primary bacteremia, these catheters should be placed aseptically and closely monitored.

Intravenous infection sets should always be suspected when the patient appears to be bacteremic. Symptoms include fever, shaking chills (rigors), sweating, abrupt onset, and hypotension. Phlebitis at the IV site is present in more than half of the IV-associated bacteremias (8). Bacteremia in a patient with an indwelling IV catheter can be most closely associated with the catheter if the blood culture and the IV tip culture correspond, the febrile episode is resolved after removal of the catheter, and other primary sites of infection have been ruled out (11).

Gram-positive skin organisms such as staphylococci, Candida, and *Corynebacterium* sp. can colonize the catheter site and subsequently the catheter. Bacterial colonization of the IV catheter appears to be an important factor in the development of primary bacteremia (12).

Organisms of the tribe Klebsielleae (*Klebsiella, Enterobacter, Serratia*) have been associated with contaminated IV fluid (13).

## Suppurative Phlebitis

One of the must serious complications of IV therapy is suppurative phlebitis, which can be fatal, especially in burn patients. Local signs of infection may be absent, and signs of sepsis may not appear for 2–10 days after the catheter has been removed (14). Suspicion of this complication requires immediate antimicrobial therapy and quite frequently surgical intervention to excise the purulent segment of vein.

## Septic Shock

Septic shock is caused in most cases by gram-negative enteric bacteria. It generally occurs in persons with severe underlying diseases (diabetes, chronic liver disease, blood dyscrasias) or immunosuppressive drug therapy and is often preceded by a manipulative procedure.

Septic shock is characterized by inadequate tissue perfusion as a consequence of tissue anoxia, pooling of blood, diminished cardiac output, and increased peripheral vascular resistance. Along with shaking chills, the patient has fever and warm extremities; cardiac output is increased in this early phase, which is followed by arterial vasoconstriction and a reduction in cardiac output, pooling of blood, and decrease in effective blood volume. Symptoms of shock then follow: hypotension, tachycardia, tachypnea, confusion. Progression of shock leads to respiratory insufficiency, heart failure, coma, and death (15). Treatment is based on support of body systems and immediate surgical intervention to remove or incise and drain the source of infection. Prevention is based on early recognition and treatment of primary infection or of septic shock when it occurs, including the monitoring of intravenous devices.

## Specimen Collection

The methods by which blood specimens are obtained and processed are critical for valid results. The recovery of a microorganism from a blood culture in a patient without clinical signs of bacteremia may indicate contamination at some point in the system of collecting, culturing, or processing blood (16,17). Unlike a urine specimen, for example, where the microbiology laboratory can detect and rule out contamination (e.g., <1000 diphtheroids), it is difficult to interpret the results of cultures positive for normal skin flora which may be causing certain patients infections.

Specimens first of all should be taken by personnel trained in venipuncture. The contamination risk is much higher, as would be expected, when personnel are not well trained in the aseptic method of obtaining a blood culture specimen.

The skin prep is very important, in order that skin flora do not contaminate the specimen. As with other preps, mechanical friction is the most important factor; there is no instant antisepsis by wetting the site with a solution. Alcohol followed by a vigorous prep with an iodophor, or an iodophor alone, remaining for at least a minute, will provide good antisepsis. Tincture of iodine, followed by removal with alcohol, is an excellent prep.

Specimens should be drawn if possible during the febrile episode; the physician needs to make decisions concerning when and how many blood cultures should be drawn (18).

Solutions thought to be contaminated should be cultured. If the IV is suspected as the primary site of infection, it should be removed. Reports conflict on the value of culturing the catheter tip. The CDC recommends a thorough skin prep, aseptic removal of the catheter, and sterile removal of the tip for culture (19). Maki (20) also recommends catheter culture, and outlined a method for culturing catheter tips that was semiquantitative and correlated well with the development of complications. Cooper et al. describe Gram staining of the distal catheter tip as a simple, inexpensive, accurate, and rapid method of diagnosing colonization of intravascular catheter tips (21).

Others state, however, that the presence of an organism on a catheter tip does not indicate the presence of bacteremia; a catheter tip can be colonized but not in enough numbers to seed the bloodstream. Alternately, the bloodstream can be primarily infected and subsequently seed the catheter; therefore, a positive culture from both blood and the tip does not necessarily indicate that the bacteremia was caused by the IV catheter and should be evaluated with clinical symptoms (22). A positive catheter tip without a positive blood culture may well be an indication, however, of impending bacteremia, especially if the IV has been in place longer than 48 hours.

## Portals of Entry

Epidemics have been traced to a variety of sources and sites in the IV and arterial setup. Possible portals of entry of bacteria are shown in Figure 12-1, and the reader is again referred to the review of epidemics by Maki and his associates (8,9). Intravenous solutions can become contaminated during the manufacturing process. In one instance, a large outbreak involving solutions contaminated during production led to the recall of the implicated product (23,24). Other outbreaks from intrinsically contaminated IV solutions have also been reported (25–29).

Hairline cracks in IV bottles or minute punctures in plastic bags can allow bacteria to enter the solution. Contamination can occur at almost any time during the IV setup: when additives are mixed with the solution; when the bottle or bag is attached to the administration set; during manipulation of a stopcock; during injection of medications into the system; and when manipulation of the insertion site occurs, during regular care or IV site care.

Insertion of the IV catheter can be the source of a bacteremic episode, if the insertion is performed under emergency conditions or using poor technique. The catheter can also become contaminated secondarily, as previously mentioned, by bacteremia that originated at another site; the colonized catheter can then lead to a local infection or can itself become a source of recurring bacteremia.

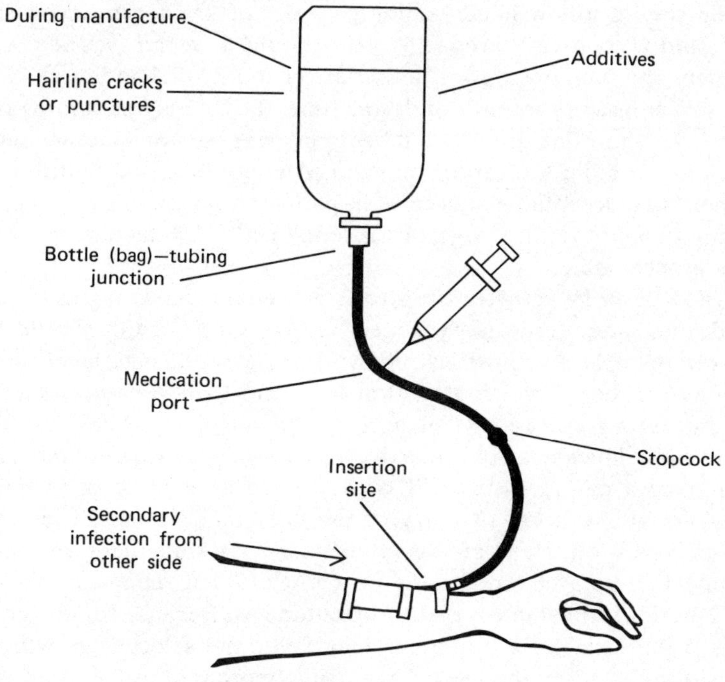


*Figure 12-1*
*Potential areas through which microorganisms can enter an IV system.*

## INFECTION CONTROL

The ICP must ensure that the hospital has specific written guidelines for the insertion and care of intravascular needles and catheters (30). Additionally, the ICP should monitor the use of IV and other intravascular devices for outbreaks of infections as well as breaks in technique. Teaching is again important, to reinforce the practices that are vital to minimize the risk of IV-associated infections.

Specific referenced guidelines for the prevention of intravascular infections are available from the CDC (19). They include hyperalimentation, arterial pressure monitoring devices, and insertion and care of IV catheters. First, intravascular devices should not be placed unless clinically indicated; if oral therapy can be used, IVs should be avoided and the use of keep-open IVs should be discouraged. Meticulous aseptic technique during IV insertion should be maintained. Lines inserted during emergency situations should be removed and restarted, if needed, when the patient's condition stabilizes. The insertion should follow handwashing by a person trained in intravenous insertion, and a good skin prep. The skin should be clean (washed with soap and water) and then prepped with tincture of iodine (2% iodine in 70% alcohol). After at least 30 seconds of drying time, the tincture should be removed with 70% alcohol. The prep should be done using friction and moving in concentric circles, from the center outward. Alcohol followed by the use of an iodophor is an acceptable alternate. In patients who cannot tolerate tincture of iodine or an iodophor, vigorous rubbing with 70% alcohol for at least 1 minute is acceptable.

Insertion of an IV catheter is a sterile procedure, requiring use of a sterile field, drapes, and sterile gloves. Steel (scalp-vein) needles should be used whenever possible and practical. Shaving is not indicated, since very small infections can begin in irritated skin and lead to a greater risk of IV site infection; cutting the hair when necessary is adequate. After insertion, the catheter should be anchored and a dressing applied. Because of the possibility that skin flora or organisms will be deposited at the site of insertion and gain access at the point of entry of the catheter, the use of an antiseptic or antibacterial ointment at the insertion site is sometimes recommended and appear to be of greatest value for catheters that remain in place longer than 72 hours and catheters placed by cutdowns. Because some studies have indicated that antibiotic ointments may favor the selected growth of fungi and resistant bacteria, the use of an antiseptic ointment such as an iodophor should be considered, if any is used (31). The date of catheter insertion should be charted.

Once started, all parenteral solutions should be completely used or discarded within 24 hours. The IV site should be evaluated daily for catheter-related complications. This can be accomplished by gently palpating the insertion site through the gauze dressing or palpation and visual examination through transparent polyurethane dressings. Pain or tenderness at the insertion site or unexplained fever warrants removal of the dressing and inspection of the site. Sites should be rotated and dressings changed every 48–72 hours. The tubing setup from the bottle to the needle or catheter hub should be changed every 48 hours. New data show that it may be safe and more cost-effective to change tubing every 72 hours (32). Careful charting or labeling of the setup is necessary to determine how long each IV has been in place on a busy ward.

The use of membrane filters has been suggested to eliminate any bacteria in the IV system; a 0.45-$\mu$m filter removes almost all bacteria and fungi except some *Pseudomonas*, and a 0.22-$\mu$m filter will block all bacteria. The use of filters, however, has not yet been shown to be effective in reducing infection and may require pumps in order to insure flow of the solution (19).

Solutions that are suspected to be contaminated from the manufacturer should be held and the name and lot number noted. Rather than wasting time culturing IV solutions, suspected solutions should be removed from the shelves and the CDC or FDA notified. Every bottle should be routinely inspected for cracks and plastic bags gently squeezed to detect punctures. Any fluid that is visibly turbid should not be used.

Programs within the hospital for adding materials to IV solutions should follow strict policies and procedures. Mixtures, such as those used for parenteral hyperalimentation, that are made up in the hospital pharmacy should be prepared under a laminar airflow hood to reduce airborne contamination. Techniques in the handling and preparation of these solutions should be closely reviewed by the ICC. Many solutions, from manufacturers, after admixture, and following manipulation during setup or care, become contaminated with microorganisms. The practice of routinely changing the entire setup every 24 hours ensures that those organisms present will not have enough time to multiply to numbers large enough to cause infection. Breaks in technique at any stage, however, can allow contamination or growth of organisms that may lead to a catheter-associated infection. Hyperalimentation or total parenteral nutrition (TPN) is included in the CDC hyperalimentation and admixture section of the vascular-related infection guidelines (19). The TPN solution, if containing crystalline amino acids, does not support the growth of microorganisms except Candida, but a variety of gram-negative bacilli grow rapidly when the solution contains lipids (19).

The placement of the catheter should be performed as a sterile procedure using sterile gloves and drapes. The solution should be used within 6 hours of preparation or refrigerated. Solutions may be refrigerated up to 1 week as long as refrigeration is continuous and initiated immediately after admixing. Catheter sites need not be changed except as necessary, as long as they are subclavian or jugular. Dressing and tubing changes are the same as those governing non-TPN vascular devices, but greater emphasis is placed on sterile technique to control skin and catheter colonization.

The ICP has the responsibility for monitoring the use of IV catheters as potential sources of nosocomial infection. Although in most cases there is prompt resolution of IV-associated bacteremia following removal of the catheter, in some instances complications occur, with serious results. Through monitoring, developing and reviewing policies and procedures, and teaching, the ICP can minimize the risk of infection associated with this vital procedure.

## REFERENCES

1. McCabe WR, Wolff SM, Bennett JV: Incidence of gram-negative bacteremia. *N Engl J Med* 292 : 111, 1975.

2. McGowan JE, Barnes MW: Bacteremia at Boston City Hospital: Occurrence and mortality during 12 selected years, with special reference to hospital acquired cases. *J Infect Dis* 132 : 316, 1975.

3. Centers for Disease Control: National nosocomial infection surveillance, 1983. *CDC Surveillance Summaries* 33(2SS) 9SS, 1984.

4. Spengler RF, Greenough WB: Hospital costs and mortality attributed to nosocomial bacteremias. *JAMA* 240(22) : 2455, 1978.

5. Haley RW, Schaberg DR, Crossley KB, et al: Extra charges and prolongation of stay attributable to nosocomial infections: *A prospective inter-hospital comparison. Am J Med* 70 : 51, 1981.

6. McCue JD: Improved mortality in gram-negative bacillary bacteremia. *Arch Intern Med* 145 : 1212, 1985.

7. Dixon RE: Nosocomial bacteremia: Etiology, diagnosis and prevention. *Hosp Physician,* July 1985.

8. Maki DG, Goldmann DA, Rhame FS: Infection control in intravenous therapy. *Ann Intern Med* 79 : 867, 1973.

9. Maki DG: Nosocomial bacteremia. *Am J Med* 78 : 719, 1981.

10. Moncrief JA: Femoral catheters. *Ann Surg* 147 : 166, 1958.

11. Smits H, Freedman LR: Prolonged venous catheterization as a cause of sepsis. *N Engl J Med* 276 : 1229, 1967.

12. Sheth NK, Franson TR, Rose HD, et al: Colonization of bacteria on polyvinyl chloride and teflon intravascular catheters in hospitalized patients. *J Clin Microbiol* 18(5) : 1061, 1983.

13. Maki DG, Rhame FS, Mackel DC, et al: Nation-wide epidemic of septicemia caused by contaminated intravenous products: epidemiologic and clinical features. *Am J Med* 60 : 471, 1976.

14. Stein JM, Pruitt BA: Suppurative phlebitis—a lethal iatrogenic disease. *N Engl J Med* 282 : 1452, 1970.

15. Shubin H, Weil MH, Carlson RW: Bacterial shock. *Am Heart J* 94(1) : 112, 1977.

16. McNeil MM, Davis BJ, Anderson WJ: Mechanism of cross-contamination of blood culture bottles in outbreaks of pseudobacteremia associated with nonsterile blood collection tubes. *J Clin Microbiol* 22(1) : 23, 1985.

17. Centers for Disease Control: False-positive blood cultures associated with automated blood-culture analyzers—Massachusetts. *Morbidity and Mortality Weekly Rep* 31(40) : 550, 1982.

18. Neu HC: Cost effective blood cultures—is it possible or impossible to modify behavior? *Infect Control* 7(1) : 32, 1986.

19. Simmons BP, Hooton TM, Wong ES, et al: Guidelines for prevention of intravascular infections. Hospital Infections Program, Atlanta, Centers for Disease Control, 1981.

20. Maki DG, Weis MS, Sarafin MS: A semiquantitative culture method of identifying intravenous-catheter-related infections. *N Engl J Med* 296(23) : 1305, 1977.

21. Cooper GL, Hopkins, CM: Rapid diagnosis of intravascular catheter—associated infections by direct gram staining of catheter segments. *N Engl J Med* 312(18) : 1142, 1985.

22. Stillman RM, Soliman F, Garcia L, et. al: Etiology of catheter-associated sepsis: correlation with thrombogenicity. *Arch Surg* 112 : 1479, 1977.

23. Centers for Disease Control: Follow-up on septicemias associated with contaminated Abbott intravenous solutions—United States. *Morbidity and Mortality Weekly Rep* 20(11) : 91, 1971.

24. Centers for Disease Control: Follow-up on septicemia associated with contaminated intravenous fluid from Abbott Laboratories. *Morbidity and Mortality Weekly Rep* 20(12) : 110, 1971.

25. Phillips I, Eykyn S, Laker M: Outbreak of hospital infection caused by contaminated autoclaved fluids. *Lancet* 1 : 1258, 1972.

26. Contaminated drip fluid. *Br Med J* 1 : 707, 1972.

27. Centers for Disease Control: Follow-up on septicemias associated with contamination of intravenous fluids. *Morbidity and Mortality Weekly Rep* 22(14) : 124, 1973.

28. Goldmann DA: Intravenous fluid contamination, aegean-style. *Infect Control* 5(10) : 469, 1984.

29. Matsaniotis NS, Syriopoulou VP, Theodoridou MC, et al: Enterobacter sepsis in infants and children due to contaminated IV fluids. *Infect Control* 5(10) : 471, 1984.

30. *Accreditation Manual for Hospitals 1986: Infection Control.* Chicago, standards adopted by the Board of Commissioneers of Joint Commission on Accreditation of Hospitals, 1985.

31. Maki DG, Bond JD: A comparative study of polyantibiotic and iodophor ointment. *Am J Med* 70 : 739, 1981.

32. Josephson A, Gambert ME, Sierra MF, et al: The relationship between intravenous fluid contamination and the frequency of tubing replacement. *Infect Control* 6(9) : 367, 1985.

# 13

# Other Nosocomial Infections

About 10–15% of nosocomial infections found during total hospital surveillance activities fall into the category of "other nosocomial infections." They include skin and subcutaneous infections, central nervous system infections, gastroenteritis, and endometritis, as well as any other nosocomial infection not previously categorized. The ICP should become familiar with these other kinds of infections that can occur among hospitalized patients.

The evaluation of each infection and the decision whether it is nosocomial should be based on the same general criteria as used with other sites and should include documentation that the patient did not have the infection on admission and evidence that the infection occurred during the hospitalization. As with the other nosocomial infections, clinical impressions or the physician's diagnosis should be accepted in preference to laboratory or x-ray film results in determining the presence of infection.

## SKIN AND SUBCUTANEOUS INFECTIONS

The skin is one of the body's primary defenses against bacterial invasion. Any break in the skin can result in infection, if technique is poor or if host susceptibility is high. Skin infections include those resulting from intramuscular injections (1,2), dermatitis, decubitus ulcers, and other local infections of the skin or underlying tissues.

The skin is normally colonized with a variety of microorganisms, among them *Staphylococcus epidermidis*, diphtheroids, and nonhemolytic streptococci. Skin in the area of the perineum or nose and mouth may have many of the microorganisms that are colonized in these sites. The development of boils, blisters, or purulence, with induration, redness, or pain, indicates the presence of infection. In some cases of cellulitis there may not be purulent drainage; therefore, other clinical signs as well as laboratory results are important in the diagnosis.

Cultures are best taken with a needle and syringe to get an aspirate of drainage, especially if anaerobes are present. The air should be expelled from the syringe and the needle capped or put into a rubber stopper; the specimen should be transported to the laboratory immediately. Open draining skin lesions can be cultured using a sterile swab, although it is difficult to ensure that the pathogen can be identified if the wound is open, because of the other organisms present.

Isolation may be warranted for a patient with an infected dermatitis. If the drainage cannot be contained by a dressing because it is so widespread, contact precautions are necessary. Control of the infection is based on the contact (direct and indirect) route of transmission; therefore, good handwashing, adequate antiseptic prep before skin procedures, and general skin care for hospitalized patients are necessary.

## CENTRAL NERVOUS SYSTEM INFECTIONS

One infection of the central nervous system (CNS) is bacterial meningitis, which can occur in hospitalized patients after neurosurgical manipulation, insertion of shunts, ventriculostomy and intracranial pressure monitoring devices (3), or as sequelae of infections at other sites. Signs and symptoms include fever; signs of meningeal irritation such as headache or stiff neck; disturbances in mental functioning, including lethargy, confusion, delirium, stupor, or coma; and other neurologic abnormalities such as seizures or focal neurologic signs (4). In certain patients such as neonates and the elderly or debilitated, classic neurologic signs may be absent: in neonates, lethargy, vomiting, and subnormal temperature may be present; in the elderly, a sudden change in mental status may be the only indication of a CNS infection.

Organisms isolated from the normally sterile cerebrospinal fluid (CSF) include skin organisms, such as *S. epidermidis* and *Propionibacterium acnes*, especially in shunt infections (5). Additionally, organisms causing infections at other sites in the compromised host can cause meningitis. Signs and symptoms combined with a positive CSF culture are diagnostic.

The role of the ICP in the prevention or control of meningitis is mainly in the area of surveillance. Any unusual increase in this relatively rare nosocomial infection should alert the ICP to begin an investigation of patient care products or procedures, particularly in the operating room setting.

## GASTROENTERITIS

Gastroenteritis, including vomiting and diarrheal illnesses, can occur in hospitals and is readily spread, in certain hospital units, among patients and personnel (6,7). Although many bacterial and viral gastroenteritis illnesses are self-limited and mild, they can be life-threatening among chronic debilitated or immunocompromised patients.

The lower gastrointestinal tract is heavily colonized with microorganisms; organisms that cause gastroenteritis are those that do not normally colonize the bowel; such organisms include *Shigella* sp., *Salmonella* sp., *Escherichia coli* (enteropathogenic), and certain viruses.

The definition of infection for surveillance purposes, is the onset of symptoms and a culture or toxin assay positive for an organism (*Salmonella* sp., *Shigella* sp., Camplyobacter, *C. difficile,* or enteropathogenic *E. coli*) known to cause gastroenteritis in a patient previously without symptoms and with a hospitalization longer than an incubation period. The definition of viral gastroenteritis, for surveillance purposes, is the onset of signs and symptoms with or without viral or serological studies, after hospitalization longer than the incubation period.

Enteric precautions are necessary against gastroenteritis, and a single room is required, especially if the patient is incontinent and has many diarrheal stools; an individual evaluation of the need for isolation may be warranted. Because of the smaller inoculum size needed to be ingested by infants or small children, outbreaks in nurseries or pediatric wards are more common, and stricter measures may be needed. In pediatric or nursery units, patients with suspected infectious diarrheal illnesses should be isolated on admission, until infectious etiologies have been ruled out.

During outbreaks, or when there is evidence that transmission has occurred, cohorting nurses into different groups may contain the outbreak. Nurses are separated into groups: "clean," who are themselves uninfected or not colonized and who care only for babies without the infection; "possibles," who care for babies whose culture results are pending or who have been exposed and may or may not develop disease (this could be two groups, since the "pending" group could be new admissions, without exposure); and "dirty," who care for babies who are ill with the outbreak infection. Minimizing the contact that others, such as house staff and laboratory, radiology, and dietary personnel, have with babies will also help to contain an outbreak of nosocomial gastroenteritis.

The role of the ICP is to monitor this nosocomial infection and intervene quickly if transmission occurs, especially in a pediatric setting. The ICC should have a protocol that outlines authority and actions for this situation;

by having this protocol before a problem develops, the decisions made during an outbreak of this kind will be greatly simplified.


# ENDOMETRITIS

Postpartum endometrial infections are typically caused by genital bacteria carried into the endometrial cavity by gloved hands in the course of rectal or vaginal examinations during labor and at delivery, with extensive manipulation from forceps, manual breech extraction, and placenta removal.

Endometritis is defined, for data collection purposes, as the development, after a patient's admission, of a purulent cervical discharge with either a positive culture or systemic manifestations of infection (8). Since many microorganisms normally colonize the lower genital tract of females, a significant culture is one that has predominant growth of a pathogen, such as *S. pyogenes* Group A, or a pure or predominant culture of *Bacteroides fragilis*, along with a positive blood culture for the same organism.

Because of the problems in the past with "childbed fever," obstetric patients were segregated from other patients in the hospital. This trend is slowly changing, because of the impracticality of separate housing and staffing as well as the better understanding of the epidemiology of nosocomial infections. Suggestions have been made for combined housing of obstetric and noninfectious gynecologic patients, without increased infection rates resulting from this practice (9,10). On the basis of these data, State Public Health Codes contain guidelines for combined units for housing obstetrical, noninfectious gynecologic, and some types of clean surgical patients (11).

The ICP should monitor the endometritis rate in the hospital and intervene quickly if there is an outbreak of infections in this population. The rates should be low, unless a problem in technique occurs or there is a change in patient population, such as an increase in the number of patients with high-risk pregnancies who have been referred to the hospital. Isolation is not generally warranted, except perhaps during outbreaks. Good handwashing is essential for all nursing personnel caring for postpartum patients and their newborns. The changing trend toward family-centered birthing units and sibling visitation on postpartum units, reflecting the changes from strict regulations governing newborn and obstetrical patients, has not resulted in increased postpartum infection rates.

There are other nosocomial infections that may come under review by the ICP or ICC. The reader is referred to other texts and the literature to determine the etiologies and methods of prevention and control for these infections.

# REFERENCES


1. Greenblatt DJ, Allen MD: Intramuscular injection site complications. *JAMA* 240(6) : 542, 1978.

2. Gremillion DH, Mursch SB, Lerner CJ: Injection site abscess caused by *Mycobacterium cheloni. Infect Control* 4(1) : 25, 1983.

3. Mayhall CG, Archer NH, Lamb VA: Ventriculostomy-related infections. *N Engl J Med* 310(9) : 553, 1984.

4. Cluff LE, Johnson JE (eds): *Clinical Concepts of Infectious Diseases.* Baltimore, Williams & Wilkins, 1972, p 231.

5. Everett ED, Eickhoff TC, Simon RH: Cerebrospinal fluid shunt infections with anaerobic diphtheroids (*Propionibacterium* species). *J Neurosurg* 44 : 580, 1976.

6. Pickering LK: Institutional salmonellosis. *Asepsis* 4(3) : 4, 1982.

7. Heard SR, O'Farrell, Holand D: The epidemiology of *C. difficile* with use of a typing scheme: Nosocomial acquisition and cross-infection among immunocompromised patients. *J Infect Dis* 153(1) : 159, 1986.

8. American Hospital Association: *Infection Control in the Hospital,* ed 4. Chicago, American Hospital Association, 1979, p 192.

9. Klimek JJ, Burchell C, Russo JN, et al: Safety and efficacy of combining obstetric and noninfectious gynecologic patients. *Obstet Gynecol* 50 : 431, 1977.

10. Klemas BW, Beck MP, Klimek JJ: A practical approach for the implementation of a combined obstetric and gynecologic facility. *APIC J* 7(2) : 12B, 1979.

11. Connecticut State Department of Health: The Public Health Code of the State of Connecticut. Sec 19-13-D 14A, 1980, p 267.

# PART THREE

# SURVEILLANCE, PREVENTION AND CONTROL OF NOSOCOMIAL INFECTIONS

# 14

# Surveillance of Infections Among Patients

As discussed briefly in Chapter 4, surveillance includes data collection, tabulation, analysis, and reporting. Surveillance has been and continues to be one of the main activities in an infection control program. Surveillance includes the monitoring of patients, personnel, and the environment for nosocomial infections and risks, community-associated infections in some institutions, and communicable (reportable) diseases. The purpose of surveillance is to establish endemic rates, identify risk groups, control epidemics, and identify problem areas. These activities result in the development of policies, procedures, and educational programs that impact on the primary goal of the ICP: to reduce and control nosocomial infections. This chapter discusses methods for surveillance, analysis, and reporting of information on nosocomial infections among patients. It describes various types of surveillance: incidence, prevalence, site specific, periodic, unit-directed, outbreak, and rotation.

Subsequent chapters will deal with surveillance of personnel, the environment, and a discussion of communicable disease surveillance and reporting.

Methods for collecting these data are discussed in this chapter, as well as the analysis, interpretation, and reporting of these data. The method chosen in each hospital depends on the age of the program, the size of the institution, the number of ICPs, and the philosophy of the ICC.

## SURVEILLANCE, ANALYSIS, AND REPORTING METHODS

The earliest method of surveillance in hospitals was some form of "infections card" that was filled out by nursing or medical personnel on each unit when a patient had or developed an infection (1). Thoburn and his colleagues reported from the Johns Hopkins Hospital that this method resulted in under-reporting of infections; in 1965 they employed a nurse epidemiologist to provide more complete surveillance of infections. At about the same time, other institutions were coming to similar conclusions about this passive form of infection surveillance (1). In 1965 the Hospital Infections Section at the CDC initiated a pilot program in six community hospitals to determine the nature, frequency, and epidemiology of nosocomial infections (2). The methodology of this program is still a baseline for any discussion of this aspect of infection control practice. The following is a detailed description of their method, fol-lowed by a discussion of other surveillance methods, some of which use CDC guidelines or are based on the CDC method.

## Traditional Surveillance Methodology

Components of the traditional surveillance program originated by the CDC include definitions, information on nosocomial infections, a place for recording information, the actual process of gathering pertinent information, and a record of each infection.

### *Definitions*

Nosocomial infections are defined as infections appearing in hospitalized patients that were not present or incubating at the time of admission. When the incubation period is unknown, the infection is called *nosocomial* if it appears any time after admission. A physician's comment on the patient's chart that a nosocomial infection has developed is sufficient criterion to establish the infection as nosocomial. An infection related to a previous hospital admission can be defined as nosocomial, even if it is present on a subsequent admission to the same hospital.

Community-associated infections are those that are not related to hospitalization and do not satisfy any of the guidelines that are presented below.

"Guidelines for determining presence and classification of infection" have been outlined by CDC and include specific criteria for defining nosocomial infections. These guidelines are reproduced in their entirety below (3).

GUIDELINES FOR DETERMINING PRESENCE AND CLASSIFICATION
OF INFECTION

A. *Urinary Tract Infections*
   1. Asymptomatic Bacteriuria: This term is applied to those persons having colony counts in urine of greater than 100,000 organisms/ml without previous or current manifestations of infection; such asymptomatic UTIs should be classified as nosocomial if an earlier urine culture was negative at a time when the patient was not receiving antibiotics. If a

patient is admitted to the hospital with a UTI, subsequent culture of a new pathogen in numbers greater than 100,000 organisms/ml should be regarded as a nosocomial infection.

2. Other Urinary Tract Infections: The onset of clinical signs or symptoms of urinary tract infection (fever, dysuria, costovertebral angle tenderness, suprapubic tenderness, etc.) in a hospitalized patient in conjunction with one or both of the following factors developing after admission is sufficient for the diagnosis of nosocomial urinary tract infections.

   a. Colony counts of greater than 10,000 pathogens/ml (a carefully collected midstream urine specimen is adequate for examination) or visible organisms on a Gram smear of unspun fresh urine.

   b. Pyuria of greater than 10 WBCs per high-power field in an uncentrifuged specimen, with a urinalysis negative for pyuria on admission.

A patient with a prior negative urinalysis and/or culture who develops clinical symptoms of urinary tract infection while hospitalized, and neither urinalysis nor urine culture have been repeated, should be considered to have a nosocomial UTI. Also, as described above, the appearance in culture of new organisms in an existing UTI together with clinical continuation or deterioration constitutes a new nosocomial urinary tract infection.

B. *Respiratory Infections*

1. Upper Respiratory Infections: This category includes clinical manifest infections of the nose, throat, or ear (singly or in combination). The signs and symptoms vary widely and depend on the site or sites involved. Coryzal syndromes, streptococcal pharyngitis, otitis media and mastoiditis are all included in this category; although these diverse entities have been grouped together, the specific diagnosis should be entered on the line listing form to allow separate analysis, if desired. The majority of these infections will be viral or of uncertain etiology. Careful attention must be paid to the incubation period in order to separate community-acquired infections that develop after admission and nosocomial infections.

2. Lower Respiratory Infections: Clinical signs and symptoms of a lower respiratory infection, (cough, pleuritic chest pain, fever, and particularly purulence) developing after admission are regarded as sufficient evidence to diagnose respiratory infection, whether or not sputum cultures or chest x-rays are obtained. When there is evidence of both upper and lower respiratory infections, concomitantly, entries should be made for both sites on the line listing form.

Other conditions that may result in similar signs or symptoms (congestive heart failure, postoperative atelectasis, pulmonary embolism, etc.) may often be differentiated by the clinical course of the patient. However, even if such entities are suspected to be present, the diagnosis of lower respiratory infection is made in the presence of one or more of the following: purulent sputum (with or without recognized pathogen on sputum culture) or suggestive chest x-ray. Suprainfection of a previously existing respiratory infection may result in a new nosocomial infection when a new pathogen is cultured from sputum and clinical or radiologic evidence indicates that the new organism is associated with deterioration in the patient's condition. Care must be used in distinguishing supracolonization from suprainfection.

## C.  *Gastroenteritis*

Clinically symptomatic gastroenteritis having its onset after admission and associated with a culture positive for a known pathogen is regarded as nosocomial gastroenteritis. If the incubation period for the pathogen is known (i.e., salmonella, shigella, etc.), the interval between admission and the onset of clinical symptoms must be greater than the incubation period. Alternatively, nosocomial gastroenteritis may be diagnosed if a prior stool culture or cultures, obtained on or after admission from a patient with gastroenteritis, were negative for the pathogen in question. Nosocomial gastroenteritis of viral etiology also occurs—in this instance, the main criteria should rest on epidemiologic data indicating likelihood of cross-infection.

## D.  *Skin and Subcutaneous Infection*

1. Burn Infections: Colonization of burn surfaces with bacteria is nearly universal, and the simple isolation of pathogenic organisms is not sufficient in itself to allow the diagnosis of infection. Purulent drainage from the burn site and/or clinical evidence of bacteremia in a patient hospitalized for treatment of a burn should lead to a diagnosis of burn infection. Such infections are often caused by organisms carried by the patient on admission; nonetheless, such infections should be regarded as nosocomial if the clinical onset occurs after admission, as nearly all of them do. Suprainfection of burns should be regarded as a separate, new nosocomial infection.

2. Surgical Wound Infections: Any surgical wound that drains purulent material, with or without a positive culture, is considered to be the site of a nosocomial infection. The source of the organisms, whether endogenous or exogenous, is not considered.

3. Other Cutaneous Infections: Any purulent material in skin or subcutaneous tissue first developing after admission is regarded as indicating a

nosocomial infection whether or not a culture is positive, negative, or has not been taken. This category includes nonsurgical wounds as well as various forms of dermatitis and decubitus ulcers. In patients who are admitted with skin or subcutaneous infections, a change in pathogens cultured from the infected site is regarded as a nosocomial infection if continuing purulent drainage can be attributed to a new pathogen. Cellulitis caused by bacterial agents is usually not accompanied by purulent drainage; in such instances primary reliance must be placed on clinical judgment, which may be confirmed by cultures of tissue fluid aspirates.

E. *Other Sites of Infection*

1. Any culture-documented bacteremia that develops in a hospitalized patient who was not admitted with evidence of bacteremia is regarded as a nosocomial infection, unless the organism has been judged to be a contaminant. Such nosocomial bacteremias may occur in the absence of recognized underlying infections, or originate from a site of nosocomial infection, or from manipulation of a site that was infected at the time of the patient's admission (i.e., catheters, drains, incision and drainage, etc.).

2. Purulent drainage from the site of an intravenous catheter or needle is regarded as nosocomial infection, even if no cultures are obtained. Inflammation of such sites, without purulent material or strong clinical evidence of cellulitis is not regarded as an infection unless a positive culture is obtained from the catheter tip or from aspirates of tissue fluid.

3. Purulent cervical discharge accompanied by either a positive culture for pathogens or systemic manifestations of infection is regarded as nosocomial endometritis if the onset occurs after admission.

4. Many other possible sites of nosocomial infection must sometimes be considered. Application of the general principles outlined above, however, will generally make classification of these infections possible. It must be reemphasized that *clinical impressions and diagnosis* (if available) always supersede laboratory or radiologic data.

F. *Intra-abdominal Infections*

1. Appendicitis, cholecystitis, and diverticulitis should not be coded as infections unless a secondary infectious complication is noted. Abscess formation, peritonitis, and cellulitis are examples of such complications. The infectious complications will generally be classified as community acquired.

2. If a wound infection develops following surgery for uncomplicated appendicitis, cholecystitis, or diverticulitis, the infection should be classified as nosocomial. Surgical wound infection following surgery involving any infectious complication of the above can be classified as nosocomial only if there is clear anatomic and/or temporal separation of the infectious processes.

Although these guidelines are specific, there are still instances when an infection is hard to define. In such cases, it is crucial that the ICP make a decision, with or without consultation with the ICC chairperson, and be consistent in that decision, should a similar infection occur.

### Information on Nosocomial Infections

There are several items of information the ICP needs to collect about patients with nosocomial infections—for example, demographic data: patient's name, hospital identification number, age, and sex. Information concerning the hospitalization includes date of admission, ward, service, responsible physician, diagnosis and underlying disease, surgery or possible predisposing procedures and dates, preinfection antimicrobial or other therapies, and any other events occurring before the onset of the infection. Information on the infection itself should include the date of onset, the site and characteristics of the infection, pathogens or culture results, and antibiograms if available. Finally, information on the outcome is useful, such as whether the patient was isolated, whether therapy was given, infection resolved, or if it caused or contributed to death, date of discharge or death, and autopsy results. Table 14-1 summarizes some of the information that can be collected.

**Table 14-1**
INFORMATION ON NOSOCOMIAL INFECTIONS

| Demographic Data | Preinfection Hospitalization | Infection | Results |
|---|---|---|---|
| Name | Admission data | Date of onset | Isolation or other control measures |
| Age | Service | Site | |
| Sex | Ward | Pathogens | Therapy |
| Hospital ID | Diagnosis | Antibiograms | Discharge date or date of death |
| | Underlying diseases | | |
| | Antimicrobials | | Autopsy results |
| | Other therapies | | Comments |
| | Surgical or other procedures (and dates) | | |
| | Responsible physician | | |

### Forms for Recording Information

The ICP needs some form on which to record infection data. There are many forms that ICPs have developed for collecting pertinent information, from 3 × 5 file cards to detailed information sheets. Examples are given in Figures 14-1 and 14-2. Figure 14-1 shows an 8 × 11-inch sheet that gives preinfection information at the left and data on the infection itself and the outcome at the

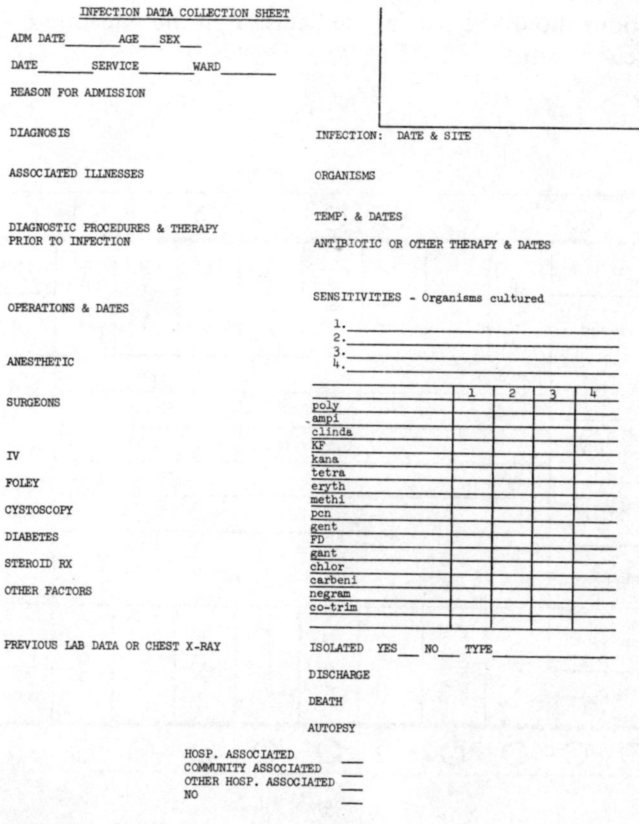

*Figure 14-1*

*An 8 × 11 infection data collection sheet is easily carried in a notebook; this example has a carbonless copy, so that after the month's data are collected and tabulated, the copy can be carried by the ICP during rounds, if the patient in question is still in the hospital.*

right. Figure 14-2 shows a McBee 5 × 8-inch keysort card, overprinted with specific hospital information (i.e., ward names), with spaces for desired infection data. A keysort card is useful for collating and retrieving information, since information can be punched on the edge of the card. A long, slender rod can be pushed through a stack of cards at a certain information point, and those that have been punched through at that point will fall out (Figs. 14-3 and 14-4). In this way information about a certain ward, site, service, pathogen, or any other variable collected can be retrieved at a later date without the need to go through each infection data form manually.

Regardless of the form selected or designed, the ICP should use a data-collection device that will ensure the gathering of similar data for all infections. Data need to be tabulated and sometimes retrieved at a later date. These considerations should be part of the decision in the selection of an infection data collection form.

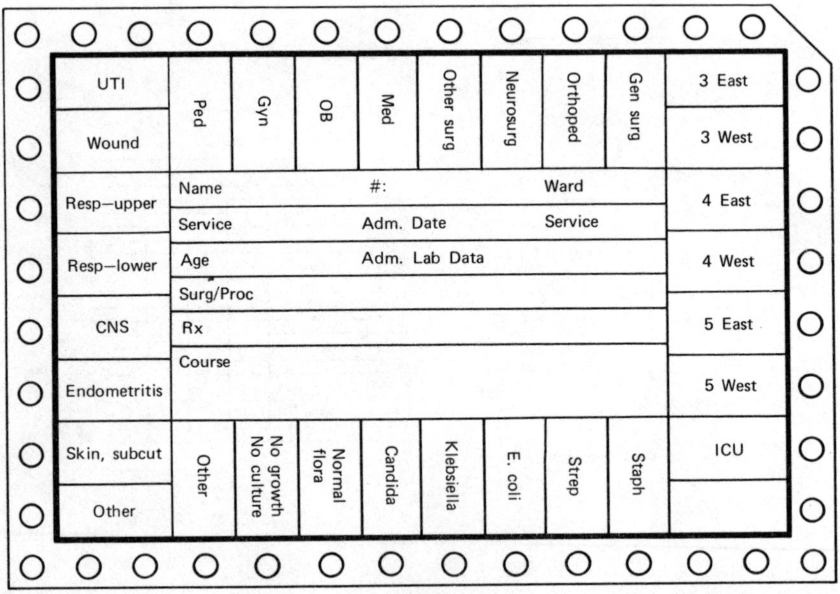

*Figure 14-2*

*A keysort card can have any information overprinted on it. This example has demographic data and information on the infection in the center. The pieces of information around the sides of the card correspond with the holes; information that the ICP may want to retrieve is noted and the corresponding hole is punched out to the edge: ward, service, organism, and site of infection.*

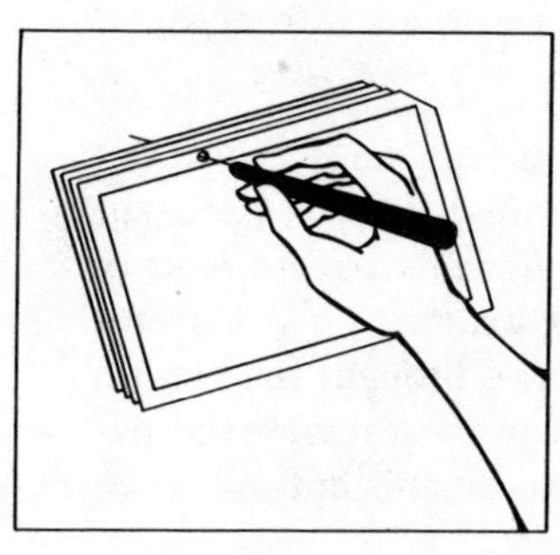

*Figure 14-3*
*The keysort cards are stacked, and the needle is pushed through the hole corresponding with the information desired for retrieval.*

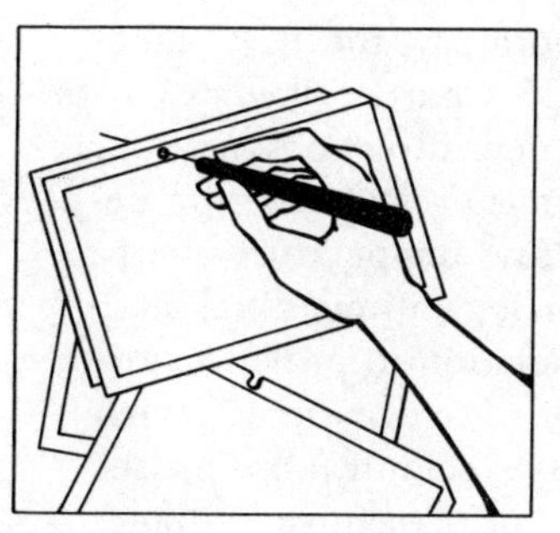

*Figure 14-4*
*The stack is lifted and shaken, and any cards that have been punched at that particular hole will fall out. An example would be a search for all surgical service patients who, during the last 6 months have had a urinary tract infection, from which a Proteus sp. has been isolated in culture.*

### *Gathering Pertinent Information*

The main activities of the CDC surveillance method are the actual monitoring of the hospital for nosocomial infections and the data collection. Because infections tended to be underreported on the cards filled out by each nursing unit's personnel, the role of the ICP was developed to include the detection of nosocomial infections, making surveillance an active rather than a passive activity.

The ICP discovers infections by several means. First, a review of daily results from the microbiology laboratory gives the ICP an indication of the number of patients who have positive cultures, as well as certain patients with negative cultures.

EXAMPLE. According to the CDC guidelines, a patient can have a nosocomial wound infection without a positive culture, provided there is purulent drainage. The ICP receives a culture result from the microbiology laboratory of "no growth at 48 hours" from a surgical patient's wound. This is useful information, because it indicates that someone may have thought the wound was infected and therefore had it cultured. The ICP can then review the patient's chart or talk to the nurses in order to follow up on this culture, even though the result was negative.

These culture results are the basis for further review and follow-up; the results alone are not sufficient to determine the presence of a nosocomial infection.

Using the information from the microbiology laboratory, the ICP makes ward rounds at varying intervals, from daily to weekly. Chart review, discussions with nursing and medical personnel, and sometimes direct observations (especially of wounds) can provide more information necessary for the determination of a nosocomial infection. The ICP also uses temperature charts, medication Kardexes (to locate patients who are receiving antimicrobial medications), and census lists that indicate patients in isolation to provide more clues about patients with possible nosocomial infections. An occasional review of all the charts on a particular unit may be helpful to detect infections missed by using the other means and to determine accuracy of present surveillance system.

Additional methods of finding nosocomial infections include review of clinic records, which may reveal cases of postdischarge infections; review of autopsy reports; medical records reviews; and contact with outpatient clinics for identification of postdischarge infections.

Through these methods, an attempt is made to find and record pertinent information on all nosocomial infections among the hospital's patients. The thoroughness, accuracy, and depth of investigation will depend on the size of the hospital and the personnel time available.

### *Record of Each Infection*

The ICC chairperson may review each infection with the ICP by going over each data form filled out during surveillance rounds. In other settings, the ICP is responsible for determining the presence of a nosocomial infection and consults the chairperson only as needed. This information is then transcribed from the data collection form onto a line listing; Figure 14-5 is an example. The ICP keeps the data collection form as a daily worksheet and updates it as needed. Since a patient may be hospitalized for several months, this individual patient form may be carried in a notebook or card file; therefore, the information needs to be entered on a line listing for a permanent record that can be used for data tabulation and analysis at the end of the month. The line listing also gives a quick indication of current locations of patients with nosocomial infections that may be useful in showing clusters or development of antibiotic resistance.

---

### *NOSOCOMIAL INFECTIONS: LINE LISTING*

| Patient Data | Date of Onset | Ward | Service | Infection | Organism | Antibiogram | Comments |
|---|---|---|---|---|---|---|---|
|  |  |  |  |  |  |  |  |

---

**Figure 14-5**

*The line listing is a daily record of infections as they are detected through surveillance activities.*

In order to perform these surveillance activities, the CDC recommends one full-time ICP be employed for every 250–300 hospital beds.

### *Data Tabulation*

To achieve the goals of the infection control program the data gathered during surveillance must be tabulated and reported to key people, including members of the ICC, hospital administrators, physicians, and quality assurance or risk management committees.

Tabulation of data to provide meaningful information must be accurate and reflect infections of patients in populations at risk. How this is accomplished is determined by the availability of information in each institution. The numbers of admissions and discharges should be available for time intervals such as months or accounting periods as well as on an annual basis. Numbers of patients admitted to and discharged from each service and numbers and types of surgical procedures performed are also useful denominators for tabulation of infection rates.

The number of patients infected in a population at risk is expressed as a rate. These rates can be readily calculated by the ICP who receives the information listed above from admissions or accounting departments in the institution. The number of infections in each ward or service for a certain period is not meaningful without knowledge of the population at risk of acquiring an infection; that is, the rate must be calculated.

EXAMPLE. During the month of January, two patients in a medical unit were determined to have a nosocomial infection. In February, four patients had infections. The ICP found that the number of admissions to the unit were 100 and 200 for January and February, respectively. Therefore, the *rate* of infection was the same, 2% for both months. Although more patients became infected during February, since more patients were admitted, the rate had not actually increased.

The denominator used in the calculation of infection rates should be the number of patients at risk of acquiring an infection. For the entire hospital or individual wards, the number of admissions *or* discharges can be used. Each will reflect the number of patients housed in the unit or in the institution who were at risk of acquiring an infection. Whether the number of admissions or discharges is used as the denominator, it is important that each month's rates be calculated consistently. Additional consideration should be given to special care units.

EXAMPLE. A surgical intensive care unit had 10 cases of nosocomial infections during January, which were found through the surveillance activities of the ICP. Admission data revealed, however, that only eight patients were admitted to the unit. Since nearly all patients housed in the unit had been transferred postoperatively from surgical wards, admission data did not supply a meaningful figure as a denominator (nor did the discharge data, since nearly all patients were transferred out rather than discharged). Information from the admissions office about transfers as well as admissions to the unit supplied the ICP with a figure to use as the denominator for calculating the infection rate.

Just as the denominator can be selected from different sources, the numerator varies from hospital to hospital. Some ICPs calculate infection rates from the number of *patients* who acquire infections, whereas others use the number of *infections* as the numerator. Each source of denominator used to calculate rates will have some built-in bias, but this is unavoidable. Rates are used to observe trends indicating problem areas or potential outbreaks and a small amount of bias will not appreciably affect these rates.

EXAMPLE. In one hospital, 34 patients acquired nosocomial infections during January. One thousand patients were admitted to the facility during that month. Of the 34 patients, six developed two nosocomial infections and one developed three infections, for a total of 41 infections during January. Using the two possible numerators, number of *patients* with infections (34) and number of *infections* (41), the infection rates were calculated to be 3.4 and 4.1%, respectively.

There may be justification for the use of either number as numerator. In general, however, it may be more appropriate to compare similar variables—*patients* with infections to *patients* at risk. Whichever numerator is selected, it is critical that the data be collected and tabulated consistently in the same manner from one data collection period to the next.

Ideally, rates of infection for specific sites should be calculated using as denominators categories that most closely represent the type of patients at risk of acquiring those infections. In many cases, however, these denominators are impossible or too difficult to obtain and may not justify the time spent in trying.

EXAMPLE. Surgical wound infections can be tabulated according to the type of surgery performed. Wounds can be classified (4) in categories from clean to dirty, and infection rates can be calculated for each type of wound. Denominators should represent the number of operations performed in each category:

$$\frac{\text{Number of clean cases that became infected}}{\text{Number of clean operations performed}} = \text{clean wound infection rate}$$

When this information is not available, the denominator might be the total number of operations performed:

$$\frac{\text{Number of wound infections}}{\text{Number of operations performed}} = \text{wound infection rate}$$

The next less specific choices of denominator would be the total number of surgical patients or the number of patients on surgical wards:

$$\frac{\text{Number of wound infections}}{\text{Number of surgical patients}} = \text{wound infection rate}$$

$$\frac{\text{Number of wound infections}}{\text{Number of patients on surgical wards}} = \text{wound infection rate}$$

The first choice is certainly the most specific in terms of patients at risk; the last choice is least specific. Whichever denominator is chosen, depending on available time and how the data will be used, this same kind of denominator data must be collected for each surveillance period.

In summary, infection rates are calculated as follows:

$$\frac{\begin{array}{c}\text{Number of patients with infections}\\ \text{(specified time period)}\end{array}}{\begin{array}{c}\text{Number of patients at risk}\\ \text{(specified time period)}\end{array}} \times 100 = \text{infection rate}$$

where the number of patients with infections is divided by the number of patients at risk during the same time period. This number, multiplied by 100, gives an infection rate in the form of a percent. This expression can be called an *infection rate,* an *attack rate,* or an *incidence rate,* since it is the number of patients who acquire infections, over a specified time period, from a population at risk of acquiring infection.

The ICP can determine, with the committee members and chairperson, what infection rates should be calculated for the monthly infection report. Table 14-2 shows some of the additional rates that could be generated from this

**Table 14-2**
POSSIBLE INFECTION RATES FROM SURVEILLANCE DATA

1. Total hospital

$$\frac{\text{Number of patients with infections (time period)}}{\text{Number of patients in the hospital (time period)}} \times 100$$

2. Ward

$$\frac{\text{Number of patients with infections on that ward (time period)}}{\text{Number of patients on that ward (time period)}} \times 100$$

3. Service

$$\frac{\text{Number of patients with infections on that service (time period)}}{\text{Number of patients on that service (time period)}} \times 100$$

method of surveillance. Worksheets have been designed by CDC personnel as an aid in calculating these rates, and similar sheets are shown in Figures 14-6, 14-7, and 14-8.

---

**A** = Number of patients with nosocomial infections during the surveillance month

**B** = Number of hospital discharges during the surveillance month

**C** = Ratio (A/B)

**D** = A/B × 100 = infection rate

---

*Figure 14-6*

*This worksheet can be used for calculating the total hospital infection rate, with the number of patients discharged as the denominator.*

(Month, Year)

NOSOCOMIAL INFECTION RATES BY WARD

WORKSHEET

| Ward | Number of Infections (A) | Number of Discharges (B) | Attack Rate (A/B × 100) |
|------|--------------------------|--------------------------|-------------------------|
|      |                          |                          |                         |

*Figure 14-7*

*Infection rates for separate wards can be calculated by using totals from surveillance data and discharge data.*

___________________

                                        _______________
                                        (Month, Year)


NOSOCOMIAL INFECTION RATES BY SERVICE

WORKSHEET

| Service | Number of Infections (A) | Number of Discharges (B) | Attack Rate (A/B × 100) |
|---|---|---|---|
| Medical | | | |
| General surgery | | | |
| Urology | | | |
| Orthopedics | | | |
| Other surgical specialties | | | |
| Obstetrics | | | |
| Gynecology | | | |
| Pediatrics | | | |
| Newborn | | | |

**Figure 14-8**

*Infection rates for services can be calculated by using totals from surveillance data and the number of discharges for each service.*


___________________

                                        _______________
                                        (Month, Year)


NOSOCOMIAL INFECTION SITES BY SERVICES

| Service | UTI | Resp | Wound | Bacteremia | Other | Total |
|---|---|---|---|---|---|---|
| Medical | | | | | | |
| General surgery | | | | | | |
| Urology | | | | | | |
| Orthopedics | | | | | | |
| Other surgical specialties | | | | | | |
| Obstetrics | | | | | | |
| Gynecology | | | | | | |
| Pediatrics | | | | | | |
| Newborn | | | | | | |
| Total | | | | | | |

**Figure 14-9**

*Information on the sites of infection for each service can be presented to the ICC in tabular form.*

(Month, Year)

NOSOCOMIAL INFECTION ORGANISMS BY SITES

| Organism | UTI | Resp | Wound | Bacteremia | Other | Total |
|---|---|---|---|---|---|---|
| | | | | | | |

**Figure 14-10**
*Information on the organisms isolated in each nosocomial infection site can be presented to the ICC.*

In addition to rates calculated from infection data, other pieces of information can best be analyzed by using tables. Figures 14-9 and 14-10 are examples of the tabulation of site–service and site–pathogen data. Clusters may be seen by looking at information presented in this form, where absolute numbers are small but clusters may still be evident.

The tabulation and analysis of data is usually done at the end of each data collection period. Since the results of cultures taken on the last day of a month may not be available for 48 hours or longer, there is a delay beyond the end of the calendar month until all that month's data can be interpreted. The rates and tables are devised with the help of the line listing, which neatly presents each variable to be analyzed.

### Data Reporting

Data collection and tabulation are useful only when this information is reported to the appropriate people in the hospital. The tabulations can be presented in a monthly report, using a compilation of Figures 14-6–14-10 as well as a line listing, for dissemination to department heads, service chiefs, head nurses, and administration. Presentations of data in the form of maps or graphs for particular areas of the hospital may also be useful. This information is first reported to the ICC; then all or part of it is disseminated to selected people in the hospital.

Results of this traditional form of surveillance are available from the CDC through their studies of hospitals of different types and sizes. The National Nosocomial Infections Study (NNIS) was begun in January 1970, and hospitals all over the country have since participated by collecting information in a consistent manner and submitting it to the CDC. From this study, infection rates have been generated based on the size and type of hospital as shown in Table 14-3 (5). Figure 14-11 shows a breakdown of the frequency of each type of infection found in those hospitals.

**Table 14-3**
NOSOCOMIAL INFECTION SUMMARY: NNIS HOSPITALS
BY HOSPITAL CATEGORY

| Hospital Category | Infections | Discharges | Rate (per 100) |
| --- | --- | --- | --- |
| Nonteaching | 6,845 | 281,122 | 2.4 |
| Small teaching | 7,875 | 255,601 | 3.1 |
| Large teaching | 13,528 | 328,559 | 4.1 |
| Total | 28,248 | 865,282 | 3.3 |

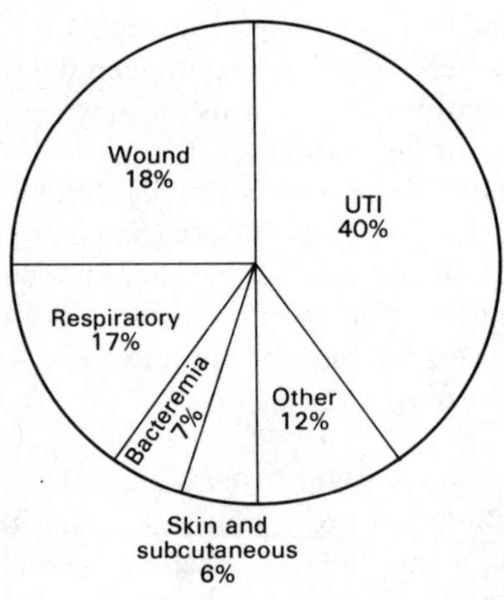


*Figure 14-11*
*The NNIS hospitals surveyed in 1983 reported this analysis of the distribution of noso-*
*comial infections.*

### *Data Analysis*

Many ICPs spend much of their time collecting, recording, tabulating, and reporting data and comparatively little time on data analysis. The purpose of surveillance as outlined in this chapter is to determine nosocomial infection rates, identify high-risk population groups, and monitor and resolve outbreak situations. Assessment of the data indicates accomplishments of these goals and pinpoints problem areas that may need attention in the form of education or control measures to achieve the primary goal of infection reduction.

## Periodic Surveillance Method

In 1978, Chelgren and LaForce reported that periodic surveillance of nosocomial infections resulted in more time for infection control activities such as education (6). Their method used the CDC guidelines for determining the presence and classification of infection, as well as the recommended method of obtaining, recording, tabulating, analyzing, and reporting infection data.

Their methodology was unique in that full surveillance was only performed for one month out of every 3-month period, or for a total of 4 months per year. The remaining 2 months of each quarter were devoted to problem solving based on the results of surveillance data or problems from other sources. The review of patients with positive blood cultures continued as the only form of formal monitoring during these months, called "limited surveillance" months.

Their results showed that, in a 440-bed hospital, 50% of the ICP's time was spent on data collection and analysis during full surveillance, whereas only 5% was spent during limited surveillance. The reverse was true for time spent in educational, supervisory, and policy-procedure review activities. The nosocomial infection rate for the hospital, shown in rates for each surveillance month, decreased from January 1974, when this surveillance method was begun, to February 1977, the end of the reported study period.

Other hospitals have had equally good experience with this method, especially in an established infection control program, when the ICP has become known as a consultant, and when baseline infection rates for different areas and services have been established.

## Prevalence Survey Method

Prevalence surveys provide information on the prevalence rate of infections, as opposed to the incidence rate. Prevalence in this case is defined as the proportion of patients in the hospital with infections at one given point in time. The most frequently used protocol for prevalence surveys is that developed by the CDC and adopted by others (7,8).

The objectives of a prevalence survey are outlined by CDC as follows:

1. To determine the magnitude and characteristics of infections among hospitalized patients at a given point in time.
2. To assess the accuracy and efficiency of a routine surveillance program.
3. To allow a direct comparison of infections and other factors among hospitals.
4. To determine patterns of antimicrobial usage.
5. To determine the frequency with which infections are cultured.

During the prevalence survey day (more than 1 day may be needed, depending on the size of the hospital and the number of personnel available for the survey) each ward is visited, and all available charts are reviewed. Similar methods are used to determine the presence of infection as those recommended for the traditional surveillance method. Infections are defined and classified using the same guidelines the CDC issued for the traditional surveillance methodology.

Infections are listed directly on a line listing; an example is shown in Figure 14-12. Nosocomial infections are listed as N+ if active during the survey; infections are listed as N− if not active during the review.

EXAMPLE. During a prevalence survey, an ICP sees admission culture data and a culture result that is 3 weeks old, indicating a nosocomial urinary tract infection. The patient subsequently received antimicrobial therapy, and a repeat culture taken 48 hours after antimicrobial therapy had ended showed no growth. The ICP recorded the infection as "N−" on the line listing.

The data collected in a prevalence survey will include more infections than would be recorded during traditional surveillance, since all nosocomial infections, whether they occurred during the calendar month or not, are recorded.

Analysis and reporting forms for site–service and site–pathogen can be the same as those used in the traditional surveillance methodology (Figs. 14-9 and 14-10). Prevalence rates can be calculated for the total hospital, for wards, and for services using other forms, as shown in Figures 14-13, 14-14, and 14-15. The figure used as the denominator for each ward is the number of charts that were reviewed. Prevalence survey results can be compared with traditional surveillance data by looking through the current and previous calendar month's data to check whether infections were missed during continuous surveillance periods. The CDC suggests calculating the efficiency of the traditional surveillance system by the following formula (7):

The number of infections found by prevalence survey that were also detected by surveillance system divided by the number of infections detected by prevalence survey times 100 equals the percent of efficiency of the surveillance system.

PREVALENCE SURVEY: LINE LISTING

| Patient Name | Hosp. No. | Age | Sex | Service | Ward | Adm. Date | Onset Date | Primary Diagnosis | Surgical Procedure | Site of Infection | Organisms | Ab Rx | N+/N− Comments |
|---|---|---|---|---|---|---|---|---|---|---|---|---|---|
|  |  |  |  |  |  |  |  |  |  |  |  |  |  |

**Figure 14-12**

*A line listing is used to record all information collected during a prevalence survey.*

Prevalence surveys can be useful in measuring the efficiency of traditional surveillance methods or the methods that are discussed below in order to determine the level of sensitivity of the method. In a program with limited personnel, or one with a heavy commitment to education, research, or aspects of infection control other than surveillance, prevalence surveys can give a quick glimpse of the infection situation at a given point in time that may be useful to the ICP and the ICC.

**A** = Number of patients with nosocomial infections
on the survey day

**B** = Number of patients in the hospital census on
the survey day

**C** = Ratio (A/B)

**D** = A/B × 100 = prevalence rate

**Figure 14-13**

*A prevalence rate for the hospital can be calculated using the data collected and the number of charts reviewed.*

PREVALENCE OF INFECTIONS BY WARD

| Ward | Number of Infections (A) | Charts Reviewed (B) | Prevalence Rate (A/B × 100) |
|---|---|---|---|
| | | | |

**Figure 14-14**

*Prevalence rates for each ward are the number of patients with infections divided by the number of charts reviewed (not the census).*

                                    

| | PREVALENCE OF INFECTIONS BY SERVICE | | |
|---|---|---|---|
| *Service* | *Number of Infections (A)* | *Charts Reviewed (B)* | *Prevalence Rate (A/B × 100)* |
| Medical | | | |
| General surgery | | | |
| Urology | | | |
| Orthopedics | | | |
| Other surgical specialties | | | |
| Obstetrics | | | |
| Gynecology | | | |
| Pediatrics | | | |
| Newborn | | | |

**Figure 14-15**

*The prevalence of infections in each type of service is also calculated, using the number of charts reviewed for each service.*

## Site-Specific Surveillance

Site-specific surveillance involves focusing surveillance on nosocomial infections from one specific site such as surgical wounds or urinary tract. Some ICPs have focused on surgical wound infection surveillance as they are the most costly site-specific nosocomial infections (9). This can be a successful and effective type of surveillance as demonstrated in the surgical wound surveillance study of Cruse and Foord (10).

## Surveillance of High-Risk Areas or Sentinel Infections

Because of limited time or personnel, some hospital committees have set up a system of surveillance of specific units for types of infections. The surveillance, using CDC guidelines, of intensive care units may provide the ICP with information only about the areas where the most compromised hosts are generally housed; most ICPs would agree that the majority of nosocomial infections in a hospital occur in or following admission to an intensive care unit.

Wenzel's surveillance data revealed that 35–45% of all nosocomial bacteremias occurred among patients in intensive care units (11). Surveillance of "sentinel" infections, such as bacteremia, may accomplish one of the goals of total hospital surveillance, that is, to identify potential problems (12).

## Kardex Review Method

In 1976, Wenzel and his colleagues reported a surveillance system based on a review of the nursing care plan (Kardex) on each ward (13). Again, based on the limited time available for surveillance activities as well as the need for other infection control activities, this system was developed as a method of monitoring nosocomial infections. The criteria used for determining the presence of an infection are slightly different from those outlined by the CDC (Table 14-4); the techniques for recording, analyzing, and reporting are similar.

**Table 14-4**
### DEFINITIONS OF INFECTION USED FOR NOSOCOMIAL INFECTIONS SURVEILLANCE AT THE UNIVERSITY OF VIRGINIA HOSPITAL

| Infection Site | Criteria for Infection |
| --- | --- |
| Wound/tracheostomy site | Presence of pus |
| Blood | Positive culture |
| Pulmonary | Infiltrate on chest x-ray, not present on admission, associated with new sputum production |
| Urine | $\geq$ 100,000 colonies of bacteria/ml |
| Intestinal | Positive culture for pathogen or unexplained diarrhea for $\geq$ 2 days |
| Burns | New inflammation or new pus not present on admission<br>Alternatively $\geq 10^6$ organisms/g of biopsied tissue |
| Miscellaneous (hepatitis, upper respiratory infections, peritonitis, etc.) | Clinical picture |

SOURCE: Wenzel RP, Osterman CA, Hunting KJ, et al: Hospital-acquired infections. I. Surveillance in a university hospital. *Am J Epidemiol* 103:251–260, 1976.

The ICP begins at the Kardex on each nursing unit, which is visited weekly. A patient's chart is reviewed if the Kardex lists any of the risk factors determined by Wenzel and his associates (Table 14-5). All patient charts in intensive care units are reviewed. Data from the microbiology laboratory are used to determine the presence of infection, but these data are not used as a primary source for locating patients with infections, as in the traditional surveillance system.

Wenzel had good results when he compared this method to a prospective

**Table 14-5**
CASE-FINDING CLUES IN THE NURSING CARE PLAN (KARDEX)
THAT ALERT THE NURSE-EPIDEMIOLOGIST TO POTENTIAL
HOSPITAL-ACQUIRED INFECTIONS

Diagnoses or condition
    Leukemia, lymphoma, carcinoma, granulocytopenia, collagen vascular diseases,
      sarcoid, widespread dermatoses (conditions often requiring steroid therapy)
    Burns
    Organ transplantation
    Hepatitis (check earlier transfusions)

Operations or procedures
    Surgery estimated to take longer than 2 hours or involving infected tissue
    Tracheostomies
    Central nervous system shunts
    Bladder catheterization
    Hyperalimentation
    Respiratory assistance therapy
    Special wound or decubitus care

All patients hospitalized for 3 weeks or more

SOURCE: Same as for Table 14-4.

review of charts of all hospitalized patients (82–94% accuracy). The time
required for surveillance was cut from 25 to 16 hours per week. The accuracy
of this system depends heavily on completely kept nursing treatment records.
However, because of the trend toward documentation of the nursing process
within the medical record, including nursing care plans, use of Kardexes is
being discontinued.

## Laboratory-Based Surveillance Method

In 1979, McGuckin and Abrutyn reported the results of a surveillance method
based on data from the microbiology laboratory (14). This method of monitoring the hospital does not provide incidence or prevalence rates of infection
but gives information that may be useful in detecting epidemics. Because of
time limitations and the need for time to be spent in activities to decrease infection rates, McGuckin and her colleagues developed a system that provided
necessary and useful information for the ICC.

The first part of McGuckin's system involves monitoring the number of
isolates, each week, of a particular bacterial species found on each nursing
unit. Either the results from the microbiology laboratory or the results of tests

of isolates submitted for antimicrobial susceptibility can be used. At the end of a 26-week period, the number of isolates for each species for each week is ranked; the number of isolates that constitutes a dividing line below which 80% of the weeks' recoveries fall was determined as the *threshold value* for that species.

EXAMPLE. Over the 26-week period, the number of *E. coli* isolates were 12, 9, 8, 11, 17, 4, 6, 9, 11, 12, 3, 7, 13, 5, 8, 9, 7, 14, 10, 13, 9, 4, 7, 8, 12, and 11. Ranked in order from lowest to highest, the numbers were 3, 4, 4, 5, 6, 7, 7, 7, 8, 8, 8, 9, 9, 9, 9, 10, 11, 11, 11, 12, 12, 12, 13, 13, 14, and 17. To find the number below which 80% of the isolates fall, take 80% of 26 = 22. The twenty-second item, counted from the lowest to highest, is the threshold. The threshold number of *E. coli* isolates is 12.

Threshold values are calculated for all bacterial species, based on this 26-week experience.

The surveillance system is based on these threshold values: if the number of isolates of a bacterial species exceeds the calculated threshold value on a ward in any subsequent week, an investigation results. The investigation begins with a determination of whether the isolates were from one or several patients and a study of antimicrobial susceptibility patterns. Chart review follows if warranted by this information.

EXAMPLE. After the calculation of four isolates per week as a threshold value for *P. mirabilis* in a surgical intensive care unit, eight isolates occur during 1 week. Closer review in the laboratory reveals that these are isolates from five patients. Antibiograms of the five patient cultures are similar. An investigation results.

The threshold values calculated for this system are arbitrary and can be changed if outbreaks are missed or too many investigations are begun that are not warranted. The system serves as a way of monitoring for outbreaks only, with the assumption that an increase in the number of organisms of a particular species will occur during an outbreak of infections caused by that organism. The sensitivity of this system depends on a high culture rate for the hospital, that is, that infections are routinely cultured. Epidemics involving more than one unit or more than one organism may be missed.

Although this method provides no data on the infection rate for the hospital, McGuckin feels that it is the most efficient way to monitor the hospital for outbreaks, leaving time for other infection control activities as well.

The microbiology laboratory, in this system as well as in the traditional surveillance method, is an important source of data for the ICP. Weinstein stated that the laboratory personnel may be in a position to detect infection trends or outbreaks by the recognition of highly infectious organisms, multiply resistant isolates, or a cluster of similar isolates in different areas of the hospital or types of specimens (15).

## Surveillance By Objective

In 1984 Haley introduced the concept of surveillance by objective (SBO) to ICPs (16). This is a variation on the well-established management by objective concept. In this concept there are two kinds of objectives: process objectives and outcome objectives. Reduction of infection is an outcome objective and how this is achieved includes process objectives such as surveillance, education, policies, and procedures. Haley encourages setting outcome objectives of a predetermined and realistic nature to decrease morbidity, mortality and hospital costs to patient and using the above-mentioned process goals to accomplish this.

EXAMPLE. Surgical wound infections affect 25% of all patients having surgery in an institution. This is 7% higher than rates published in the NNIS data (5). The outcome objective is to reduce surgical wound infection rates by 7%. Process goals would include:

1. Notifying surgeons of wound infections rate as compared to NNIS data.
2. Monitor and change policies and procedures that are not optimal for wound infection reduction.
3. Notify surgeons of their infection rates.
4. Monitor and tabulate wound infections.

Process objectives achieve the outcome objective of 7% wound reduction. Added objectives would be reduced costs to surgical patients.

## Other Surveillance Methods

Many hospitals have designed variations of the methods already described in order to monitor their patient population for nosocomial infections. The variations are mostly in the data base used for finding problem areas and include systems based on the number and types of orders for antimicrobial drugs received in the pharmacy, a review of x-ray film reports, infectious disease consultations, and census information for isolation placement. A review of medical records and autopsy results has been suggested, but because it is retrospective the data may not be useful in preventing or controlling outbreaks of infections (17,18).

## USE OF COMPUTERS IN SURVEILLANCE, ANALYSIS, AND REPORTING

The goal of any surveillance system is to provide useful information to the ICP and the ICC in the least amount of time, thereby allowing adequate time for appropriate intervention. One of the problems encountered by ICPs performing routine or periodic surveillance has been the amount of data generated by these activities. Computer systems, therefore, have been developed in many hospitals to handle these data and present them in more meaningful ways.

Reports of computer programs for the collection, tabulation, and analysis of nosocomial infections are evident from the earliest days of infection surveillance (19). Currently there are commercial programs available, as well as programs developed using the facilities of particular institutions (20). Some programs are specific for infection control; the ICP or another person enters information into the computer, which provides an analysis and a report. Data collection sheets or forms in these settings are usually designed for easy transfer onto keypunch cards or direct computer entry.

An increasing number of hospitals are computerizing the entire medical record, or parts of it. In these institutions, the ICP may be able to have a program designed that can retrieve and tabulate a report directly from patient charts; following review of this information and verification of the presence of a nosocomial infection, the computer can provide summary data and, in some cases, statistical analyses of infection trends.

## LONG-TERM CARE

The methods of surveillance discussed in this chapter with little modification are adaptable to long-term care. The types of nosocomial infections that are prevalent in long-term care are urinary tract, pneumonia, and wound. Criteria for identification of these infections should be developed with emphasis placed on clinical signs and symptoms. Additionally, cultures are difficult to obtain and must usually be stored prior to transport. They are often processed by an outside laboratory, and there is a longer period of time for results to come back. The institution must assess its program and select surveillance methods for data collection, tabulation, and reporting that is of most value to prevent infection transmission.

The idea of surveillance of the patient population for nosocomial and, in some cases, community-associated infections was developed by the CDC and is supported by this group as well as by the American Hospital Association (21) and the Joint Commission on Accreditation of Hospitals (22). The traditional method of surveillance as outlined by the CDC has been, and continues to be, the basis for infection control activities in hospitals. Data provided by the NNIS study have established rates of infections that are used as standards throughout the country (5). Surveillance by objective may be the trend for the last half of this decade.

Other methods of surveillance have been developed in part to give more time to ICPs to teach and intervene in health care procedures in an attempt to lower infection rates. Baseline infection rates determined by traditional surveillance methods are useful as a "before" measure to compare with rates measured after a specific intervention. Each method and variation of surveillance may have its role and usefulness, depending on the changing priorities of an infection control program.

Daily surveillance activities bring the ICP into frequent contact with other members of the hospital staff while promoting awareness of infection control. There are as many surveillance variations as there are ICPs. No single form of surveillance is optimal for every hospital. Appropriate measures might depend on hospital size, patient population, resources, and infection control capacities. Infection Control Practitioners and ICCs must consider their priorities and select the best surveillance method for collecting, analyzing, and reporting data in accordance with their goals.

# REFERENCES


1. Thoburn R, Fekety R Jr, Cluff LE, et al: Infections acquired by hospital patients. *Arch Intern Med* 121 : 1, 1968.

2. Eickhoff TC, Brachman PS, Bennett JV, et al: Surveillance of nosocomial infections in community hospitals. 1. Surveillance methods, effectiveness and initial results. *J Infect Dis* 120(3) : 305, 1969.

3. Center for Disease Control: Outline for surveillance and control of nosocomial infections. Atlanta, U.S. Department of Health, Education, and Welfare, Public Health Service, Centers for Disease Control, 1972.

4. National Academy of Sciences, National Research Council, Division of Medical Sciences, Ad Hoc Committee of the Committee on Trauma: Post-operative wound infections: The influence of ultraviolet irradiation of the operating room and of various other factors. *Ann Surg* 160(Suppl) : 1, 1964.

5. Centers for Disease Control: Nosocomial infection surveillance, 1983. *CDC Surveillance Summaries* 33(2SS) : 9SS, 1984.

6. Chelgren G, LaForce FM: Limited, periodic surveillance proves practical and effective. *Hospitals* 52 : 151, 1978.

7. Centers for Disease Control: Protocol for prevalence survey. Atlanta, U.S. Department of Health, Education, and Welfare, Public Health Service, Centers for Disease Control, 1969.

8. Latham EK, Standfast SJ, Baltch AL, et al: The prevalence survey as an infection surveillance method in an acute and long-term care institution. *Am J Infect Control* 9(3) : 76, 1981.

9. Pinner RW, Haley RW, Blumenstein BA, et al: High cost nosocomial infections. *Infect Control* 3(2): 143, 1982.

10. Cruse PJ, Foord R: The epidemiology of wound infection: A 10 year prospective study of 62,939 wounds. *Surg Clin North Am* 60(1): 27, 1980.

11. Wenzel RP, Osterman CA, Donowitz LG, et al: Identification of procedure-related nosocomial infections in high-risk patients. *Rev Infect Dis* 3(4): 701, 1981.

12. Eickhoff TC: Nosocomial infections. *Am J Epidemiol* 101(2): 93, 1975.

13. Wenzel RP, Osterman CA, Hunting KJ, et al: Hospital-acquired infections. I. Surveillance in a university hospital. *Am J Epidemiol* 103: 251, 1976.

14. McGuckin MB, Abrutyn E: A surveillance method for early detection of nosocomial outbreaks. *APIC J* 7(1): 18, 1979.

15. Weinstein RA, Mallison GF: The role of the microbiology laboratory in surveillance and control of nosocomial infections. *Am J Clin Pathol* 69(2): 130, 1978.

16. Haley, RW: Surveillance by objective: A new priority-directed approach to the control of nosocomial infections. *Am J Infect Control* 13(2): 78, 1985.

17. Blake S, Cheatle E, Mack B: Surveillance: retrospective versus prospective. *Am J Infect Control* 8(3): 78, 1980.

18. Birnbaum D, King LA: Disadvantages of infection surveillance by medical record chart review. *Am J Infect Control* 9(1): 15, 1981.

19. Steinhauer BW, Cox F, Stobie GH, et al: A method of hospital infection surveillance incorporating the use of the computer. *Henry Ford Hosp Med J* 15: 139, 1967.

20. Berg R, Elder HA, Hierholtzer WJ, et al: The use of computers in infection control. *Conversations in Infect Control* 6(4): 1, 1985.

21. American Hospital Association: *Infection Control in the Hospital,* ed 4. Chicago, American Hospital Association, 1979, p 24.

22. *Accreditation Manual for Hospitals 1986: Infection Control.* Chicago, standards adopted by Board of Commissioners of Joint Commission on Accreditation of Hospitals, 1985.

# 15

# Surveillance of Infections Among Hospital Personnel

Each institution has a responsibility to its employees to provide immunization, when possible, against communicable diseases for which they are at risk during patient care. In addition, educational programs should be given that emphasize maintenance of good health and proper use of isolation techniques to prevent transmission of disease or infection. The institution is also responsible for follow-up treatment, prophylaxis, and counseling after exposure to infectious diseases on the job. The institution also has a responsibility to its patients that all members of the health care team, in the process of providing patient care, will not transmit any infectious diseases to these patients. The employee health service can accomplish these goals through a preemployment screening of all personnel, educational programs for all employees, and restriction from patient care when necessary. The CDC has published referenced guidelines for control of infections among hospital employees (1).

The Joint Commission on Accreditation of Hospitals (JCAH) states in its infection control standards that the ICC shall have input into the employee health program (2). This chapter discusses the role of the ICP and the ICC in the development and implementation of an employee health program. The discussion is limited to infectious disease aspects of the program; each facility's program may include more components to screen for diseases that are not communicable. Additionally, each employee health program varies from hospital to hospital, based on factors such as size and type of facility.

The ICP must have a role in the employee health program because of the ongoing responsibility for monitoring personnel and patients for infections. In larger institutions, there may be an employee health department, which should be represented on the ICC. Input may be in the form of approval of policies and procedures for employee health recommended by the committee. In smaller institutions, the ICP may be the Employee Health Coordinator and have more direct responsibilities for implementing the committee-approved program. Regardless of the degree of involvement, the infection control and employee health programs have one shared goal—to minimize the risk of infections from patients to personnel and from personnel to patients. There are two ways this goal can be achieved: one is to screen patients for communicable diseases and isolate patients with such diseases early and appropriately; the other is to minimize the number of susceptible persons in the hospital personnel population through screening and immunization (3). The first approach is covered by the infection control policies on isolation; the second approach is the employee health program.

State laws affect employee health programs in terms of employee screening and follow-up for communicable diseases. The ICP and committee members should be aware of state regulations when reviewing and approving the employee health program. The program should be complete, with policies covering all anticipated problems with patient or personnel infections. The components of employee health programs are discussed below, with reference to the interaction between employee health and infection control personnel.

## PREEMPLOYMENT SCREENING

Potential employees need some form of screening to rule out conditions that might endanger patients, other employees, or the potential employee. The most comprehensive employment screening includes a complete history and physical examination; for most institutions, however, this procedure is too costly. If a complete physical examination is not given or required at the time of employment, employees should be educated to understand the need for maintaining their own health and to seek regular health maintenance and care. In other words, a screen for selected conditions should not mislead employees into thinking that their preventive health care needs have been met. Employees should be educated regarding their risks to patients when communicable or infectious conditions are present.

The initial evaluation may include a general physical examination of employees and taking a history of any communicable diseases a potential employee may have had, such as measles, mumps, tuberculosis, chickenpox, hepatitis, diarrheal disease, and any chronic skin disease or infection. Most hospital employees will have had and will be immune to the common childhood illnesses. The small group that is susceptible, however, can acquire the disease (especially if a person who falls into such a category works in pediatrics) and can spread the illness to children, immunocompromised hosts or other susceptible employees.

### VDRL and Other Laboratory Tests

Routine testing such as blood counts, urinalysis, VDRL, chest x-ray, or pre-employment screening for enteric pathogens or nasopharyngeal carriage of organisms, such as staphylococci or streptococci, are not good predictors of employee risk to patients. Preemployment screening for rubella, hepatitis B, and tuberculosis are all beneficial to both patients and hospital employees.

### Rubella

Rubella is a common childhood disease that, because it is mild, is often disregarded. The most dangerous sequelae of the infection are the fetal complications that can occur when pregnant women get the disease during the first trimester. Rubella monitoring and immunization programs in hospitals are designed to protect the pregnant employee or patient from infection.

Some hospitals test all employees; the Public Health Service Advisory Committee on Immunization Practices recommends the following:

> All personnel (male or female) who are considered to be at increased risk of contact with patients with rubella or who are likely to have direct contact with pregnant patients should be immune to rubella (3).

This passage could be interpreted as proposing the testing of women of childbearing age assigned to the pediatric, nursery, and obstetric areas and of male employees who work in hospital areas such as prenatal clinics or departments performing diagnostic tests on pregnant patients. The extent of testing and vaccination may vary from hospital to hospital. Titers of 1 : 8 or less indicate susceptibility to the disease. Although the disease confers immunity, a history of rubella alone is not acceptable, since it is often misdiagnosed and the person's recall of exposure or disease is not reliable.

### Tuberculosis

All new employees should receive a baseline tuberculin skin test (PPD), or, if an employee is known to have a positive PPD test result, a preemployment chest x-ray film should be taken as screening for tuberculosis. Generally in the United States surveillance and control measures rather than BCG vaccination are all that are necessary (1).

### Hepatitis B

All employees who will work in areas that are at high risk for exposure to the hepatitis B virus (HBV), such as dialysis units, OR, ER, laboratories dealing with blood and body fluids, renal transplant units, blood banks, and dental clinics, should be screened for susceptibility to HBV. It may be cost-effective to prescreen before vaccination, but vaccinating immune persons does not appear to be a risk (1). It may be beneficial to know HBV status in personnel working in high-risk areas who refuse HBV vaccination.

## Education

Personnel should be educated at the time of employment on the benefits of immunization if they are placed in high-risk areas. Employees should also be made aware of health policies such as the isolation manual for protection from disease transmission, risk to patients when employees work when sick or infected, and the importance of seeking employee health services when exposure to communicable disease occurs.

## Immunizations

Employee health programs may include immunizations against a variety of diseases. The recommendations of the Public Service Advisory Committee on Immunization Practices (ACIP) should be consulted for updated information on dosage and contraindications. These guidelines can be obtained from Public Inquiries, Building 1, Room B63, Centers for Disease Control, Atlanta, GA 30333.

Diphtheria and tetanus vaccination should be offered to employees who have never been immunized or when a booster is needed, every 10 years. Primary immunization can be offered to employees against polio; measles and mumps vaccine can be offered to nonimmunized employees who will have contact with pediatric patients. In some institutions mumps vaccine is given to males only in this category.

## Rubella

Rubella vaccine, as previously stated, should be offered to all male and female employees of childbearing age with Rubella antibody titers of less than 1:8 who work in high-risk areas. Vaccine should not be given to pregnant employees. Female employees receiving the vaccine must not become pregnant during the first 3 months after immunization because of the theoretical risk to the fetus from vaccine virus crossing the placenta. Consideration should be given to administering the rubella vaccine in combination with measles and mumps where applicable. Consult current ACIP guidelines for detailed discussion on vaccine administration and side effects (4). Figure 15-1 is an example of a consent form for rubella vaccine.

---

EMPLOYEE HEALTH
RUBELLA VACCINE IMMUNIZATION
CONSENT/WAIVER FORM

I,_________________________, have been informed that my rubella titer is below 1:8. This means I am not immune to rubella (German measles). I will agree to one of the following:

_____I desire to have the rubella vaccine given to me by my private physician, and I will bring a signed statement to that effect to Employee Health.

_____I desire Employee Health to give me the rubella vaccine after a pregnancy test has been performed.

_____I refuse to be given the rubella vaccine and assume entire responsibility, absolving the _______________ hospital of any complications in the event of the disease or pregnancy.


Date:_________________Signature:_______________________________________

Witness:_________________________________________

---

**Figure 15-1**

*This consent and waiver form informs employees of their status with respect to rubella and is filled out on the basis of an employee's decision. This form is kept in the employee's health file.*


## Hepatitis B

The risk of acquiring hepatitis B from a patient is greater for an employee than is the risk to patients from infected personnel (1). Transmission occurs from contact with blood infected with HBV. Transmission may occur from sticks with dirty needles or sharps, blood exposure to hands with breaks in the skin, or mucosal absorption from blood exposure. Personnel who work in high-risk areas previously mentioned are susceptible and at risk of acquiring HBV and should receive HeptaVax (HBV vaccine). Recommendations on administration, side effects, and populations at risk outlined in the ACIP for hepatitis (5). Figure 15-2 is an example of a consent form for the HeptaVax.


## Influenza

Personnel in the Employee Health Department should be on appropriate mailing lists so that they will receive yearly updates on the nationwide status of influenza, as well as current recommendations on the immunization of hospital personnel. *Morbidity and Mortality Weekly Report,* published by the

### HEPATITIS B VACCINE INFORMATION AND CONSENT FORM

Hepatitis B vaccine appears to be safe, effective way of preventing acute infection. Field tests involving more than 6000 individuals have been carried out over the past 5 years. In these trials, the rate of hepatitis B has been reduced by more than 90%, acute side effects have not been severe (sore arm, low-grade fever), and prevention seems to last more than 3 years. The long-term side effects of the vaccine are unknown as yet.

You are considered to be at higher risk of hepatitis B because of your work in the hospital. Please complete the following questionnaire and indicate whether you wish to be immunized or not. (In either case, please complete the questionnaire and record your preference.) If you wish to be immunized, we will draw blood to determine whether or not you are susceptible to infection. Approximately 15–20% of hospital employees are already immune to this infection. If you are immune, you will not need to be immunized.

Circle appropriate response and sign.

<u>Yes</u>    I understand the risks and benefits of immunization with hepatitis B vaccine. If I am not already immune, I would like to receive vaccination.

Signed _______________________________________________________

<u>No</u>    I understand the risks and benefits of immunization with hepatitis B vaccine. Despite the potential benefits, I prefer *not* to be immunized at this time.

Signed _______________________________________________________

If you have decided to receive hepatitis B vaccine, you will need to be serologically tested. We will be in contact with you when the time and place for testing has been decided.

Please complete the following (whether your response is yes or no):

1. Name ___________________________ 2. Age _______ years.

3. Sex M _______ F _______ 4. Title of position in hospital _______________

5. Major work responsibility _______________ Department _______________

6. Duration of time at this job _______ months.

7. Frequency of contact with blood: weekly, daily, several times a day (circle one).

8. Have you had hepatitis previously? Yes _______ No _______

If yes, what type _______________

9. Are you pregnant? Yes _______ No _______

***Figure 15-2***

*This consent and waiver form informs the employee of the risk of hepatitis B and benefits of immunization.*

CDC, has the most current information and recommendations. Depending on the epidemiology of the influenza virus in the community, vaccine may be offered to high-risk employees, or there may be a need for a hospitalwide influenza vaccination program.

Other services may be offered during the preemployment screening to rule out other diseases, but these are the communicable diseases that are important to screen or immunize for from an infection control standpoint. Employees may waive all or part of the screening by presenting evidence from a private physician that the required examination and/or tests were done. Documentation in the employee's chart of waivers or evidence of screening outside the hospital will be important if complications occur and should be kept available along with other screening documents.

## FOLLOW-UP OF EMPLOYEES

In addition to the preemployment screening, the employee health program should have policies for follow-up of employees, both as a routine and in the event of employee exposure to infection. Follow-up of exposure to communicable disease is discussed later in this chapter.

### Yearly Review

Many hospitals do annual PPD skin tests on all employees whose previous tests had been negative. The conversion rate has been reported as low as 0.11% (6). The CDC has recommended that policies for repeating PPDs be in accordance with the risk of acquiring new tuberculosis infection (1). The cost of routine testing may not be justified in a hospital where the tuberculosis morbidity is low. Preemployment PPDs and testing during contact investigation may be more appropriate in this setting (1).

### Employee Illness

The ICP is responsible for reporting communicable diseases among employees as well as among patients to the appropriate health authorities. Cultures and other appropriate laboratory tests should be performed to document the presence of infection.

There should be specific policies regarding return to work for employees with communicable illnesses. Some hospitals have developed a system whereby employees who are ill for longer than a certain number of days (e.g., 3) must be cleared by their supervisor before returning to the work area. If the supervisor has any doubts about the noninfectiousness of the worker,

*General Guidelines Relating to Personnel Health and Medical Care*

This statement is intended to be a general guideline for personnel with certain infections, or who have been exposed to patients with certain specified infectious diseases. The policies set forth below apply chiefly to personnel with patient contact. It should be emphasized that employees have the right to seek advice and treatment of their choice, unless institutional liability or moral obligation dictates that the employee be evaluated and his/her treatment managed by the Personnel Health Service or by another physician. In general, pregnant employees should avoid unnecessary exposure to patients with infectious diseases. An absolute contraindication to care by pregnant employees exists in the case of patients with rubella, unless the employee is known to be immune.

*Personnel with Infection*

*Acute upper respiratory disease.* A general hospitalwide policy requiring personnel with such illness to report to Personnel Health Service or to obtain clearance before returning to work is not feasible. Personnel who have patient contact may either be sent home or to Personnel Health Service at the discretion of their supervisor. It is neither necessary nor feasible to remove all personnel with acute upper respiratory disease from their jobs. A special area, such as the premature infants center, newborn nursery, or transplant service, may develop its own special requirements in consultation with the Director of Health Service and the ICC. Personnel with documented streptococcal pharyngitis need not undergo a repeat throat culture during or after antibiotic treatment and may return to work 24 to 48 hours after initiation of appropriate chemotherapy, depending on their clinical status.

*Staphylococcal or streptococcal skin disease.* Acne is the most common skin disease in this category. Control is impossible, except in certain specialized areas; these areas should be handled as discussed above. Personnel with draining or crusted skin lesions should be referred to Personnel Health Service for evaluation and treatment. Generally, the employee should not return to work until cultures for the causative organism, usually staphylococci or streptococci, are negative or until clearance has been given by Personnel Health Service.

*Hepatitis.* Employees recovering from hepatitis must have clearance from Personnel Health Service or their physician before returning to work.

*Carriers of upper respiratory staphylococci, streptococci, meningococci, and similar infectious organisms.* Because of the ubiquity of these bacteria, a variable proportion of hospital personnel may be expected to be asymptomatic carriers of such organisms, which only rarely have general significance in the hospital. When indicated by appropriate epidemiologic circumstances, the identification, evaluation, and management of personnel carriers may be undertaken by Personnel Health Service, in consultation with the ICC, the Divisions of Infectious Disease, and the staff director of the area concerned.

*Diarrhea of uncertain etiology.* Employees with sudden onset of diarrhea should report to Personnel Health Service. Symptomatic treatment will be begun, and, when indicated, stool cultures will be obtained.

---

**Figure 15-3**
*Sample policies related to personnel with infectious diseases.*

| Disease | Work Status | Duration Off Work |
| --- | --- | --- |
| AIDS | May work with restriction | Evaluated by Employee Health and Infectious Disease |
| Draining abscess, boils, and so forth | Off | Until drainage stops, if employee has patient contact |
| Chickenpox (varicella) | Off | Until all lesions are crusted and dry |
| Diarrhea<br>Shigella<br>Salmonella | Variable | Individual, depending on extent of symptoms and cultures and evaluation by Personnel Health Service |
| Gonorrhea | May work | |
| Hepatitis A | Off | Until 7 days after onset of jaundice |
| Hepatitis B, NANB | May work | Personnel may work, but must wear gloves for procedures that involve tissue trauma or mucous membrane contact |
| Herpes simplex<br>Oral–facial | May work | Emloyee Health evaluation; may be restricted in high-risk areas |
| Genital | May work | |
| Herpetic Whitlow (fingers) | Off | Until lesions are crusted and dried |
| Herpes zoster | No patient contact | If able to work, may do so, but not in high-risk areas |
| Influenza and upper respiratory infection | Variable | Evaluation by Personnel Health Service, depending on work area |
| Impetigo | Off | No patient contact until crusts are gone |
| German measles (rubella) | Off | Until rash is cleared (minimum of five days) |
| Measles (rubeola) | Off | Until rash is cleared (minimum of four days) |
| Positive PPD conversion | May work | Evaluation and follow-up by Personnel Health Service |
| Active TB | Off | Until under treatment and 3 smears taken on 3 consecutive days are negative |
| Strep throat (group A) | Off | May work 24 hours after being placed on appropriate antibiotic and/or symptom-free |

**Figure 15-4**

*Sample guideline for employees with infections, indicating their work status and when they can return to work.*

---

### *EMPLOYEE INFECTION AND COMMUNICABLE DISEASE REPORT*

CONFIDENTIAL

***************

The Section of Epidemiology  -  Employee Health Services

---

Name of employee __________________ Area of employment _____________

Date infection noted or exposure to communicable disease occurred __________

Date employee seen _________

    Where seen? _____ EHS _____ ER _____ Other _____

Type of infection or communicable disease __________________________________

Culture taken:     Yes _____ No _____ Results: ___________________

Lab tests done:     Yes _____ No _____ Results:___________________

Treatment: _______________________________________________________

_________________________________________________________________

_________________________________________________________________

Was employee sent off duty? Yes _____ No _____

If yes, for how long? __________

Was infection control leave granted? Yes _____ No _____

Employee allowed to work with the following restrictions:

    No food contact __________      No patient contact __________

Patient contact with the following restrictions: __________________________

_________________________________________________________________

_________________________________________________________________

Signature of person completing form ____________________ Date _________

---

Epidemiologic comments: ___________________________________________

_________________________________________________________________

_________________________________________________________________

_________________________________________________________________

**Figure 15-5**

*Employee Health completes this form and sends one copy to the worker's supervisor and one to the ICP.*

that employee must report to the Employee Health Department. An example of policies of this kind is shown in Figure 15-3, with a sample guideline for employees returning to work (Fig. 15-4).

The ICP should be informed of all employees with communicable diseases in order to monitor any patient population which has been exposed. Figure 15-5 is a copy of the form used for this purpose. One copy is returned to the personnel's supervisor with work status indicated, and a copy is sent to the ICP.

## Employees Exposed to Communicable Diseases

A program should be developed to cover inadvertent exposures of employees to communicable diseases. The ICP should be involved in contact investigation and outbreak workups of this nature. Documentation of any employee exposures to infections in the form of incident reports are necessary in the event that Worker's Compensation claims must be filed. It is essential that the hospital have protocols to follow in the event of the exposure of personnel to communicable diseases. After the exposure has occurred, there is generally little time and a lot of anxiety, and carefully outlined protocols will assist in the smooth management of these situations. A form for this purpose is shown in Figure 15-6.

---

*EMPLOYEE EXPOSURE TO COMMUNICABLE OR INFECTIOUS DISEASE*

Type of exposure ______________________________________________

Patient _______________________________________________________

Date _________________________________________________________

| *Employee* | *Unit* | *Employee* | *Unit* |
|---|---|---|---|
|  |  |  |  |

---

**Figure 15-6**
*This form can be used to keep track of exposures among personnel.*

In general, the exposure of employees to infectious diseases calls for action, using the following steps (3): first, further transmission should be prevented by isolation or discharge of the infected person. Second, all contacts should be identified and their susceptibility determined. If the exposure requires documentation by a preexposure and postexposure test, such as acute and convalescent sera or baseline and postexposure PPD, the preliminary tests should be done immediately.

The third step in follow-up of exposed employees is to administer promptly the appropriate prophylaxis to the exposed persons. A fourth step involves the prevention of secondary cases, that is, exposures of personnel who may be incubating the infection and may themselves be communicable to other personnel or patients. The need for this step will depend on the epidemiology of the disease. In the case of a highly communicable disease, exposed susceptible employees may need to be sent home for the duration of their incubation period and disease. An example is chickenpox (varicella). Personnel exposed to or diseased with hepatitis B, as another example, need not be sent home during the incubation period, and need remain home only while actively diseased. They can return to work as asymptomatic carriers provided they are extremely careful about handwashing (1). Another way of approaching exposed susceptible personnel is to cohort this group, in other words, keep them together as a group so that new patients or other personnel are not exposed to the infection they carry.

The fifth step in handling employee exposures is to immunize newly admitted patients, if possible, or to immunize patients before admission, so that they are not susceptible if exposed employees are incubating the disease. Immunization of other susceptible employees will also decrease the number of people at risk of secondary disease after exposure to the employee. Protocol for employee exposure to specific diseases is discussed briefly.

### *Hepatitis*

There have been many advances in the past 10 years in hepatitis research, mainly related to the development of serologic tests and the availability of HeptaVax. Because of these advances, more information is now available about the incubation periods, length of infectivity, numbers of chronic carriers, and resulting immunity to the hepatitis diseases.

At least three clinically, epidemiologically, and serologically different diseases are recognized: hepatitis A (HAV), hepatitis B (HBV), and non-A, non-B hepatitis (NANB), which ultimately may be identified as one or more distinct diseases; each presents different risks to personnel.

*Hepatitis A.*   Hepatitis A has been called *infectious hepatitis, short-incubation hepatitis;* symbols associated with it are HAV (hepatitis A virus), HAAg (hepatitis A antigen), and anti-HA (antibody to hepatitis A) (5).

Hepatitis A often resembles a viral gastrointestinal illness. The symptoms include fever, malaise, nausea, and jaundice. The disease is generally acute and lasts 2–4 weeks. After initial exposure, the incubation period is short, 2 weeks to 2 months, with an average incubation of 28 days. The infectious period is short, beginning 12–15 days before illness. Virus is excreted in the stool, peaking at 2 weeks before onset of clinical symptoms. When jaundice appears, virus is no longer excreted in the stool. There is no chronic carrier state or chronic hepatitis secondary to infection with hepatitis A. Studies of antibody to hepatitis A have shown that this virus is not a problem among hemodialysis patients or staff (7).

Personnel who have had direct fecal–oral exposure from a patient found to have hepatitis A should be given prophylactic immune serum globulin (ISG) at a dose of 0.02 ml/kg of body weight. This dose of ISG is 80–90% effective in preventing the illness or attenuating the severity of hepatitis A. Protection lasts about one incubation period (5).

Hepatitis A in the hospital is controlled by appropriate isolation as discussed in Chapter 18.

*Hepatitis B.* Terminology associated with hepatitis B includes hepatitis B virus (HBV), hepatitis B surface antigen ($HB_sAg$), hepatitis B core antigen ($HB_cAG$), hepatitis B e antigen ($HB_eAg$), and antibodies to each of these antigens: anti-$HB_s$, anti-$HB_c$, and anti-$HB_e$. Figure 15-7 shows the location of these antigens in the virus.

Hepatitis B frequently has an insidious onset. The disease can have an acute or chronic course, including jaundice and many of the same symptoms as hepatitis A. It can also appear as rheumatoid arthritis or a skin rash. The incubation period is longer than that of hepatitis A. Four to six weeks after exposure, surface antigen appears in the serum. Clinical illness begins at about 10 weeks after exposure and lasts for about 5 weeks. Antibody to the surface antigen appears shortly after the symptoms subside. There is considerable range, however, in the time intervals seen in this disease. The incubation period can be 2–6 months. The infectious period begins before the onset of clinical symptoms as in hepatitis A but can continue on, especially if the person develops chronic disease.

A chronic carrier state can be defined as persistent $HB_s Ag$ in the blood for 6 months, regardless of liver functions. About 10 percent of the general population who get hepatitis B will become chronic carriers. In the carrier state the presence of $HB_e Ag$ or anti-$HB_e$ are thought to be indicators of infectivity (5).

In an institution, exposure of personnel to HBV usually occurs from (1)

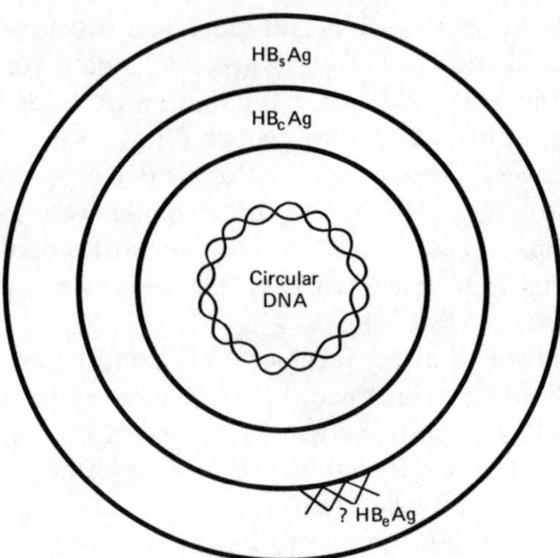


**Figure 15-7**

*Schematic representation of the hepatitis B virus; the intact virus is called the* Dane *particle. Shown schematically are the locations of circular DNA, hepatitis B core antigen (HB_cAg), surface antigen (HB_sAg), and e antigen (HB_eAg).*

direct inoculation of blood or fractions, such as serum or plasma, positive for HBV by needlesticks or cuts with sharps; (2) nonneedle percutaneous inoculation of HBV-positive blood, serum, or plasma through cuts or abrasions in the skin; (3) contact of HBV-positive blood, serum, or plasma with mucosal surfaces such as bucchal or occular mucous membranes; and (4) indirect transfer of contaminated blood from contaminated equipment or infectious waste in the hospital environment. Hepatitis B immune serum globulin (HBIG), given for exposure to HBV, is found to be more effective in HBV prophylaxis than immune serum globulin (ISG) because the concentration of antibodies to the HBV is much higher (5). In many institutions the first dose of the HeptaVax is given along with HBIG prophylaxis.

*Non-A, Non-B Hepatitis.* Non-A, non-B (NANB) hepatitis was first reported in 1974 in a series of posttransfusion hepatitis cases (8). It has now been shown that 80–90% of posttransfusion hepatitis is NANB hepatitis, and it accounts for 20% of the sporadic cases of hepatitis among adults.

Clinically, the acute phase of the disease tends to be milder than hepatitis B, but fatal fulminant hepatitis can occur. There is a chronic carrier state, although most cases are mild and seem to be resolved without chronic disease. There is, however, a 20–40% incidence of chronic disease following NANB hepatitis.

Spread is predominantly through the parenteral route, as evidenced by the high proportion of cases of posttransfusion hepatitis caused by this agent or agents. Because there are no serologic markers currently identified, it is impossible to determine whether one or more agents are involved. The incubation period seems to be between that of hepatitis A and B, at 2–12 weeks, with an average of 10 weeks. The diagnosis of NANB hepatitis is made by exclusion, when the clinical picture and serologic evidence do not match hepatitis A or B. Prophylaxis has not been investigated in depth, but ISG has been shown to be of little or no benefit in preventing NANB hepatitis after blood transfusions (9).

Hepatitis A is rarely a problem among hospital personnel. There are certain areas in the hospital where spread of hepatitis B may occur more easily. They include the emergency room, the hemodialysis unit, the laboratories, and surgery.

Exposures of employees to hepatitis should be documented by an incident report. Exposure to hepatitis B can be by direct transfusion, needlestick, or contaminated blood or blood products coming into contact with an open wound or mucous membranes (mouth, eye). The follow-up depends on the nature of the exposure and whether the source is known and can be tested for $HB_sAg$. A guideline for exposures is shown in Figure 15.8. Since there are no antigenic markers for NANB hepatitis, exposures to sources that are unknown or that are $HB_sAg$-negative are grouped together.

Because of the known risks to personnel, particularly those working in dialysis units and laboratories, and the questionable value of the current measures available for prophylaxis, prevention remains the most important aspect of infection control in this area. Personnel who become positive for $HB_sAg$ and are asymptomatic have not been shown to transmit hepatitis B to patients and therefore need not be removed from work (1).

### *Rubella*

Exposure to rubella has occurred in hospitals and may be widespread because of the frequency of illness that is not apparent. Documentation is important for medicolegal reasons. There is no evidence that postexposure immunization of persons exposed to rubella prevents subsequent disease. However, vaccination of a person who is incubating the disease is not harmful. In the event of a hospital outbreak, sera can be drawn for rubella titers, but it may be easier in a large outbreak to vaccinate exposed employees (10). Rubella titers should be drawn on any exposed pregnant employees, and counseling given to those with negative titers. Immune serum globulin given to exposed

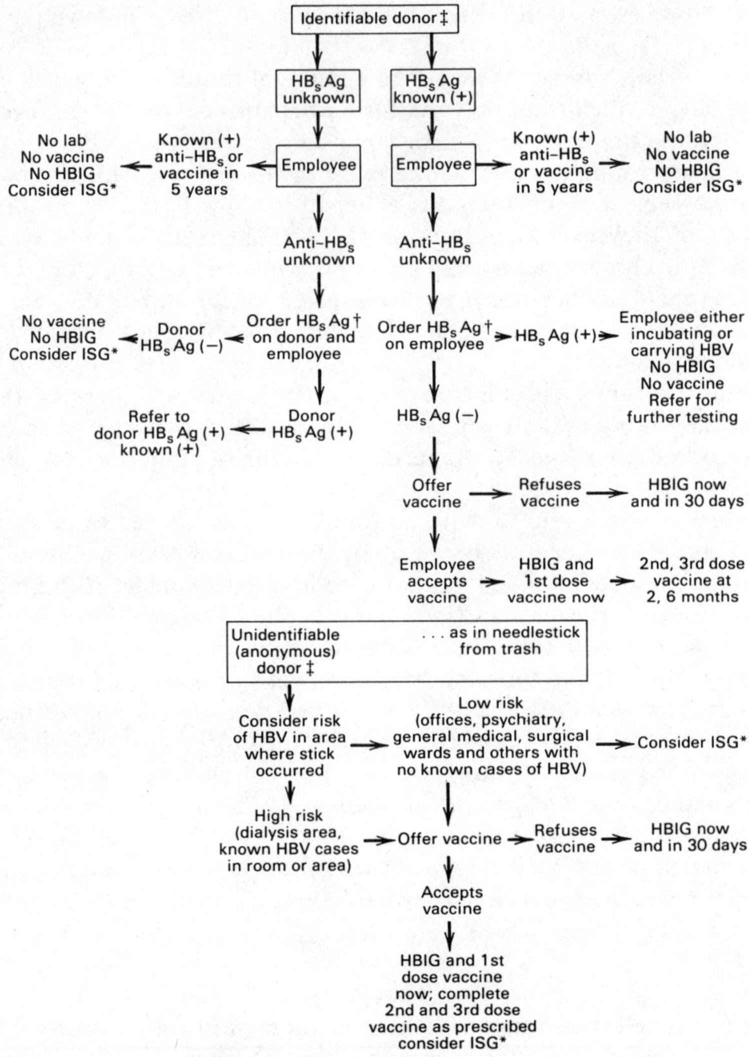


*Figure 15-8*

*This protocol for investigating needlesticks, both from known and unknown sources, is helpful in identifying and following personnel at risk of acquiring hepatitis B. (Reproduced with permission, J. J. Klimek, Hartford Hospital, Hartford, CT.)*

personnel will not prevent infection but may make the disease less severe. Immune serum globulin should generally not be given to exposed pregnant personnel, since there is a risk of congenital rubella in their infants (4).

### *Meningococcal Meningitis*

Exposure of employees to an unrecognized case of meningococcal meningitis occurs occasionally. Exposure consists of intimate contact with the patient, such as mouth-to-mouth resuscitation or other direct contact with contaminated secretions or fluids. Documentation of an exposure is necessary. Recommendations for prophylaxis are based on the amount and kind of contact with the undiagnosed and untreated patient (1).

### *Tuberculosis*

Follow-up of exposures of personnel to a patient with untreated tuberculosis who is not in isolation is based on the infectivity of the patient and the length of employee exposure. A discussion of the pathogenesis and natural history of tuberculosis may be helpful in understanding employee exposures.

Tuberculosis in caused by *M. tuberculosis* and is spread via the upper respiratory tract secretions of a person with active pulmonary tuberculosis. When this person coughs, talks, or sneezes, droplets are released into the surrounding air. The larger particles, greater than 10 $\mu$m in size, contain bacilli in a drop of water, and they will fall to a horizontal surface such as the floor. If a person is close enough to inhale these particles, the upper respiratory defense mechanisms trap the drop and carry it out of the upper airway or to the pharynx, where it is swallowed and causes the person no harm.

Smaller particles ($<5$ $\mu$m) from the person with active disease are called *droplet nuclei* and are light enough to remain airborne. Once released from the infected person, they disperse throughout a room (11). Infection occurs when another person inhales these smaller particles. The particles are small enough to bypass the upper respiratory defenses and can lodge in the alveoli. The organisms then begin to multiply; they grow slowly, multiplying once every 18–24 hours. The bacteria are spread via the lymphatics to the regional nodes at the hilus of the lung, through the thoracic duct, and into the superior vena cava. Once in the bloodstream, they are disseminated by general circulation throughout the body, seeding every organ. Without any defenses, the newly infected person develops disseminated tuberculosis.

Most people can mount a defense against the tubercle bacillus 2–12 weeks after initial implantation of the organism. The major defense is cellular immunity; sensitized lymphocytes direct the activity of other inflammatory cells, which engulf the bacilli and prevent further growth. When this acquired immunity occurs, the tuberculin skin test becomes positive. Engulfed bacilli remain dormant inside phagocytes and are impervious to further defenses.

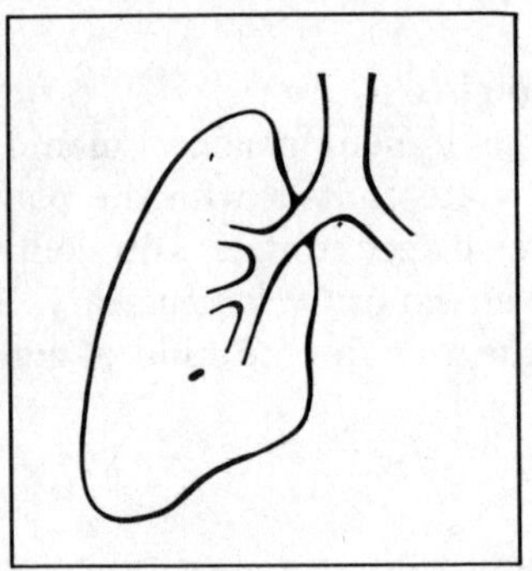

**Figure 15-9**

*Tubercle bacilli are inhaled and deposited in the alveoli.*

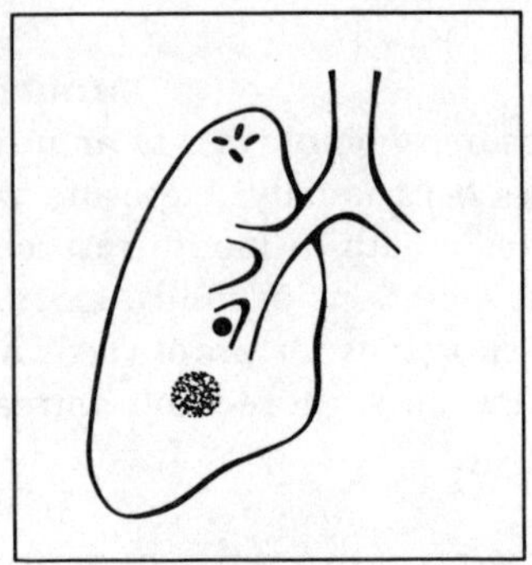

**Figure 15-10**

*Tubercle bacilli multiply in alveoli, and some are spread via lymphatics and the bloodstream to the upper lungs. Body defense mechanisms are beginning to work.*

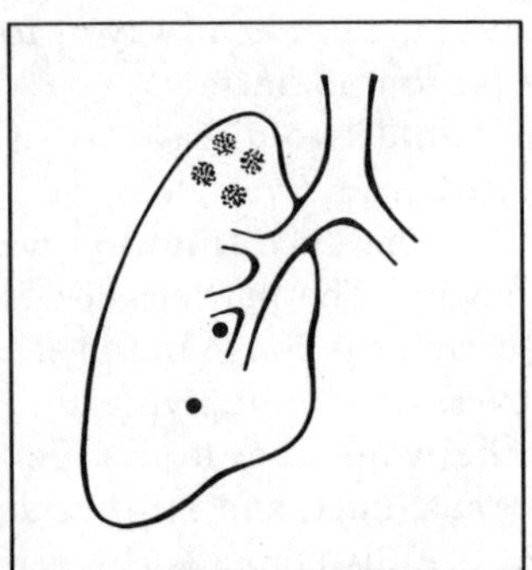

**Figure 15-11**

*The body's defenses have healed the original foci in the lower lung, hyaline nodes, and upper lung. Bacilli may still be alive, however, within these scars or elsewhere in the body.*

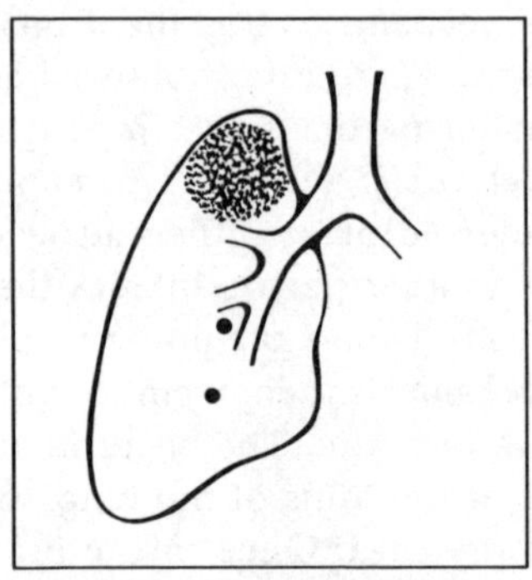

**Figure 15-12**

*Active pulmonary tuberculosis may occur weeks or years later when host defenses break down.*

This entire series of events is symptomless for the infected person. Weeks or years later, if general or local host defenses break down, the bacilli can begin to cause symptoms and disease. Therefore, a positive skin test indicates infection with the tubercle bacillus and the possible presence of live tubercle bacilli in the body, but not necessarily the presence of active disease.

The most common site for tuberculosis disease is the upper lung, and in a small number of persons, there is a relatively direct progression from initial infection to clinical illness (11). Figures 15-9–15-12 show the possible progression. Other organs are seeded, but the bacillus tends to grow best in areas of high oxygen tension; other common sites of clinical disease are in the reticuloendothelial system, serosal surfaces (peritoneum, pleura, pericardium), the apices of the lung, the renal cortex, and the epiphyses of growing bones. In a small number of people, defenses break down and a focus of infection erodes into a blood vessel, releasing large numbers of bacilli; host defenses are overwhelmed and infection of nearly all body organs occurs; this is called *miliary tuberculosis.*

There is much more information on the disease process and its treatment, culture methods, morbidity, and mortality that is well beyond the scope of this text. The reader is referred to medical texts for further information on the disease.

Patients with tuberculosis used to be housed in special institutions; because of its declining incidence and better understanding of the disease and its treatment, tuberculosis patients are now admitted to general hospitals (12). Since the initial infection is essentially symptomless, patients who come to the hospital with symptoms of disease are most often exhibiting reactivation of old infections. An additional danger in hospitals is that persons with healed foci may be admitted to the hospital for treatment of other diseases, and through involved procedures, therapies, or complications that debilitate the host defenses of these patients, old infection sites may be reactivated and become communicable. Lack of adequate chemotherapy during the first clinical episode can be an important factor in reactivation (13).

Exposure of personnel to an undiagnosed case of pulmonary tuberculosis is based on the degree of infectiousness of the patient. Since organisms must be inhaled for initial infection to occur, the person with active disease must be disseminating live tubercle bacilli via the respiratory tract. The infected person who is coughing vigorously, producing sputum, and whose sputum is positive on smear for acid-fast bacilli (AFB) is considered a probable transmitter.

In the event of a probable exposure, personnel who cared for the patient directly should be monitored by PPD (purified protein derivative) skin tests and, if needed, chest x-rays. A process of concentric circles can be used for evaluating exposures (Fig. 15-13). Since nursing service personnel generally

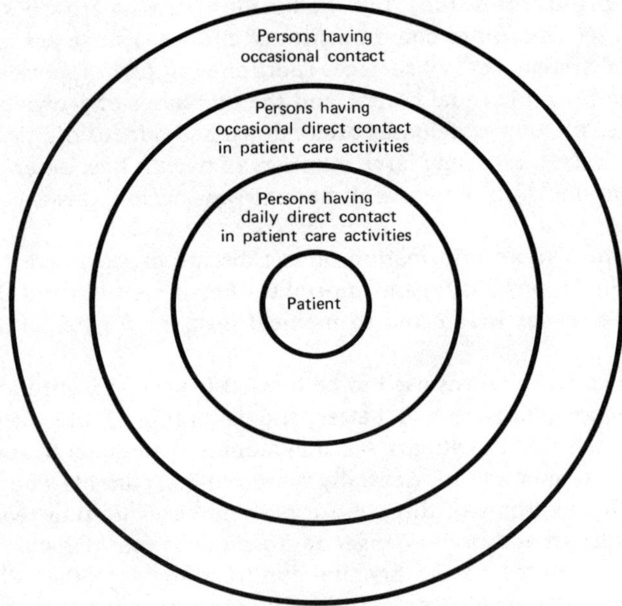


*Figure 15-13*

*Tuberculosis contact investigation can be aided by following this scheme of concentric circles: if skin-test converters are found in the center ring, the next group is tested. Moving outward according to the amount of contacts experienced by exposed persons, the investigation follows each group until no converters are found, and the investigation for new cases ends there.*

have the most contact with a patient, they are skin-tested and evaluated first, as are other patients who were roommates. If any in this group convert to a positive PPD when tested 90 days after a negative baseline test, then personnel less often involved with the infected patient are evaluated; the investigation of possible contacts expands until a group is found among whom there has been no change to a positive PPD.

Testing of previously negative but newly exposed employees should be by PPD immediately after the exposure and again at 10 weeks to detect infection. Pregnant employees may be tested at 6 weeks, if closer monitoring is desired. Care must be taken in applying the PPD to assure accurate results. The PPD is injected intracutaneously, and results are read on the second or third day after injection. The protein in the test brings out a cellular immune response in the individual who has been infected with the tubercle bacillus, when the body "recognizes" the protein. The presence of induration of 10 mm or more indicates a positive reaction. Induration of 5–9 mm indicates a doubtful result, and less than 5 mm is negative. Specific guidelines for administering and reading PPDs are available and should be followed closely (1).

Preventive prophylaxis with isoniazid may be given to employees whose skin test converts; exposed employees whose skin tests are already positive may be monitored by chest x-rays at regular intervals.

The ICP should understand the epidemiology and control of tuberculosis in the hospital (14) and may be involved in workups of exposed patients and employees. This involvement may range from identifying contacts only and working with the employee health service to, in smaller hospitals, administering PPDs and conducting the entire investigation and follow-up. The ICP in the latter setting will need further information on the booster effect of PPD skin testing, prophylaxis and contraindications, and other aspects of treatment and follow-up (1).

### AIDS

At this time, there is no known prophylaxis or treatment for exposure to personnel from patients who are infected with the HIV virus that causes the acquired immunodeficiency syndrome (AIDS). HIV is transmitted by infectious blood and through sexual contact. Exposure of personnel with infectious blood should be treated the same as hepatitis B and efforts made to identify the HIV antibody status of the donor. Employees should be counseled and monitored at periodic intervals for the development of HIV antibodies.

### Varicella

Employees who are exposed to chickenpox and for whom antibody status to varicella is unknown should have an antibody titer done as soon as possible. Incubation for varicella is 14–21 days. The disease is most contagious 2 days prior to eruption of the vesicles until 5 days after eruption, when in most cases lesions are crusted and dried. If positive varicella antibody status is not determined or status is negative, personnel should be removed from patient care or contact with susceptible employees from 10 days after exposure until day 21.

## RISKS DURING PREGNANCY

Institutions have developed fetal protection policies that restrict pregnant personnel. Those who are not immune to certain diseases are prevented from caring for patients with communicable diseases that place the fetus at risk. Such diseases are rubella, the varicella-zoster group, and sometimes cytomegalovirus (CMV), although this risk appears to be small (1,15).

## SPECIAL WORK AREAS

Employees working in special areas of the hospital may require different or more frequent follow-up by the employee health program. Personnel working in dialysis areas, for example, should have, before employment, a routine $HB_sAg$ test or HeptaVax or both. Liver function tests may also be done regularly in this area to monitor the occurrence of NANB hepatitis.

Stool samples from food handlers for enteric pathogens and routine monitoring of employees to detect asymptomatic carriers of certain microorganisms such as staphylococci, *Salmonella* sp., or streptococci are not warranted except in the investigation of an outbreak (1).

## LONG-TERM CARE

Each institution must assess the needs of its residents in incorporating policies to set standards for employee risk to residents and the exposure of infected residents to employees. Screening and immunization programs should include both residents and personnel. Personnel and residents should receive an initial tuberculin skin test: residents to detect undiagnosed TB in new resident admissions; and personnel for a screening of potential disease and as a baseline for further exposure. Influenza vaccine may be of value to both resident and personnel population. Rubella screening and immunization of personnel is probably not of value. Residents who undergo dialysis on a long-term basis should be offered hepatitis B vaccination. Personnel are not at increased risk and do not require vaccination if dialysis is done at an acute care institution.

## EMPLOYEE EDUCATION

The ICC and Employee Health Service can provide an initial screening and ongoing program to protect the employee and the patient from infections. The responsibility for total health maintenance and care, however, rests with the individual employee, as well as the responsibility for staying home and seeking care as needed when ill. The ICP can teach employees the symptoms and risks to patients if they come to work with a communicable disease, such as cold sores in nursery personnel, skin lesions among operating room personnel, and general hygiene for personnel with upper respiratory or diarrheal infections.

Additional information on risks to pregnant employees may be given if it is felt that the risks may be significant, such as in children's referral hospitals. Any additional information should include careful explanations and further instruction.

The employee health program can vary considerably from hospital to hospital. The ICC must have input into the program, especially in terms of pre-employment screening and follow-up of exposures to certain infections. The program may well cover the screening and education of all hospital employees except physicians. In university settings it is especially difficult to obtain the participation of all those who have patient contact and to develop a mechanism for accomplishing this, since many physicians and students rotate from service to service or to other hospitals. Private community hospitals, even those with a stable medical staff, have similar difficulties in obtaining physician compliance with the employee health program. The solution to this problem lies with the executive committee, where department chairpersons agree to require participation from their staff.

# REFERENCES


1. Williams WW: Guidelines for infection control in hospital personnel. Hospital Infections Program, Atlanta, Centers for Disease Control, 1983.
2. *Accreditation Manual for Hospitals 1986: Infection Control.* Chicago, standards adopted by Board of Commissioners of Joint Commission on Accreditation of Hospitals, 1985.
3. Gardner P, Oxman MN, Breton S: Hospital management of patients and personnel exposed to communicable diseases. *Pediatrics* 56(5): 700, 1975.
4. Immunization Practices Advisory Committee: Recommendations on rubella prevention. *Morbidity and Mortality Weekly Rep* 30: 37, 1981.
5. Advisory Committee on Immunization Practices: Recommendations for protection against viral hepatitis. *Morbidity and Mortality Weekly Rep* 34(22): 313, 1985.
6. Vogler DM, Burke JP: Tuberculosis screening for hospital employees. *Am Rev Respir Dis* 117: 227, 1978.
7. Limon SM: Type A viral hepatitis: New developments in an old disease. *N Engl J Med* 313(17): 1059, 1985.
8. Prince AM, Brotman B, Grady GF, et al: Long-incubation post-transfusion hepatitis without serological evidence of exposure to hepatitis B virus. *Lancet* 2: 241, 1974.
9. Hoofnagle JH, Gerety RJ, Tabor E, et al: Transmission of non-A, non-B hepatitis. *Ann Intern Med* 87: 14, 1977.

10. Rubella in hospital personnel and patients—Colorado. *Morbidity and Mortality Weekly Rep* 28(28): 325, 1979.

11. American Lung Association: Transmission and pathogenesis. In *Diagnostic Standards and Classification of Tuberculosis and Other Mycobacterial Diseases*. New York, American Lung Association, 1974, p 9.

12. Sencer DJ: Management of tuberculosis in the general hospital. *Proceedings of an Institute on the Control of Infections in Hospitals*. University of Michigan, 1965, p. 119.

13. Geboes K, Bossaert H: Reactivation of tuberculosis in old age. *J Am Geriatr Soc* XXV(7): 318, 1977.

14. Centers for Disease Control: Guidelines for prevention of TB transmission in hospitals. Atlanta, U.S. Department of Health, Education, and Welfare, Public Health Service, 1974.

15. Valenti W: Infection control and the pregnant health care worker. *Am J Infect Control* 14(1): 20, 1986.

# 16

# Surveillance of Communicable Diseases

In this chapter the processes of surveillance, analysis, and reporting of diseases and conditions to public health authorities are discussed. Certain conditions may be *communicable* but not *reportable,* and vice versa.

EXAMPLE. Two patients are housed together in a semiprivate room, and both have Foley catheters in place. One has an *Escherichia coli* urinary tract infection. The infection is communicable to the other patient, especially via hands of nursing personnel who empty the catheter bag at the end of the shift or care for the catheter without washing their hands. The infection, however, is not reportable to the health department.

By contrast, animal bites and foodborne outbreaks are reportable, but the infections or conditions they represent may not actually be communicable, as in the bite of a nonrabid animal, or a foodborne outbreak of illness from chemical contamination.

The terms *communicable* and *reportable,* however, are used interchangeably in this chapter to indicate diseases or conditions that require public health department notification.

Traditionally, the reporting of communicable diseases has been the responsibility of the physician. State laws require that physicians notify appropriate health authorities of any reportable disease that comes to their attention (1). In a hospital setting, however, this responsibility may be less clear. Because of the number of physicians on a particular service and the ongoing rotation of house staff and students among services and hospitals within a university complex, this responsibility may be lost. Additionally, these personnel may not be familiar with current state requirements for what to report and to whom.

The ICP is in a good position to detect communicable diseases in the hospital and in many areas has assumed the responsibility for reporting these diseases to local and state health departments, for several reasons. First, the ICP must know if there is a problem in the community that might affect the hospital.

EXAMPLE. Officials in the local health department contacted the ICP because they had just detected a measles (rubeola) outbreak in the city. The ICP talked to the head nurses in the pediatric units, and through increased awareness the personnel were able to recognize the onset of measles symptoms in a recently admitted child and put him into isolation; no other cases occurred in the hospital.

A good working relationship with local and state health departments is critical for the ICP in the event of an outbreak of infections within the hospital. Many Epidemiologic Intelligence Service (EIS) officers from the CDC are located in state health departments around the country and are available to help in outbreak investigations.

Infection control practitioners in Denver, Colorado hospitals have agreed to be responsible for reporting communicable diseases from their respective institutions. Local health departments and the Colorado State Health Department personnel use the ICP as a liaison between the institution and the health department. The ICP serves as a stable contact within the hospital for obtaining further information or notifying hospital personnel of a problem in the community. The following description of the Denver system can serve as an example of the surveillance, analysis, and reporting activities of the ICP with respect to reportable diseases.

## SURVEILLANCE

### Criteria for Determining the Presence of a Reportable Disease

As in the case of nosocomial surveillance, the correct surveillance of communicable diseases is based on specific definitions and criteria. Table 16-1 is the guideline developed by the Colorado State Health Department for diseases reportable to public health authorities. These guidelines may vary from state to state, in terms of what diseases require a report, the time interval, and the information needed by the health department for follow-up. These variations are based on the differences in disease frequency and in conditions from one region to another.

## Table 16-1
### REPORTING COMMUNICABLE DISEASES: A GUIDE FOR HEALTH DEPARTMENTS, NURSES, PHYSICIANS, HOSPITALS, AND SCHOOLS

| Disease | Type of Report[a] | Immediate Telephone Report | Criteria for Initial Report | Laboratory Procedures | Public Health Response |
|---|---|---|---|---|---|
| AIDS | 2 | Yes | Clinical diagnosis: presence of immunocompromised disease | HIV antibody test | CDC surveillance form |
| Amebiasis | 2 | No | Laboratory confirmation | Required: examination of stool specimen for cysts or trophozoites of *E. histolytica* | Epidemiologic investigation optional |
| Animal bites | 1 | No | Clinical diagnosis | | Epidemiologic investigation optional |
| Anthrax | 2 | Yes | Clinical diagnosis[b] | Required for final report: isolation of *B. anthracis* | Epidemiologic investigation mandatory |
| Botulism | 2 | Yes | Clinical diagnosis | Optional: isolation of toxin in blood or suspect food; mouse inoculation for typing | Epidemiologic investigation mandatory final diagnosis for reporting purposes will be made in consultation with public health physician |
| Brucellosis | 2 | No | Clinical diagnosis[b] | Required for final report: isolation of *Brucella* organisms from blood, or diagnostic titer of specific serum agglutinins | *CDC surveillance form;* epidemiologic investigation mandatory |

**Table 16-1**(Continued)

| Disease | Type of Report[a] | Immediate Telephone Report | Criteria for Initial Report | Laboratory Procedures | Public Health Response |
|---|---|---|---|---|---|
| Chickenpox | 1 | No | Clinical diagnosis | Optional: isolation of virus or fourfold increase of serum antibodies to specific virus | Epidemiologic investigation optional |
| Colorado tick fever | 1 | No | Clinical diagnosis with history of tick exposure | Optional: blood examination for presence of virus, or fourfold increase of serum antibodies to specific virus | Epidemiologic investigation optional |
| Diphtheria | 2 | Yes | Clinical diagnosis[b] | Required for final report: isolation of toxin-producing *C. diphtheriae,* or association of clinical case with an epidemic | CDC surveillance form; epidemiologic investigation mandatory |
| Encephalitis, viral (primary and postinfectious) | 2[c] | No | Clinical diagnosis | Optional: virus isolation, or fourfold rise of specific antibodies (virus isolation or serology *required* for confirmation of arboviral encephalitis) | CDC annual report form; epidemiologic investigation optional; differentiation of primary and postinfectious encephalitis to be made in consultation with public health physician |
| Foodborne disease (see "Group outbreaks," below) | | No | | | |

| Giardiasis | 1 | No | Clinical diagnosis | Optional: examination of stool or duodenal aspirate for cysts or trophozoites | Epidemiologic investigation optional |
| Group outbreaks (e.g., gastroenteritis, streptococcal epidemics) | 2 | Yes | Clinical diagnosis of an illness occurring in a geographic or temporal cluster | | Epidemiologic investigation mandatory |
| Hepatitis A | 2 | No | People with clinical or laboratory evidence of acute hepatitis who are (1) $HB_sAg$-negative, (2) involved in a common source outbreak or an epidemiologic chain of person-to-person spread, or (3) younger than 15 years with no history of transfusions or intravenous drug use | Optional: $HB_sAg$ test; liver function tests (required in absence of clinical symptoms) 1. bilirubin 2. SGOT or SGPT | CDC surveillance form; epidemiologic investigation optional |
| Hepatitis B | 2 | No | People with clinical or laboratory evidence of acute hepatitis who are $HB_sAg$-positive | Required: $HB_sAg$ test; liver function tests (required in absence of clinical symptoms) 1. bilirubin 2. SGOT or SGPT | CDC surveillance form; epidemiologic investigation optional |

**Table 16-1**(Continued)

| Disease | Type of Report[a] | Immediate Telephone Report | Criteria for Initial Report | Laboratory Procedures | Public Health Response |
|---|---|---|---|---|---|
| Hepatitis, unspecified | 2 | No | People with clinical or laboratory evidence of hepatitis who are 15 years or older, on whom no $HB_sAg$ determination has been made, and who are not epidemiologically related to a known hepatitis-A case | Optional: liver function tests (required in absence of clinical symptoms)<br>1. bilirubin<br>2. SGOT or SGPT | CDC surveillance form; epidemiologic investigation optional |
| Influenza, confirmed | 1 | No | Laboratory confirmation | Required: isolation of influenza A or B virus or fourfold increase of serum antibodies to specific virus | Epidemiologic investigation optional |
| Influenzalike illness | 1 | No | Clinical diagnosis | | |
| Legionnaires' disease | 2 | No | Clinical diagnosis | Required: fourfold increase of serum antibody or direct fluorescent antibody (FA)-positive tissue specimen | Epidemiologic investigation mandatory |
| Leprosy | 2 | No | Laboratory confirmation | Required: acid-fast stain of smear, or biopsy section | CDC surveillance form; epidemiologic investigation mandatory |

| Leptospirosis | 2 | Yes | Clinical diagnosis[b] | Required for final report: isolation of leptospira organism in urine or blood or from source, or fourfold increase of serum antibodies to specific leptospira | CDC surveillance form; epidemiologic investigation mandatory |
| Malaria | 2 | Yes | Clinical diagnosis[b] | Required for final report: visualization of malaria organism on blood smear | CDC surveillance form; epidemiologic investigation mandatory |
| Measles (rubeola) | 2 | Yes | Clinical diagnosis | Optional: isolation of virus or fourfold increase of serum antibodies to specific virus | State surveillance form; epidemiologic investigation mandatory |
| Meningitis, aseptic | 2[c] | No | Clinical diagnosis | Optional: CSF–normal sugar, increased protein, increased cells (mononuclear), or isolation of virus; or fourfold increase of serum antibodies to specific virus | CDC annual report form; epidemiologic investigation optional |
| Meningococcal meningitis | 2 | Yes | Clinical diagnosis[b] | Required for final report: isolation of *N. meningitidis* from blood or CSF, or gram-negative diplococci on Gram stain of CSF | Epidemiologic investigation mandatory |

**Table 16-1**(Continued)

| Disease | Type of Report[a] | Immediate Telephone Report | Criteria for Initial Report | Laboratory Procedures | Public Health Response |
|---|---|---|---|---|---|
| Mumps | 1 | No | Clinical diagnosis | Optional: isolation of virus or fourfold increase of serum antibodies to specific virus | Epidemiologic investigation optional |
| Pertussis syndrome | 2 | No | Clinical diagnosis | Optional: isolation of *B. pertussis;* presumptive diagnosis by fluorescent antibody testing | Epidemiologic investigation optional |
| Plague | 2 | Yes | Clinical diagnosis[b] | Required for final report: diagnostic stained smears, or isolation of *Y. pestis* from clinical material | Epidemiologic investigation mandatory |
| Poliomyelitis, paralytic | 2 | Yes | Clinical diagnosis[b] | Required for final report: isolation of polio virus from clinical material, or fourfold increase of serum antibodies to specific virus | CDC surveillance form; epidemiological investigation mandatory |
| Psittacosis | 2 | No | Clinical diagnosis[b] | Required for final report: isolation of Chlamydia organisms from sputum or blood, or fourfold increase of serum antibodies to *C. psittaci* | CDC surveillance form; epidemiologic investigation mandatory |

| Disease | | | | | |
| --- | --- | --- | --- | --- | --- |
| Q fever | 2 | No | Clinical diagnosis[b] | Required for final report: isolation of organism from sputum or blood, or or fourfold increase of serum antibodies to *C. burneti* | Epidemiologic investigation mandatory |
| Rabies in animals | 2 | Yes | Clinical diagnosis[b] | Required for final report: fluorescent antibody-positive brain impression | Epidemiologic investigation mandatory for domestic animal rabies |
| Relapsing fever | 2 | No | Clinical diagnosis[b] | Required for final report: positive blood smear demonstrating spirochetes | Epidemiologic investigation mandatory |
| Reye's syndrome | 2 | No | Clinical diagnosis | Required for final report: any preexisting viral illness; supporting laboratory data | CDC surveillance form; epidemiologic investigation optional |
| Rheumatic fever | 2 | No | Clinical diagnosis[b] | Required for final report: evidence for preceding streptococcal infection, including isolation of Group A streptococci or antibodies (e.g., ASO) indicating recent strep infection; satisfaction of Jones criteria | Case follow-up at discretion of public health physician |

**Table 16-1**(Continued)

| Disease | Type of Report[a] | Immediate Telephone Report | Criteria for Initial Report | Laboratory Procedures | Public Health Response |
|---|---|---|---|---|---|
| Rocky Mountain spotted fever | 2 | No | Clinical diagnosis[b] | Required for final report: fourfold increase of serum antibodies to RMSF group antigen; Weil–Felix reactions may support a diagnosis | Epidemiologic investigation mandatory |
| Rubella (German measles) | 2 | Yes | Clinical diagnosis | Optional: isolation of virus, or fourfold increase to specific virus | State surveillance form; epidemiologic investigation mandatory |
| Rubella, congenital syndrome | 2 | No | Clinical diagnosis[b] | Required for final report: if neonate, isolation of virus or fourfold increase of serum antibodies, or presence of IgM specific antibodies | CDC surveillance form; epidemiologic investigation mandatory; final diagnosis for reporting purposes to be made in consultation with public health physician |
| Salmonellosis | 2 | No | Laboratory confirmation | Required: stool culture | Epidemiologic investigation optional |
| Shigellosis | 2 | No | Laboratory confirmation | Required: stool culture | Epidemiologic investigation optional |
| Streptococcal infection (see "Group outbreaks," above) | 2 | No | | | |

| Disease | | | | | |
|---|---|---|---|---|---|
| Tetanus | 2 | No | Clinical diagnosis | | CDC surveillance form; epidemiologic investigation mandatory |
| Toxoplasmosis | 2 | No | Clinical diagnosis[b] | Required for final report: isolation of the protozoan from body fluids, or specific serology | Epidemiologic investigation optional |
| Trichinosis | 2 | Yes | Clinical diagnosis[b] | Required for final report: specific serology or positive biopsy specimen from patient or implicated meat | CDC surveillance form; epidemiologic investigation mandatory |
| Tuberculosis | 2 | Yes | Clinical diagnosis | Contributory tests: x-ray, isolation of *M. tuberculosis*, positive sputum smear, tissue biopsy specimen | Epidemiologic investigation mandatory; final diagnosis for reporting purposes to be made in consultation with public health physician |
| Tularemia | 2 | No | Clinical diagnosis[b] | Required for final report: isolation of *F. tularensis* from clinical material, or positive serum agglutinins | Epidemiologic investigation mandatory |

Table 16-1(Continued)

| Disease | Type of Report[a] | Immediate Telephone Report | Criteria for Initial Report | Laboratory Procedures | Public Health Response |
|---|---|---|---|---|---|
| Typhoid fever | 2 | Yes | Clinical diagnosis[b] | Required for final report: isolation of *Salmonella typhi* from clinical material; serum agglutination reactions may suggest a diagnosis but are usually inadequate for confirmation | Epidemiologic investigation mandatory |
| VD—gonorrhea | 2 | No | Laboratory confirmation | Required: appropriate Gram-stained smear, or culture results | Epidemiologic investigation optional |
| VD—syphilis, early (primary, secondary, early latent [<1 year]) | 2 | yes | Laboratory confirmation | Required: serologic tests for syphilis, or darkfield examination | Epidemiologic investigation mandatory; cases to be confirmed by State Department of Health |

[a] Type of report: (1) report by number only—report county of residence when available; (2) report by name, age, sex, address, and responsible physician; additional information such as telephone number and laboratory results are helpful.

[b] A clinical diagnosis is acceptable in order to initiate the mandatory epidemiologic investigation. Final reporting, by a public health department, will follow laboratory confirmation.

[c] Report patient's initials, age, sex, county, and viral isolates or serologic tests, pending or completed.

SOURCE: Colorado State Department of Health: Reporting of Communicable Diseases: A guide for health departments, nurses, physicians, hospitals and schools. By permission.

## Case Finding

There are several ways in which the ICP can find cases of communicable diseases within the hospital. These include the microbiology laboratory, surveillance rounds, outpatient areas, head nurses, and physicians.

Personnel in the microbiology laboratory should have and be familiar with the reporting guidelines. When a reportable isolate is identified, the ICP or a designated substitute should be called if the isolate requires a 24-hour telephone report. In institutions where the laboratory report is computerized, the word "Reportable" can be printed on the slip.

Depending on the method of nosocomial infection surveillance performed, the ICP may be able to detect reportable diseases during regular rounds. Since some types of conditions are not cultured by the microbiology laboratory, the ICP can take advantage of this opportunity to detect these diseases.

Many communicable diseases are seen in the clinics and emergency area of the hospital. Guidelines for reporting such cases should be available to all personnel in these areas. The ICP can set up a reporting system in which clerks are responsible for filling out reporting forms. Using daily logbooks and the guidelines, clerks can fill out most or all of the required information, with help from and supervision by the head nurse.

Head nurses in all areas, both inpatient and outpatient, can be a source of case-finding information for the ICP. These people should have available the state guidelines for dealing with reportable diseases. Personnel in charge of nursing units during evening, night, and weekend shifts should be made aware of their existence and use. Physicians can also alert the ICP to the presence of a patient with a communicable disease. Infectious disease physicians, if this service is available, should have the guidelines for reporting and may share this responsibility with the ICP, especially since this service covers weekends and nights.

## Data Collection

Figures 16-1 and 16-2 represent examples of a data-collection form for communicable diseases and a specific form for reporting hepatitis. The report forms should be designed so that the person who files the report can provide all the necessary information easily.

## ANALYSIS AND REPORTING

All data-collection forms, whether filled out in outpatient areas by clerks or in inpatient areas by the ICP, should be collected and reviewed weekly by the ICP. Any trends in or clusters of cases of infection should be noted for follow-up with health department personnel or for discussion with the ICC.

---

COMMUNICABLE DISEASE REPORT

Date______________Clinic (or)____________Responsible physician_________________

                       inpatient unit____________

Patient's name______________________          Infection

Chart number________________________

Birth date____________Sex___________

Address________________________________      Laboratory results      Rx

___________________________________________

___________________________________________

Phone number________________________                      Yes______

County________________________________     Phoned to Health Dept.

                                            No______Date______

---

***Figure 16-1***
*An example of a communicable disease report form.*

EXAMPLE.  The ICP in one hospital reports to three health departments in the city. During one week she noticed an increase in the number of *Salmonella* isolates, from the pediatric inpatient and clinic areas, in reports going to all three local health departments. She discussed this phenomenon with personnel in the epidemiology section of the State Health Department, who followed up and found that there was a common day-care center where transmission of the disease may have occurred, even though the patients resided in different health department regions.

The reports then are sent to the appropriate health department each week; a written report of diseases phoned in is submitted, should any have required an immediate telephone report. The forms in Figures 16-1 and 16-2 have an original and a carbonless copy, and the copy is kept in a 5 × 8 file box in the infection control department.

The ICP serves as liaison between hospital and local and state health departments, should they need more information. The information, filed alphabetically by the patient's name, can be retrieved easily for this purpose. Because certain conditions require an immediate telephone report, the ICP and ICC must devise a contingency plan to cover reporting during the times when the ICP is not available. A specific person, such as the infectious disease physician on call or the nursing service supervisor, can be designated as the responsible person during these times. Since the need for a telephone report to the health

---

HEPATITIS REPORT

Date_____________Chart number_________  Diagnosis  Hepatitis A_____________

Patient's name_________________________             Hepatitis B_____________

Birth date_______________Sex___________             Unspec./Unk_____________

Address_______________________________             Other___________________

_______________________________________  Onset of symptoms_______________

_______________________________________  Lab Results

Phone number___________County_________  HAA+____−____Not Tested_________

                                                             Unk._______________

Clinic/inpatient unit___________________

Responsible physician__________________  SGOT

Occupation/school________ _____________  Bilirubin

Address_______________________________  Alkaline phosphatase

                                          Other

**Figure 16-2**
*An example of a hepatitis report form.*

department is relatively rare, the contingency situation will not occur often, but there must be some provision for such a situation in the infection control policies and procedures.

Surveillance, analysis, and reporting of communicable diseases should be part of the infection control program in every hospital. The ICP must know when reportable diseases occur in the institution and who is the logical person to serve as a liaison between the hospital and public health authorities.

## REFERENCES

1. Benenson AS (ed): *Control of Communicable Diseases in Man,* ed 12. Washington DC, American Public Health Association, 1975, p. xxiii.

# 17

# Surveillance of the Hospital Environment

Environmental surveillance is a necessary part of the infection control program, and this aspect of infection control practice has probably undergone the greatest change in the past 10 years. In the past, more emphasis was placed on the role of the environment in the transmission of infections; therefore, culturing areas and objects in the inanimate environment was one of the main activities of the ICP.

In the late 1950s and early 1960s, in reports of air and surface sampling in hospitals, it was proposed that the hospital environment played a part in the spread of nosocomial disease. In 1977, Mallison (1) reviewed the history of hospital environmental surveillance up to 1964, when the CDC published methods for surface sampling, and to the mid-1960s, when researchers began to publish guidelines for the interpretation of environmental sampling (2,3).

By 1970, many infection control programs were largely environmental sampling programs with lots of data but little in the way of meaningful interpretation. In 1970, the CDC began to reconsider its position on environmental sampling, as did the American Public Health Association, American Hospital Association, and certain individuals, for example (4–7).

Although it is now felt that most infections are spread through contact or droplet routes, or contact with contaminated articles in the hospital environment, some environmental surveillance is still necessary.

## CULTURES OF THE INANIMATE ENVIRONMENT

### Routine

In 1973, the Committee on Infections Within Hospitals, of the American Hospital Association, issued a statement indicating that routine culturing of inanimate objects in the hospital environment was not a useful activity (6). Because of the lack of correlation between culture data and infections in patients or personnel, this information did not prove to be useful to the ICP or the ICC in making appropriate interventions. Additionally, few criteria were proposed for environmental cultures; for example, limits to the acceptable numbers or kinds of organisms in a particular sample were not set. Therefore, routine sampling is now discouraged as a time-consuming activity of little value to infection control practice.

### Suspected Outbreaks

In the event of an outbreak, the microbiology laboratory personnel may be the first to be made aware of the problem by a staff member bringing environmental cultures to the laboratory. The ICP should be designated to screen all such environmental cultures so as to be notified of potential outbreaks and to ensure that personnel time and money will not be spent on unnecessary cultures. The ICP also can provide vital data to the personnel who take the cultures.

EXAMPLE. A medical technologist called the ICP after swab samples from various sites in the delivery suite were brought to the microbiology laboratory for culture. The ICP found, from the people who took the samples, that there was a growing concern about the number of patients who were developing postpartum endometritis. These personnel had been instructed by the physicians to "take some cultures of the delivery rooms to find the cause of the problem."

The ICP investigated the suspected outbreak and found that the number of cases of endometritis was coupled with an increase in the total number of deliveries and cesarean sections performed and that the actual infection rate had not increased. In a combined meeting of OB/Gyn physicians and nursing personnel, the ICP presented these data, as well as information on the low likelihood of an environmental source of infection for obstetric patients. The personnel were relieved to know that an outbreak was probably not in progress, and a general discussion of infection control priorities in the delivery suite took place.

The environmental cultures were held in the laboratory until this information was known, then discarded; no personnel time or supplies were used.

In the event that an outbreak is suspected and an environmental source is likely, cultures should be taken by the ICP or the person responsible for the outbreak investigation. The kind of culture taken depends on the information desired; the ICP must work closely with the microbiology personnel in order to collect the specimen appropriately. Swabs moistened with trypticase soy broth or transport media are best for evaluating environmental sources in outbreaks where a single organism is responsible. The ICP must be aware, however, of the epidemiology of certain infections and infectious agents; in other words, the ICP must know or find out when it is appropriate to suspect a human, versus an environmental, source.

EXAMPLE. In the case of an outbreak of streptococcal wound infections following surgical procedures, the ICP would look for a human source of the infecting organism. By contrast, in an outbreak of pneumonias caused by *A. calcoaceticus* in a surgical intensive care unit, the ICP would consider environmental sources.

The kind of culture to be taken must be decided before the cultures are obtained. This will save both time and money.

When a commercial product is suspected as an environmental source in an outbreak, all suspected lots of the product should be removed from the shelves and held. The ICP should notify the state health department and through them the CDC and/or the FDA. The suspected product should not be cultured in the hospital; it should be turned over to the CDC and the FDA. Because of the difficulties in culturing a packaged item in the hospital laboratory and the possibility of introducing contamination during the culturing process, the results obtained in this way are generally not reliable. Therefore, when a product is contaminated and there is a need for nationwide recall, valuable time could be lost by such in-hospital testing. The ICP should notify the state health department immediately of a suspected problem and then after consulting with that agency, institute the recall and collection of the suspected product within the hospital.

## Teaching and Research

Environmental sampling is acceptable for teaching or research purposes because, although the results have not been well correlated with patient or personnel disease, the comparison of "before" and "after" cleaning cultures may make a great impression on housekeeping personnel. Minimal time and supplies should be used, however, since the microbiology laboratory time is needed for evaluation of clinically significant cultures.

In summary, routine culturing of inanimate objects in the hospital environment has not been shown to be of value in monitoring or reducing the infection rate in hospitals. Sampling the environment during outbreaks is warranted if an environmental source is suspected but should be done in close consultation with the microbiology laboratory personnel. Sampling for teaching or research purposes is acceptable but again must be done carefully, with advance planning, to provide the most useful information.

## STERILIZER MONITORING

The JCAH requires testing of all-steam sterilizers weekly (8). The JCAH further recommends the monitoring of ethylene oxide (EO) sterilizers for every load. Testing the sterilizers in a hospital is the responsibility of the department heads responsible for operating these machines. The ICP should periodically monitor for compliance with JCAH standards.

Sterilizers are tested with live spores, usually *Bacillus stearothermophilus* or *B. subtilis*. Generally, an ampule containing spores and media in separate compartments is placed in the sterilizer in a central area. Ideally, an additional ampule should be placed inside a pack. Following a normal sterilization cycle, the ampule is crushed, allowing the spores to contact the media. A control ampule, taken from the same lot, is processed in the same way without undergoing the sterilization cycle. Figure 17-1 serves as an example of a

---

AUTOCLAVE STERILITY TEST

| *Sterilization Test Data* | *Results* |
|---|---|
| Department__________________________ | Date ampule was cultured____________ |
| Date of test________________________ | Test ampule was +________ −________ |
| Sterilizer_________________________ | Control ampule +________ −________ |
| Type of autoclave<br>  Gas________Steam________ | |
| Temperature<br>(Dial thermometer)________°F | Should test be repeated?<br>  Yes________ No________ |
| Thermometer<br>(Recording thermometer)________°F | |
| Exposure period________ minutes | Signature_____________________________ |
| Test conducted by__________________ | Date_________________________________ |

---

*Figure 17-1*

*A small envelope is printed with information on the sterilizer and cycle run. The ampule is placed inside the envelope and sent to the laboratory; in this way, the ampule and the information related to the test will not be separated.*

AUTOCLAVE STERILITY TESTS

Month________________

| Area | | | | | |
|---|---|---|---|---|---|
| Operating room | | | | | |
| 1. steam | | | | | |
| 2. steam | | | | | |
| 3. steam | | | | | |
| 4. steam | | | | | |
| 5. steam | | | | | |
| 6. ethylene oxide | | | | | |
| Central service | | | | | |
| 1. steam | | | | | |
| 2. steam | | | | | |
| 3. steam | | | | | |
| 4. ethylene oxide | | | | | |
| Delivery suite | | | | | |
| 1. steam | | | | | |
| 2. steam | | | | | |

**Figure 17-2**

*A sample report form for results of sterilizer monitoring tests. This report would be sent for review to the ICC along with the other infection control reports.*

data collection sheet for pertinent information such as department, sterilizer tested, information about the cycle, and results of the culture. This information is printed on an envelope and can hold the ampule as it is delivered to the laboratory, to make sure each ampule is kept together with the information about that machine.

The ampules are then incubated at 40 °C, and the results are read after 48 hours. Under normal circumstances the control ampule will be positive for growth, since it did not go through the sterilization process. The tested ampule(s) should be negative for growth. A negative control ampule indicates that the test should be repeated, and possibly the lot of ampules should be discarded, since the validity of "no growth" on the test ampules is in question. Spore strips may be used instead of ampules.

Growth in a spore test may indicate failure of the sterilizer but may also indicate other problems. If a sterilizer is packed too tightly, if the packs are too big, or if the wrong kind or amount of wrapping is used, the steam or gas may not be able to penetrate and kill the spores (9). Positive test results, therefore, are reason to evaluate all variables in packaging and sterilizing in addition to the machine itself. In the event of a malfunctioning sterilizer, the ICP and the department head should be prepared to consider recalling all items sterilized by that machine since the time of the last negative test. This decision, made by the ICP, the ICC and the department head, will depend on the nature of the items sterilized, the feasibility of locating and resterilizing all items, and the occurrence of disease related to the malfunctioning machine.

The envelopes suggested for use are returned to the ICP; positive results are phoned to the ICP and the responsible department head. The results are summarized and reported to the ICC; Figure 17-2 shows a sample report.

## GENERAL ENVIRONMENTAL SURVEILLANCE

During nosocomial infections rounds, the ICP should be aware of the environment and potential infection hazards. Environmental surveillance can be conducted by a "rounds committee" on a regular basis. These rounds can monitor adherence to infection control policies such as appropriate isolation, labeling and dating of sterile solutions or multidose vials, rotation of sterile supplies and removal of outdated sterile supplies, adequate and functioning handwashing dispensers, and appropriate storage of clean linen and removal of soiled linen. They can observe that the area is well cleaned and that waste material, including infectious waste, has been removed. The rounds committee should include the Administrator, the ICP, the Housekeeping Manager, the Engineering Manager, the Pharmacist, the Nursing Assistant Director, and a representative from Fire and Safety. These management members can initiate action if infractions of acceptable standards are present. Feedback to departments with identified deficiencies should be done to facilitate corrective action. These rounds also serve to increase the awareness of administration regarding the importance of infection control in the institution (10). The ICP and the ICC together determine appropriate cleaning, disinfection, and sterilization procedures for the inanimate environment; and follow-up to ensure that these procedures are carried out properly is the responsibility of the ICP.

Additionally, the ICP cooperates with specific departments such as Maintenance and Housekeeping in formulating policies and procedures related to the environment.

EXAMPLE. The ICP works with the Maintenance Department to make sure that there are an adequate number of air exchanges per hour in key areas such as the operating room and that hazardous areas such as the microbiology laboratory are properly vented.

The ICP works with the Housekeeping Department to devise safe policies and procedures for the handling and disposal of needles; even if they are ultimately disposed of outside the hospital, they are still the responsibility of the ICP and the ICC.

The ICP works with the Dietary Department on cleaning procedures and makes sure they have an adequate ongoing program for vector control.

The ICP becomes involved in environmental concerns of all areas and departments in the hospital. It is beyond the scope of this text to discuss each area in detail; the reader is referred to the JCAH guidelines (8) and a manual that discusses infection control policies and procedures related to the environment in different hospital departments (11). Although the environment is now much less emphasized in the transmission of infections than in previous years, the ICP must monitor and intervene appropriately when the environment poses a real or potential threat of becoming a source of infectious organisms.

## REFERENCES


1. Mallison GF: Monitoring of sterility and environmental sampling in programs for control of nosocomial infections. In Cundy KR, Ball W (eds): *Infection Control in Health Care Facilities*. Baltimore, University Park Press, 1977, p. 23.

2. Pryor AK, Vesley D, Shaffer JG, et al: Cooperative microbial surveys of surfaced in hospital patient rooms. *Health Lab Sci* 4 : 153, 1967.

3. American Public Health Association: Guidelines for hospital operating and delivery room air conditioning systems. *Am J Public Health* 57 : 1053, 1967.

4. Garner JS, Favero MS: Guideline for handwashing and hospital environmental control. Atlanta, Centers for Disease Control, 1985.

5. American Public Health Association: Environmental microbiologic sampling in the hospital. *Health Lab Sci* 12 : 234, 1975.

6. American Hospital Association: Statement on microbiologic sampling in the hospital. *Hospitals* 48 : 125, 1974.

7. Eickhoff TC: Microbiologic sampling. *Hospitals* 44 : 86, 1970.

8. *Accreditation Manual for Hospitals 1986: Infection Control*. Chicago, standards adopted by Board of Commissioners of Joint Commission on Accreditation of Hospitals, 1985.

9. Goodlad RL: Biological indicators, a discussion of products, techniques, and philosophies. *Infection Control Rounds*, Minnesota, 3M Company, 2(1) : 1978.

10. Ajemian E: Environmental rounds. *Asepsis* 5(1) : 22, 1983.

11. Craig CP, Reifsnyder DN: *Departmental Procedures for Infection Control Programs*. New Jersey, Medical Economics Company, 1977.

# 18

# Isolation Techniques

The practice of isolating one group of people from another to avoid cross-transmission dates back to the 14th century when ships sailing the Mediterranean had to undergo 40-day periods of isolation of the ship, cargo, passengers, and crew when the ship came from a port that had certain epidemic diseases or there was unusual illness among the passengers or crew.

Isolation had no scientific foundation until the late 1800s, when the causative agents and modes of transmission of many of the important epidemic diseases were discovered. Much of this practice was initiated in health care institutions just prior to the U.S. Civil War. In the early 1870s the first training programs for nurses were established and isolation practices were based on historical precedent with overuse of the segregation tactic of single rooms for all, regardless of disease transmission (1).

The Public Health Act of 1944 stated that the causes and means of propagation and spread of diseases of humankind should be studied along with the development of methods of prevention and control and standardization of isolation practices. Over the years, as the epidemiology of disease became more clearly identified, practices of isolation progressed through standards outlined by the Public Health Service (2). A handbook, *Control of Infectious Disease in General Hospitals*, lists a table of communicable and infectious diseases as a basis for management of these patients in the hospital (3). However, fear of contamination from an isolated patient still remains today and is a problem that challenges the ICP.

The ICP is involved in all aspects of isolation, in all areas of the institution. The purpose of isolation is to prevent the transmission of disease. Historically, all patients with infections were totally isolated. Through recent developments in and understanding of infectious diseases, isolationhas become a much more specific set of practices: the disease is isolated, based on the organism and its means of transmission, but the patient is not totally sealed away from human contact.

Isolation can be seen in varying degrees in many areas of a hospital. An operating room, for instance, is in some ways an isolation unit. In order not to transmit infecting organisms to patients in the operating room, various controls have been instituted: a controlled access to the operating room; the use of special clothing in the area; extensive washing of a patient's surgery sites and personnel hands and arms; and the use of sterile equipment and supplies.

Some hospitals have isolation wards, which house all patients with communicable diseases; others isolate patients with infections in whatever unit they would normally be. There are advantages and disadvantages to each method of handling communicable diseases.

In an isolation ward, personnel are specially trained to minimize the risk of acquiring or transmitting infecting organisms. Whereas there is a risk of cross-infection within the unit, the infected patients are, both in terms of personnel and environment, geographically distant from uninfected susceptibles, such as patients just out of surgery, immunosuppressed patients, or those with immunodeficiency diseases. This may be a safe way of housing patients who have communicable illnesses. However, the most communicable stage of an infection is frequently the early stage, at the onset. If the infection is not recognized early on the general unit, transmission may occur, especially if other hospital personnel are not accustomed to taking care of patients with infections and recognizing early signs and symptoms.

The education of personnel in areas other than the isolation unit is therefore an important consideration. Because overtly infected patients are in the unit, there may be a feeling outside the unit that infecting organisms can't be spread, since no infections are present. As outlined in Chapter 6, potential pathogens are carried as normal flora on all people, and the presence of intrusive devices such as Foley catheters, tracheostomy tubes, and IVs make inoculation of these organisms from a carrier who is not overtly infected a real risk.

In the other situation, where isolated patients are housed throughout the hospital, the advantages may include a more general infection control awareness among all personnel. But having overtly infected patients in rooms near susceptible patients and the possibility of poor or careless nursing techniques (in multiple patient encounters by the same personnel) may result in transmission of infection.

Both types of institutional organization can provide adequate isolation care; neither ensures that transmission will not occur. What remains the most important criterion in evaluating an isolation setup is the education and awareness level of all hospital personnel in terms of the early recognition of infection, understanding mechanisms of transmission, and appropriate isolation techniques to interrupt transmission.

Chapters 5–8 discussed causes of infection. Prevention of infection occurs when transmission of the infectious agent is interrupted. This chapter focuses on methods of disrupting this transmission.

The most popular reference of the ICP for isolation practices was the CDC handbook, *Isolation Techniques for Use in Hospitals* (4). It went through many revisions and printings and topped the best seller list of the Government Printing Office (5). This isolation manual gave specific instructions for isolation requirements.

The manual grouped diseases with similar isolation requirements together into categories. The major categories of this system were strict, wound and skin, respiratory, and enteric. All diseases or infections were placed in one of these categories except minor wound or skin infections; other minimal body fluid infections were placed in one of two categories—drainage or secretion precautions. This category isolation system was easy to administer and teach to personnel; all they needed to do was recognize the color coded card for the category and follow the printed list. Figure 18-1 is an example of one such category.

The category system of isolation has been so popular and effective that it is one of two systems included in the new CDC guidelines for isolation precautions in hospital (6). The category system has expanded to include seven categories: strict, respiratory, tuberculosis, enteric, contact, drainage and secretion, and blood and body fluids. Its disadvantages are cost and overuse of supplies. There are variations in diseases, and lumping them within a category may involve overuse of isolation material and personnel time without any added benefit. This has prompted the CDC to offer a new system of isolation called *disease-specific isolation*. Both of these systems are discussed in this chapter, and detailed information can be found in the CDC isolation guidelines (6).

---

### STRICT ISOLATION

*Visitors Must Stop at Nursing Station Before Entering Room*

1. Masks are worn by all persons entering room.
2. Gowns are worn by all persons entering room.
3. Gloves are worn by all persons entering room.
4. Articles contaminated with infectious material require special handling.

---

**Figure 18-1**
*Signs hung outside the patient's door such as this one give instructions to personnel and visitors.*

# ISOLATION OF PATIENTS WITH COMMUNICABLE INFECTIONS

## Correct Isolation Procedures

Supplies to be used in isolation should be in a cart outside the patient's door (Fig. 18-2). Ideally, this cart is specially designed or purchased for isolation use, with the following as suggested parts:

- Drawers for gowns, gloves, or masks
- A pole on the side of the cart to hang outdoor coats or lab coats
- Ample room on top to set food tray, medical technician's supply basket, or other items that should not be taken into the isolation room
- Wheels for easy maneuvering

Newer isolation units sometimes have built-in shelves or closets outside each patient cubicle for isolation supplies.

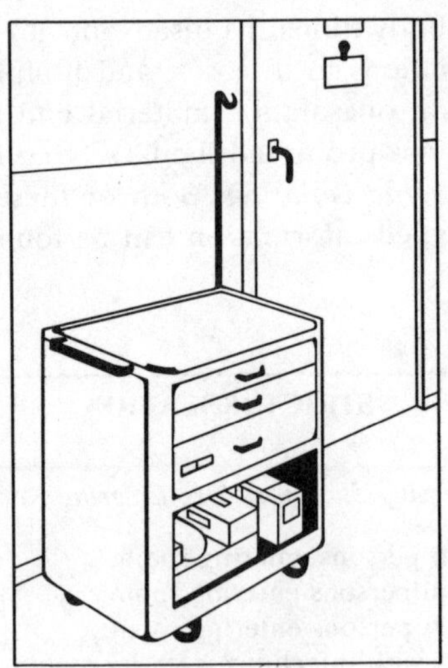

*Figure 18-2*

*The isolation cart, outside the patient's room should contain all the necessary equipment, plus an area where things can be left that do not enter the isolation room.*

# CATEGORY-SPECIFIC ISOLATION

The category-specific isolation system divides isolation into seven basic types, according to both the communicability of the agent and the mode of transmission of the disease. In this way, patients are isolated only as needed to stop the transmission of their disease, and patient contact and care are not unnecessarily limited. Through the use of isolation cards hung on the patient's door, the requirements for each type of isolation can easily be seen by each person entering the patient's room.

## Strict Isolation

Strict isolation is required for patients with diseases that are highly communicable and are spread by contact, including direct, indirect, and droplets, and are airborne. Examples of such diseases are plague, Lassa fever, smallpox, and diphtheria. Varicella (chickenpox) requires isolation, since the disease can be spread by upper respiratory droplets or the draining lesions characteristic of the disease and localized zoster in immunocompromised patients or patients with disseminated disease.

There is another important indication for strict isolation: suspected illnesses during the diagnostic period. If more than one disease is suspected, and more than one means of transmission is possible (e.g., respiratory isolation for meningococcal meningitis and excretion precautions for viral meningitis), strict isolation may be warranted to avoid transmission by airborne and contact routes until a diagnosis is established.

In order to prevent airborne transmission, the patient is housed in a private room with the door shut as much of the time as possible. Personnel wear gowns and gloves to enter and have contact with the patient and a mask to avoid mucous membrane contact with infective droplets, through inhaling or swallowing. All articles in the patient's room must be handled appropriately before leaving the room. Handwashing after contact with this patient and before contact with other patients is essential.

Whenever possible, patients in strict isolation should not leave their rooms. Any patient who must be transported must be adequately covered and handled to prevent disease transmission during transport or in another area of the hospital.

## Respiratory Isolation

Respiratory isolation is used for patients with an infection transmitted by respiratory droplets via the airborne route; infection occurs by inhalation of viable organisms. Diseases requiring respiratory isolation include epiglottitis; pneumonia in children and meningitis caused by *Hemophilus influenzae;* meningococcal diseases such as meningitis, bacteremia, and pneumonia; erythema infectiosum; and some of the common childhood illnesses, such as measles, mumps, and pertussis. Since the contact route (direct or indirect) is not important for these diseases, attention should be focused on the patient's respiratory tract products as the infection source. The patient should be in a private room, but the door need not be shut since respiratory droplets travel only a few feet. All people entering the room must wear masks (unless they are immune to the disease, as might be the case for measles, for example).

Articles contaminated with respiratory tract secretions should be disinfected or disposed of in the patient's room. The infecting organisms must be inhaled to infect a host. Since there is a possibility of aerosolizing organisms from heavily contaminated respiratory therapy equipment or soiled tissues, adequate handling of these materials is necessary.

Patients in respiratory isolation can leave their rooms if necessary, provided they wear masks appropriately.

## Tuberculosis Isolation

Tuberculosis isolation is necessary for patients with or suspected of having pulmonary or laryngeal tuberculosis. Isolation may be initiated on the basis of a positive sputum smear of acid-fast bacilli (AFB) or a chest x-ray highly suggestive of disease or presence of clinical signs and symptoms. A private room is indicated with ventilation to the outside because small droplet nuclei can be transmitted via recycled air. Masks are indicated for all persons entering the room. Laryngeal tuberculosis rapidly disseminates organisms through talking. Patients should wear masks or cover their mouths when outside the room. The door to the room should be kept shut to prevent spread of droplet nuclei to the corridor.

## Enteric Precautions

When the infecting organisms are transmitted via fecal material, enteric precautions should be taken. These infections occur after ingestion of the organisms; therefore, the contact route (direct and indirect) is important in the transmission of the organism from the host to a susceptible person.

Diseases spread in this manner include infectious diarrhea caused by cholera, *Salmonella, Shigella, Campylobacter, Cryptosporidium,* amebic dysentery, *Yersinia,* enteropathogenic *E. Coli,* enterocolitis caused by *Staphylococcus aureus* and *Clostridium difficile,* and viral agents known to cause diarrhea. Other diseases that shed organisms in the fecal material and can be transmitted by the fecal–oral route are echovirus, poliomyelitis, coxsack-ievirus, hepatitis A, herpangina, and viral agents causing pericarditis or my-ocarditis. Acute diarrhea of unknown etiology in a hospitalized patient should be assumed to be communicable and precautions should be taken. Patients should be isolated at the same time a sample is taken for culturing; it is unwise to wait for culture results, since the identification of *Salmonella* and *Shigella*, for instance, can take 72 hours.

Patients should be housed in separate rooms, if hygiene is poor and/or fecal contamination of the environment occurs. Otherwise, they do not need single rooms. Because of the mode of transmission, several factors should be con-sidered. Patients sharing facilities should be taught to wash their hands after using the commode. Since the fecal–oral route is required for transmission, roommates should also be instructed to wash their hands after using shared bathrooms and before eating. Single rooms may be necessary on a pediatric unit because of the age and the habits of children (e.g., putting objects in their mouths) and the fewer numbers of organisms required as a sufficient innoculum size to cause infection.

People caring for the patient in enteric isolation should wear gowns and gloves to avoid picking up the organism on uniforms or hands. All articles coming in direct contact with fecal material should be considered contami-nated and handled appropriately before leaving the room.

The patient can be transported to other departments as long as fecal material is contained.

## Contact Isolation

This type of isolation is required for patients who have a disease or infection that is highly contagious and spread primarily by close or direct contact. This category includes extensive skin or burn wounds, viral respiratory infections in young children (e.g., pharyngitis and pneumonia), *Staphylococcus aureus* and group A streptococcal pneumonia, rabies, rubella, scabies, pediculosis, staphylococcal scalded skin syndrome, vaccinia, and multiply resistant bacte-ria from any body site. Weinstein et al. found that contact isolation of patients with multiply drug-resistant organisms markedly decreased the incidence of these organisms in "epi" centers such as intensive care units (7).

The infective material can be respiratory secretions, wound drainage, or other body fluids. The criteria for isolation of a patient with an infected wound is primarily the amount of purulence present. Any wound or skin infection that is purulent and cannot be covered by a dressing, or one that drains so heavily that the dressing must be changed twice in a 4-hour period, requires single-room isolation.

It is most important to emphasize the criterion of purulence rather than the culture results. There are several reasons for this: the culture results are useful primarily for systemic or topical antimicrobial therapy; waiting for culture results could mean 48–72 hours during which virulent organisms may be spread from the nonisolated infected patient; inappropriate culture techniques or specimen handling could result in false-negative results. Regardless of the infecting organism, a purulent, heavily draining wound is the site of many virulent organisms and requires precautions. A culture should be taken, however, at the time infection is diagnosed, for epidemiologic and therapeutic purposes.

The infective material may be respiratory secretions, wound, or other body fluid drainage. The patient should be placed in a single room, and persons coming close to the patient should wear masks. Gowns should be worn if soiling of clothes is likely and gloves are necessary when touching infected drainage, secretions, or contaminated articles.

## Drainage Secretion Precautions

This is a new category designed to prevent infections that are transmitted by direct or indirect contact with minimal purulent drainage from wounds or other body sites. Wound drainage is usually contained by a dressing and presents risk of transmission only during dressing changes. Patients do not require single rooms, but close attention must be paid to disposal of all infectious waste. Gloves should be worn during contact with infective material. If soiling of clothes is likely, gowns should be worn. Minor skin, wound, and burn infections as well as conjunctivitis are included in this category. As with contact isolation, special handling of articles contaminated with infectious material is required. Contaminated articles that are disposable should be disposed of in plastic bags marked "isolation waste." Reusable articles must be cleaned, disinfected, or sterilized before reuse.

## Blood and Body Fluids Precautions

Patients who have diseases that result in infected blood or body fluids are placed on precautions to prevent transmission. Some diseases in this category, such as malaria, are transmitted only by blood, while other diseases, such as hepatitis B and acquired immune deficiency syndrome (AIDS), can also be transmitted by other body fluids, including semen, and possibly urine, saliva, or tears, although these have shown low risk for transmission (8). Diseases requiring blood and body fluid precautions are dengue, yellow fever, Colorado tick fever, hepatitis B and NANB hepatitis, malaria, leptospirosis, rat-bite and relapsing fever, AIDS, and primary and secondary syphilis with skin and mucosal lesions.

Patients whose hygiene is good do not require a single room but do require

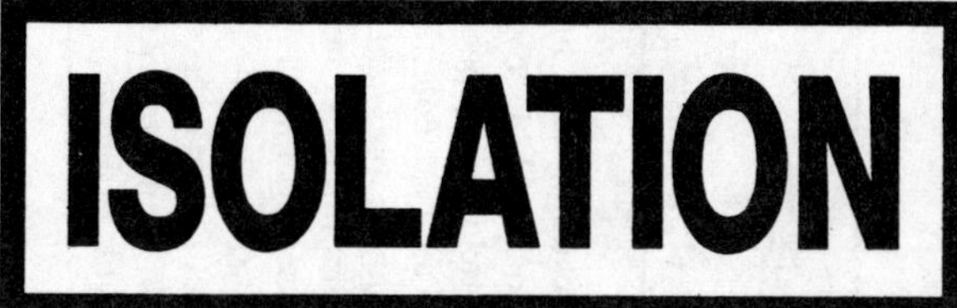



**Figure 18-3**

*This disease-specific isolation card allows personnel to fill in appropriate instructions for handling the patients or articles.*

**Table 18-1**
DISEASE-SPECIFIC ISOLATION PRECAUTIONS

| Disease | Precautions indicated | | | | Infective Material | Apply Precautions How Long? | Comments |
|---|---|---|---|---|---|---|---|
| | Private room? | Masks? | Gowns? | Gloves? | | | |
| Hepatitis, viral Type B ("serum hepatitis"), including hepatitis B antigen ($HB_sAg$) carrier | No | No | Yes if soiling is likely | Yes for touching infective material | Blood and body fluids[a] | Until patient is $HB_sAg$-negative | Use caution when handling blood and blood-soiled articles; take special care to avoid needlestick injuries; pregnant personnel may need special counseling Gowns are indicated when clothing may become contaminated with body fluids or blood |

[a] All laboratory specimens of blood and body fluids should be labeled "Isolation—Blood Precautions" in red.

SOURCE: Adapted from CDC guidelines for isolation precautions in hospitals (6).

education on the importance of handwashing to prevent transmission. Gowns are necessary when soiling of clothing is likely to occur during patient contact. Gloves are always worn when touching infective blood or body fluids and when touching articles contaminated with infective material.

When drawing blood or giving injections, care should be taken to avoid needlestick injuries. Needles should not be cut, broken, or capped. They should be disposed of in an impervious container at the bedside. Blood and body fluid spills should be cleaned up with an adequate disinfectant (8).

## DISEASE-SPECIFIC ISOLATION

The disease-specific isolation system deals with each infectious disease or type of infection individually. Attention is focused on infective material and barrier precautions that will interrupt disease transmission. The advantages of disease-specific isolation are the cost savings from more appropriate use of isolation supplies such as gown, masks, and gloves. Single rooms are utilized less frequently for isolation. Patients may be more appropriately isolated, and compliance of isolation requirements is better if isolation is not in excess but is nonetheless effective. It also allows the isolation card to be marked with individual needs. Specific requirements are determined by identifying the disease from an alphabetical table. The table indicates which barrier precautions are necessary as shown in Table 18-1. An isolation card shown in Figure 18-3 illustrates the system and also shows a place for indicating any special precautions such as pregnancy or indication of any special handling, for instance, when all laboratory slips must be marked "blood and body fluid isolation" to alert laboratory personnel. The infective material is listed on the isolation card and is a constant reminder to all personnel as to the source of contamination.

## SPECIFIC ISOLATION PROCEDURES

In the previous sections the barrier precautions required by personnel caring for infected patients have been described briefly. These procedures are discussed in greater detail below (9); the education of personnel in these techniques and the enforcement of policies related to isolation are primarily the responsibility of the ICP in conjunction with the inservice director and department heads.

### Gowning, Gloving, and Masking

All the supplies required for entering the isolation room should be conveniently located outside the patient's door. Depending on the kind of isolation, gowns, gloves, and/or masks will be worn. After washing hands, a fresh, clean

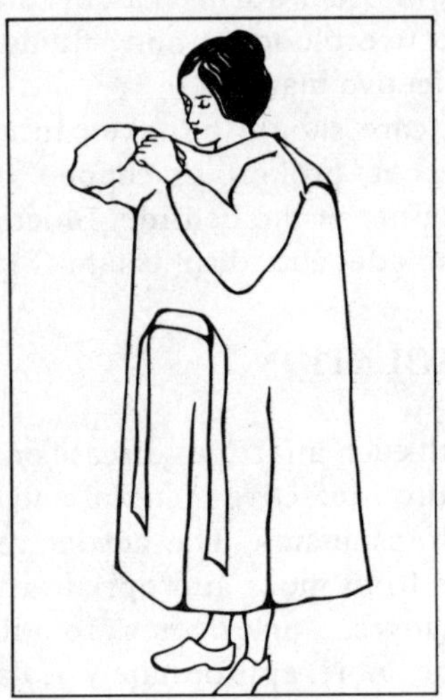

**Figure 18-4**
*The gown is large enough to cover the uniform and should have long sleeves.*

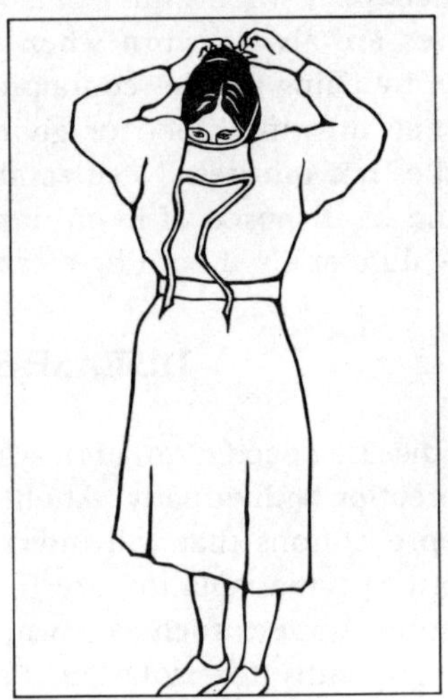

**Figure 18-5**
*The mask should fit snugly.*

gown is put on, with the opening at the back, and is tied securely at the waist and neck. The gown should be long enough to cover the clothes and should have long sleeves, as shown in Figure 18-4. The gown may be paper or cloth. Cloth will not be effective if wet. There are paper gowns that are impervious to moisture.

The mask should be tied high on the head so that it does not slip during care (Fig. 18-5). The best masks are of heavy paper or cloth. One type of paper mask has a metal band that can be molded over the bridge of the nose for a snug fit. Most masks are no longer effective after they become moist, usually after 20 minutes of use.

Gloves should be pulled over the ends of the gown sleeves, as shown in Figure 18-6. They need not be sterile, unless care is given to a site that requires asepsis such as a central line dressing change, and should be disposable. If paper gowns are worn, the thumb can be pushed through the end of the sleeve, thereby holding the sleeve end inside the glove during arm movement. Gloves should be strong enough to resist being torn during normal patient care. Rings and jewelry with sharp edges should not be worn under gloves for this reason. If the patient's room does not have a clock available, personnel can use a plastic bag to hold a watch which may be necessary for calculating the patient's vital signs.

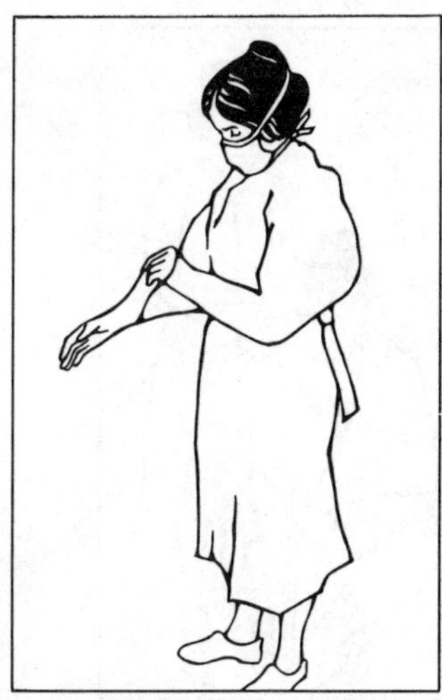

*Figure 18-6*
*The gloves should be pulled over the sleeve*
*of the gown.*

## Transporting the Infected Patient

Protection of other patients and personnel from the patient with a communicable disease who is being transported is based on the same principles as those used in the isolation room. The difference is that the infectious patient is out in the open rather than in a separate area. To avoid contact (direct and indirect) routes of transmission, the patient is wrapped in a clean sheet as a barrier (Fig. 18-7). If the droplet or airborne routes of transmission are important, patients, whenever possible, wear masks while outside their rooms. The mask contains the respiratory droplets, and gown, gloves, and cover sheet are not necessary.

It is essential that nursing personnel notify the department of the type of isolation required for the patient being transferred. Personnel in the receiving department should wear appropriate isolation attire if the patient removes the mask or is removed from the clean sheet and has direct contact with them. The sheets used in transport are discarded with the other isolation linen (if the contact route is important in transmission) in the patient's room; gowns and gloves used by personnel in the receiving department during contact with the patient should be handled appropriately in that area. Because the patient is clothed as a protection for others, there is no need for the transporting personnel to wear isolation clothing during the transport itself (Fig. 18-8). Gowns, gloves, and/or masks used in preparing the patient for transport

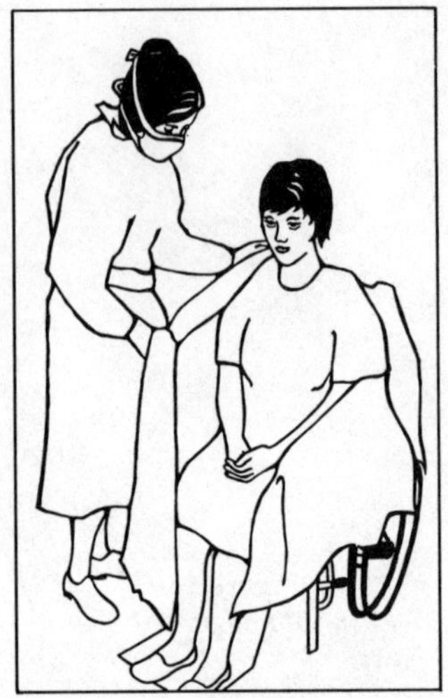

**Figure 18-7**

*A sheet is placed on the wheelchair, and the patient is wrapped in it before being transported.*

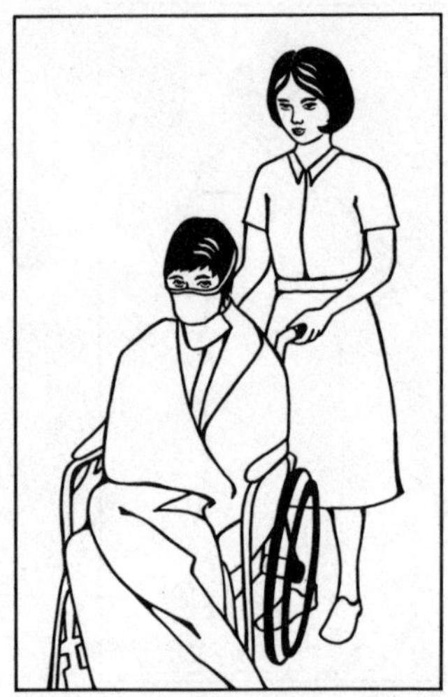

**Figure 18-8**

*While outside the isolation room, the patient wears protective clothing; personnel transporting the patient leave their isolation clothing inside the room.*

should, in fact, be discarded in the patient's room. Adequate preparation of the patient for transport will make it unnecessary for others to wear protective clothing until they arrive at the receiving department.

## Handling Contaminated Materials

In isolation rooms where the contact (direct and indirect) route of transmission is important, patient care equipment and supplies may become heavily contaminated with the infecting organisms. These items must be prepared in the same way that the patient is prepared for transport, in order to protect other patients and personnel from these potential sources of infecting organisms. The procedure used, however, will depend on the destination and final outcome of the contaminated material.

### *Nondisposable Patient-Care Equipment*
Supplies that will be returned to the Central Supply Department for sterilization or disinfection must be cleaned of all visible gross contamination before

leaving the patient's room. Soap, water, and a good scrub are all that is necessary to prepare the item, which then should be bagged (as described later) for transport to Central Supply. Similarly, nondisposable dietary utensils that may be contaminated should be washed (food and liquids can be flushed down the commode) and bagged to be sent back to the Dietary Department. Cleaning these items, in almost all cases, is adequate protection for personnel of the receiving departments, and bagging provides an extra safeguard.

### Linen

Linen may be grossly contaminated with infecting organisms and obviously cannot be washed in the patient's room. It should be gathered in an impermeable bag inside the room and sealed. The process of double-bagging is then used; the first bag is the one used and sealed inside the room. A ("clean") person stands outside the door with a clean, impermeable bag opened, with the end folded over the hands in a large cuff. The person inside the isolation

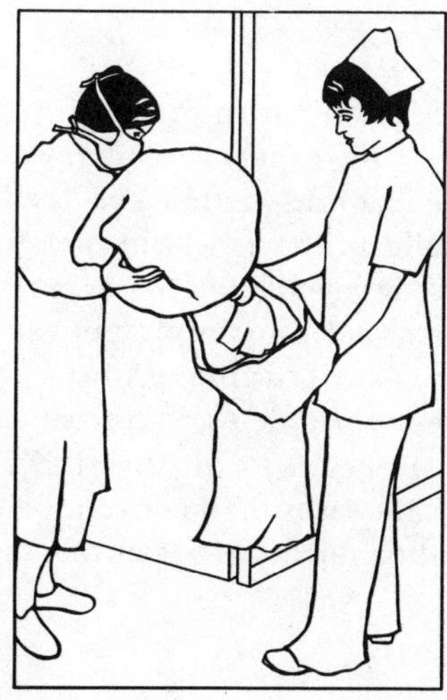

**Figure 18-9**

*The person inside the isolation room, in isolation clothing, places the full, sealed bag into the clean bag. The nurse outside the door has a large cuff of the bag over her hands to avoid touching the contaminated bag.*

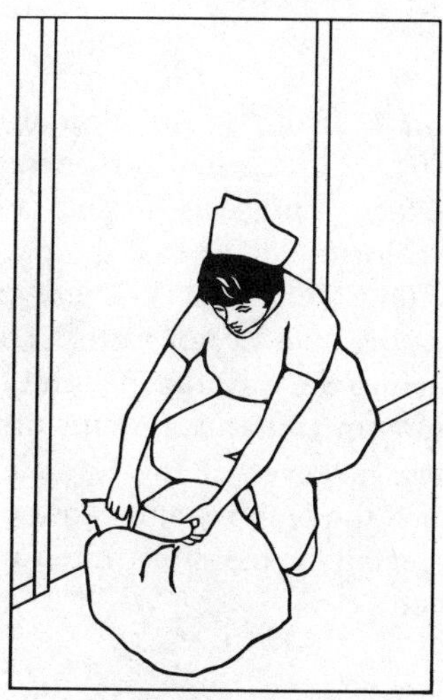

**Figure 18-10**

*The nurse unrolls the cuff, expels the air away from her face, and seals the bag.*

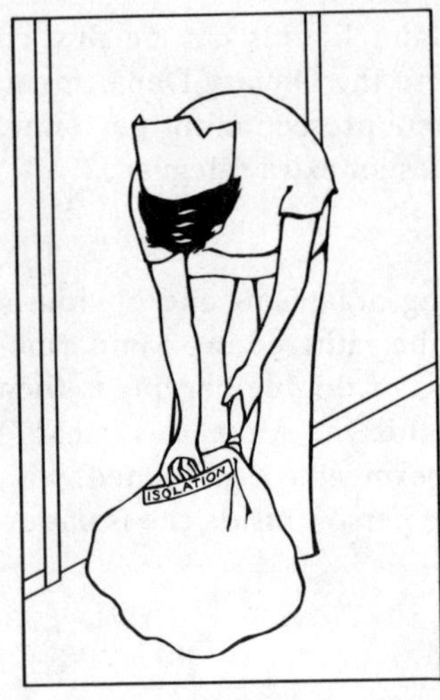


*Figure 18-11*
*The bag must be marked in some way so that other department personnel will know that the material inside is potentially hazardous.*

room ("dirty," in isolation attire) places the sealed bag in the clean bag (Fig. 18-9). The "clean" person then unfolds the cuff, expels the air (away from the face), and seals the bag (Fig. 18-10). The bag must be marked "Isolation" or color-coded so that the personnel who collect the bag will be alerted to its contents (Fig. 18-11). There are some linen bags available for use in isolation that dissolve in hot water. The laundry personnel can simply put the entire bag into the washing machine, thus eliminating any possible risk from opening and emptying the contents of the bag. There are problems with some of these bags, however, if the linen is wet. They may begin to dissolve before they reach the laundry and cause more problems and risks than conventional bags, especially since moist linen may in fact harbor far more organisms than dry linen.

### *Trash*

Trash is double-bagged in the same way as linen. A comparative study of single- and double-bagging of trash from isolation rooms indicated double bagging is unnecessary (10). In the future, this may not be done, although some state agencies still require double-bagging for linen and trash. For the most efficient operation, trash is "bagged out" once or twice during each shift, in succession, for all isolated patients in a unit.

### *Disposal of Needles*

For patients with diseases requiring blood and body fluid precautions, needles should be disposed of in the patient's room. An old IV bottle can be used to hold discarded used needles; several types of commercial needle boxes, designed specifically for this use, are available. If possible, these needles should be terminally disinfected or sterilized prior to disposal.

### *Toys, Books, and Personal Items*

Items used in an isolation room should be evaluated in terms of the amount of their contact with infectious material and the degree of infectivity of the organism causing the disease. Clothes can be sent home in a plastic bag with instructions to wash in hot water and tumble dry or hang in sunlight. Specific instructions for laundering clothes of patients in strict isolation are found in CDC guidelines for isolation precautions in hospitals (6). Personal items, including toys, should be kept to a minimum in the hospital isolation room, but the psychological well-being of the patient should also be kept in mind. No toys or personal supplies or equipment of any kind should be shared among patients. With the exception of visible soilage with secretions, these items do not require special handling for most isolation cases. Cleaning the gross contamination will depend on the material it is made of.

## Leaving the Isolation Room

### *Removing the Gown, Gloves, and/or Mask*

In order to remove isolation attire correctly, it is important to know which parts are considered clean and which are considered contaminated. The entire front of the gown has probably come into contact with infecting organisms during patient care, as have the gloves; the front of the mask, if worn, is also considered contaminated, as shown in Figure 18-12. The back of the gown is considered possibly contaminated only from the waist downward, and the neck and mask ties are clean (Fig. 18-13).

The gown and gloves are removed so as to prevent contamination of the uniform while doing so. After the waist ties are untied (Fig. 18-14), the gloves are removed (being reversed in the process) (Fig. 18-15); this procedure minimizes hand contact with the contaminated side of the gloves and adds a safeguard for trash handlers should the bag of trash accidentally open. The mask, if worn, can easily be removed by untying the strings, holding it by the strings only (Fig. 18-16), and discarding it in the appropriate container. For certain highly communicable airborne diseases, a special container for discarded masks should be placed outside the patient's closed door so that the mask need not be taken off inside the patient's room along with the other isolation attire. The neck ties are untied and the gown is slipped off in such a

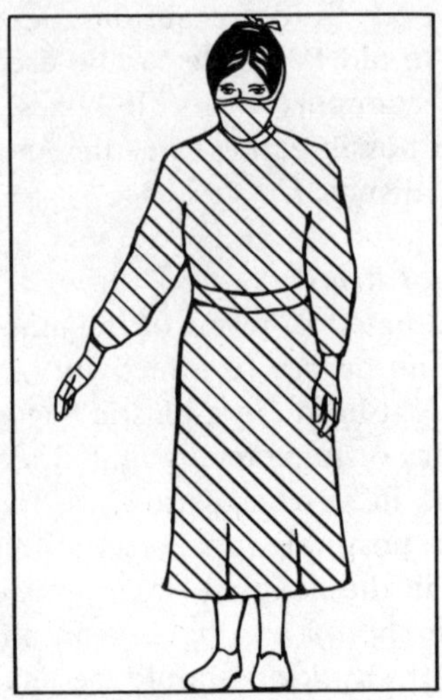

**Figure 18-12**
The shaded areas show the areas of contamination: the entire front of the gown, the mask, and all parts of the gloves are considered contaminated.

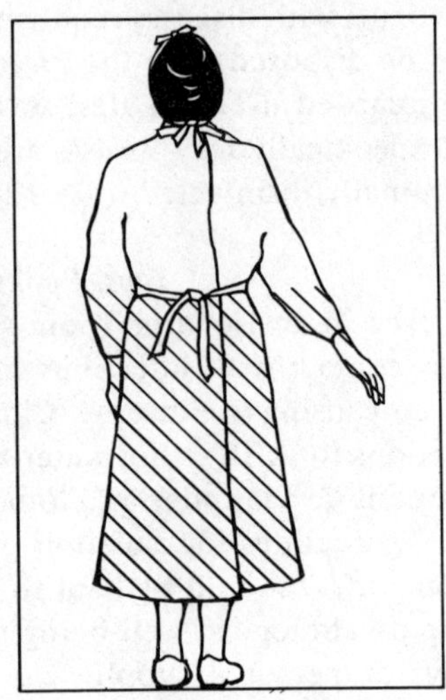

**Figure 18-13**
In the back, the gown from the waist down is considered contaminated; the neck ties and the mask ties are clean.

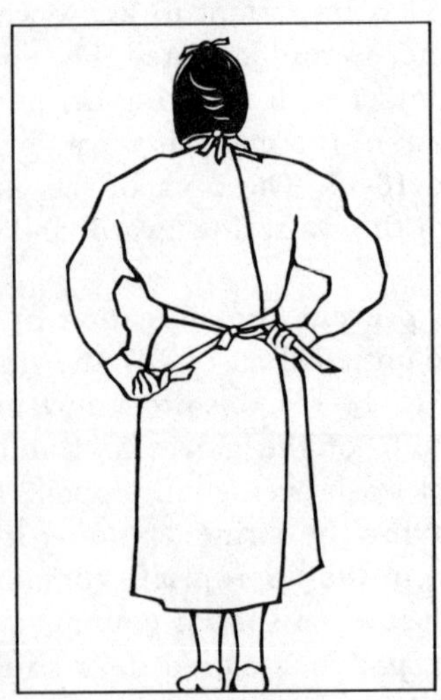

**Figure 18-14**
The waist ties are untied first.

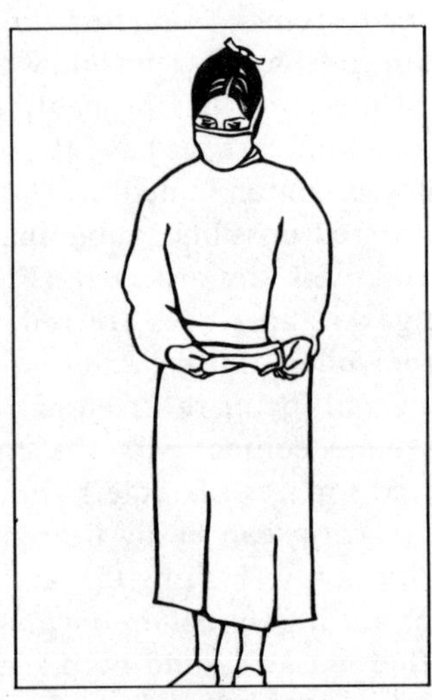

**Figure 18-15**
The gloves are removed without contaminating the hands.

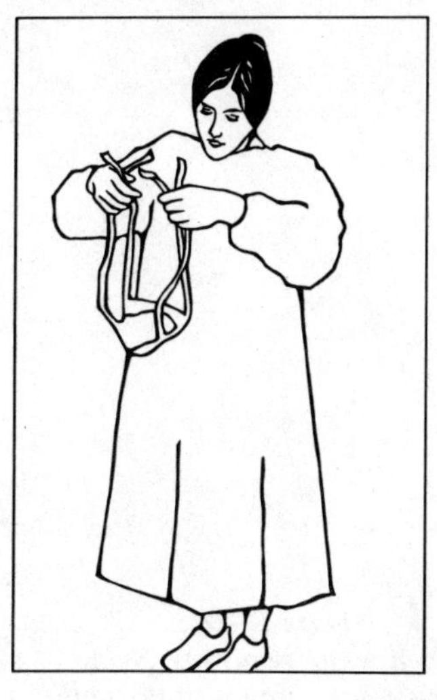

Figure 18-16
The mask is removed by holding it by the ties.

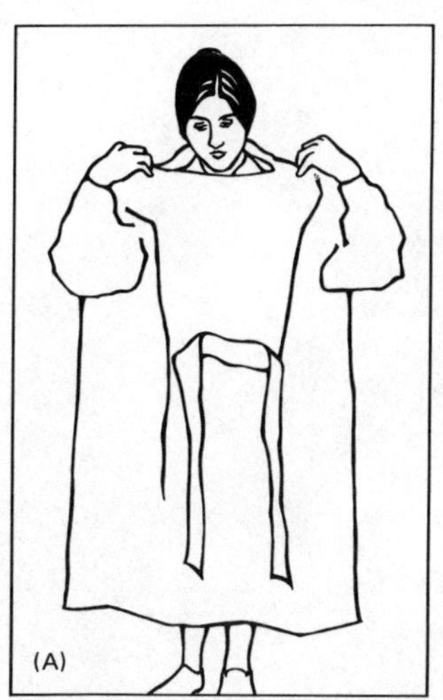

(A)
(B)
Figure 18-17
The gown is slipped off the shoulders (A) and pulled off (B).

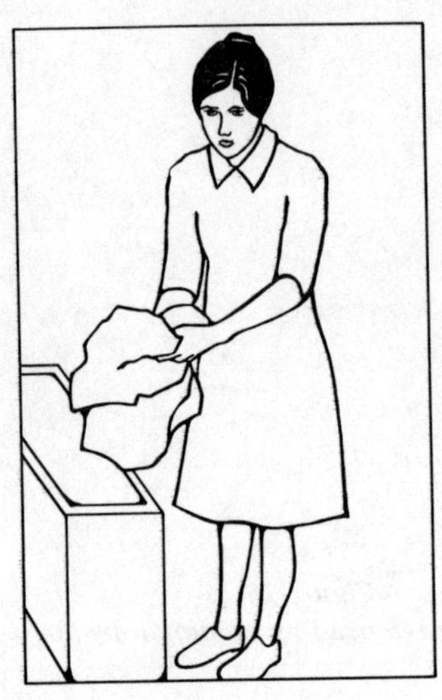

*Figure 18-18*
*Care is taken while removing the gown so that the gown does not touch the uniform.*

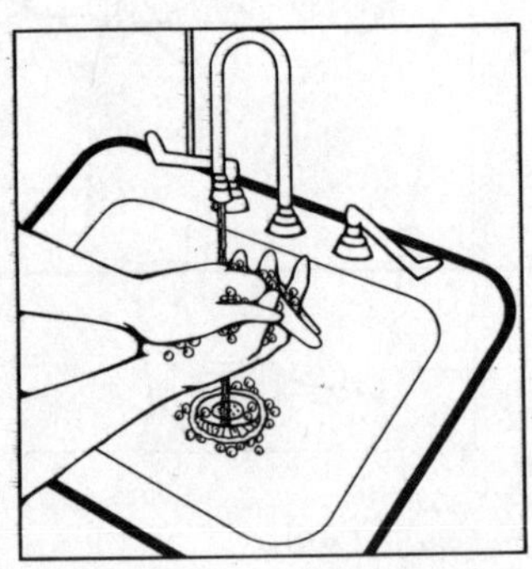

*Figure 18-19*
*Handwashing is critical after the isolation clothing is removed.*

manner as to avoid contact with the uniform, as shown in Figures 18-17 and 18-18. Gowns should be worn only once and discarded.

The last step to be taken when leaving the isolation room is handwashing (Fig. 18-19). The correct technique is discussed below.

## Handwashing

Handwashing is the single most important means of preventing the spread of infections in hospitals. It is the first step in any patient care procedure and the last step after patient care or leaving an isolation area. There are different procedures for handwashing depending on the degree of contamination and the reason for decontaminating the hands. Scrubbing before surgery is quite different from washing before dispensing oral medications, and the types of solutions and the time spent in scrubbing will differ depending on the procedure planned.

The purpose of handwashing for general patient care is to remove potentially pathogenic organisms. These organisms have many different sources: organisms from a patient's infected wound may be carried on the hands of personnel to another patient; organisms from infected urine, picked up during routine emptying of Foley catheter bags, may be deposited on the next patient's catheter bag and, through retrograde movement, may cause infection; organisms from the bowel may be picked up on the hands when one is using the toilet and then may be transmitted to a patient's IV insertion site. Handwashing serves to remove potential pathogens from these and other sources; there is no need to sterilize the hands before general patient care activities.

There are three essential parts of a good handwash: friction, soap, and warm running water. Friction must be used to remove gross contamination, dead skin, and other particles that may contain potentially pathogenic organisms. Soap helps to remove such matter by emulsifying skin oils that tend to hold these particles. There is much controversy about the relative merits of different types of soap—powders, liquids, bar soap, leaflet, and so on—and institutions differ in their preferences. Most important, from the ICP's viewpoint, is to motivate personnel to wash their hands, and to do it often. A mild soap that is easy to use and makes a good lather is best for general patient care (11).

An antimicrobial handwashing preparation should be used when invasive procedures are done such as central line placement and cutdowns for arterial lines. Additionally, personnel who work in high-risk areas such as intensive care, neonatal, transplant, or hemodialysis units may wish to use an antimicrobial handwashing preparation (12). There is controversy over the efficacy of this action, and some organisms seem to develop resistance to the antimicrobial handwashing preparations (13,14).

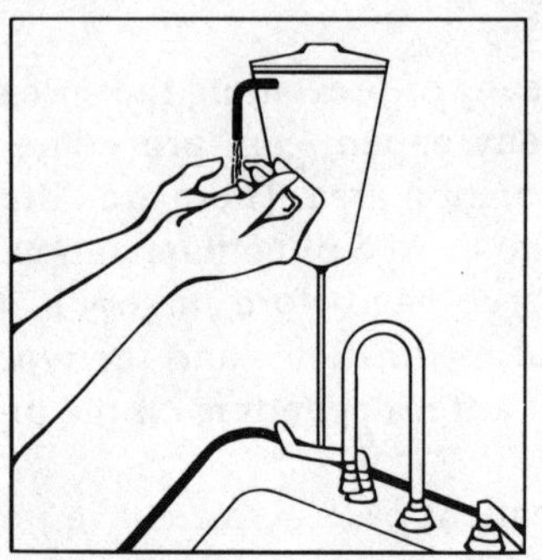

**Figure 18-20**

*The use of a mild soap and warm running water is important for handwashing before or after general patient care.*

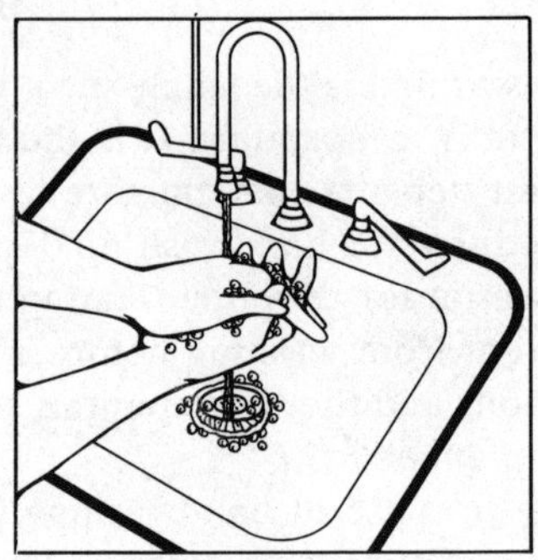

**Figure 18-21**

*Friction is the most important part of the handwashing procedure.*

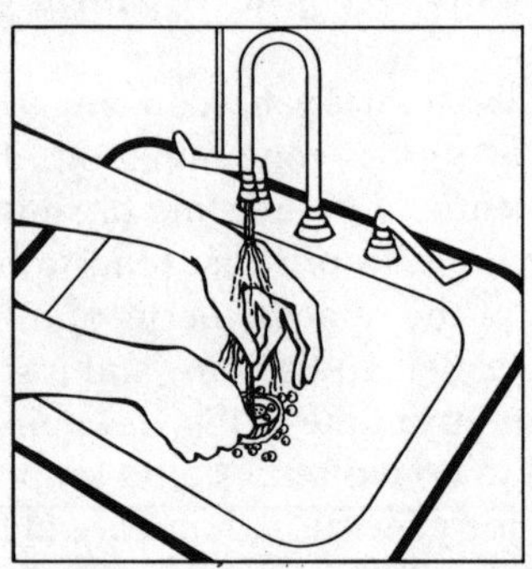

**Figure 18-22**

*The hands are rinsed while they are held downward.*

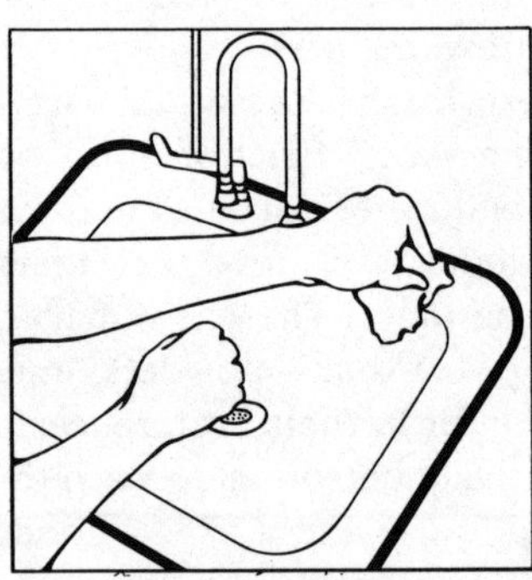

**Figure 18-23**

*Turning the water faucets off with a paper towel will prevent recontamination of the hands.*

The correct handwashing procedure is shown in Figures 18-20–18-23. Warm running water will facilitate the action of the soap and will rinse away loosened debris. Standing water in a basin is unacceptable because it is a good medium for bacteria, leading to the possibility of adding more bacteria to the hands rather than removing them. Turning off the water faucets with a paper towel will prevent the possible reinoculation of organisms onto the hands.

## Terminal Cleaning of an Isolation Room

When a patient is discharged or when that patient's infection is no longer communicable, terminal cleaning of the isolation room is begun by nursing personnel, who remove, in the appropriate manner, all patient care supplies that may still be contaminated with infectious material. For example, a suction bottle containing respiratory tract secretions from a patient with staphylococcal pneumonia is cleaned, double-bagged and sent to Central Supply when the patient is transferred, has expired, or has responded to treatment and is no longer infectious to others. After the patient is discharged from the isolation room, all such equipment should be handled according to previously described methods, if they are still thought to be infectious; then the Housekeeping Department should begin cleaning the room. Room cleaning in most cases should be the same for all rooms, regardless of whether their occupants were in isolation; visibly soiled walls and grossly soiled curtains should be cleaned. All beds, furniture, and floors should be cleaned routinely; the cleaning should be adequate to remove all potential pathogens from the next patient's environment. It is important to reconsider the host factors outlined in Chapter 8; the normal flora of a noninfected patient could become pathogenic in a severely immunocompromised host; therefore, cleaning procedures should be consistent and adequate after each patient is discharged. In terminal cleaning of isolation rooms, where there is much visible soilage of the patient's environment and where the contact route of infection is important, it may be necessary for housekeeping personnel to wear gowns, gloves, and/or masks.

## ISOLATION OF PATIENTS WHO ARE HIGHLY SUSCEPTIBLE TO INFECTIONS

As discussed in Chapter 8, placing certain patients because of their particular conditions, diagnoses, or therapies on so-called protective isolation using mask, gown, and gloves is costly, time-consuming, and does little to reduce their risk of acquiring nosocomial infections (15,16). Many immunocompromised patients acquire infections from their own microbial flora rather than from personnel. Protective isolation does little to decrease this risk. Most nosocomial infections in immunocompromised patients are acquired by contact transmission from organisms on the poorly washed hands of personnel and contaminated patient care articles.

Emphasis on frequent and appropriate handwashing before and after patient contact would reduce this risk (12). Motivating personnel to wash their hands enough is an ongoing problem for the ICP (17–19).

## ISOLATION IN OUTPATIENT AREAS

Outpatient areas are most difficult to control in terms of communicable disease transmission, yet it is the responsibility of the ICP to address this problem. Guidelines should be devised to minimize the spread of disease in the clinic setting.

Waiting rooms probably provide the opportunity for the closest contact among infected patients and potential hosts. Optimally, separate waiting areas for patients with suspected communicable diseases minimize the risks. There should be a mechanism for screening patients as they first register at the clinic, so that possibly infectious patients can be moved quickly into examining rooms and out of the general waiting area.

Pediatric clinics are a problem because of the closer contact between patients while waiting. Any child with a suspected communicable disease should be seen immediately; if this is not possible, the mother should be instructed to hold the child on her lap and not allow the child to play or come into contact with any of the other children. In general, toys used in common waiting areas should be of the type that are easily cleaned. Toys that have been used by a child with an infection should be washed.

## LONG-TERM CARE

Each institution must assess its capabilities for accepting communicable or infectious patients as transfers from acute care institutions. Staff members, such as aides, who will be caring for these people on a regular basis should demonstrate an understanding of disease transmission and utilize appropriate barrier precautions. The institution must have physical facilities such as adequate single rooms, when necessary, to house these patients. Patient interaction at programs and meals must be assessed when developing isolation protocols to decrease transmission risk. Decreased mental status may be a factor in patient education. Because of these factors, which are prevalent in the elderly and long-term care, more single rooms may be required or it may not be feasible to accept infectious patients from acute care institutions.

The following checklist for incoming patients may be helpful:

1. Has this patient been isolated for an infectious process?
2. Has this patient been treated for an infectious process?
3. Has the site of infection been cultured? When?
4. What are the culture results?
5. Are the organisms resistant to antibiotics?
6. Has the infection resolved?
7. What type of isolation was used for this patient?

These simple questions will allow assessment of infectious conditions of the patient prior to admission and enable staff to use appropriate isolation precautions to prevent exposure to employees and other residents. Protocol for employees who are sick or infectious and follow-up of exposure to infectious residents should follow procedures discussed in this chapter.

## ROLE OF THE INFECTION CONTROL PRACTITIONER IN ISOLATION PROCEDURES

The ICP may have the authority to place patients into isolation. In one study, the involvement of infection control personnel in these decisions resulted in a decrease in overisolation and a savings in charges to patients (20).

The ICP will also be involved in teaching all personnel the techniques involved in isolation care. The training is meant for personnel who care for the patient directly as well as those who simply have contact with the room or contaminated objects, if the contact route is important. Included are housekeeping, dietary, maintenance, and other groups. If the hospital is in a part of the United States where a language other than English is used, bilingual isolation signs should be available. Similarly, the ICP may become involved in developing patient information sheets or booklets that explain isolation to the patient and the patient's family. Samples of information sheets are shown in Figures 18-24–18-27.

Isolation techniques are based on the idea that infecting organisms should be restricted to the host, who is receiving various forms of treatment to eradicate the infection completely. Methods to prevent the transmission of potential pathogens, from infected patients and to susceptible hosts, are used in varying degrees throughout the hospital environment. These isolation categories represent in some ways the end point in precautionary measures;

You have an infection that may be contagious to others, so you will receive special care to prevent the spread of infection.

The germs that cause your infection are so small that they cannot be seen, but they can easily be spread through the air on hands, clothing, or even some of the things that are used to care for you. Hospital personnel will wash their hands before and after doing something for you or touching anything in your room. They will probably be wearing gowns, masks, and gloves. You can help the nursing staff by asking them to take care of as many of your needs as possible when they are in your room. You will be in a room by yourself, and the door will remain shut as much as possible. You should stay inside your room unless given permission to leave it or escorted by staff.

### Personal Belongings

Send all unnecessary clothes and supplies home. For certain illnesses, your relatives will be given instructions for washing these items. Only toilet articles may be kept in your room. However, special appliances such as hearing aids or orthopedic devices may be kept in your room.

### Patient Care Supplies

Special precautions will be necessary for instruments, dressings, and linens used during your stay in isolation.

### Visitors

Your visitors should consult with nursing personnel when visiting you in isolation so that they can be shown what precautions to take. Visitors will probably have to wear a gown, gloves, and masks, and be especially careful when they come to see you. Visitors should not sit on your bed, drink, or eat in your room. They should not bring food without permission. Visitors may be asked to leave the room temporarily while you are receiving treatment.

Visitors should be limited to two at a time and should keep your condition in mind in determining the length of their visits. If visitors are making you overtired ask a nurse to limit the number of visitors allowed and/or the length of visits. Visits should be made only by family members; your friends should wait until you are better. No children under the age of 12 are allowed.

These precautions are enforced to ensure that infections are not spread throughout the hospital. Please discuss with your nurse any questions or problems you may have during your hospital stay.

**Figure 18-24**

*Information sheets on strict isolation can be distributed to patients and their families to explain isolation procedures.*

## DRAINAGE PRECAUTIONS

You have an infection that may be contagious, so you will receive special care to prevent the spread of infection to others. You may be in a private room. If so, you should stay inside your room unless given permission to leave it or escorted by staff.

The germs that cause your infection are so small that they cannot be seen, but they can be spread on hands, clothing, or even some of the things that are used to care for you.

Please do not touch your would or dressing.

Personnel will wash their hands before and after doing something for you or touching anything in your room. They may also wear gowns and gloves when caring for you. You can help the nursing staff by asking them to take care of as many of your needs as possible when they are in your room.

### Personal Belongings

Send all unnecessary clothes and supplies home. For certain illnesses, your relatives will be given instructions for washing these items. Only toilet articles may be kept in your room. However, special appliances such as hearing aids or orthopedic devices may be kept in your room.

### Patient Care Supplies

Special precautions will be necessary for instruments, dressings, and linens used during your stay in isolation.

### Visitors

Your visitors should report to the nursing station before visiting you in isolation so that they can be shown what precautions to take. Visitors may be asked to leave the room temporarily while you are receiving treatment.

Visitors should be limited to two at a time and should keep your condition in mind in determining the length of their visit. If visitors are making you overtired ask a nurse to limit the number of visitors allowed and/or the length of visits. Visits should be made only by family members; your friends should wait until you are better. No children under the age of 12 are allowed.

These precautions are enforced to ensure that infections are not spread throughout the hospital. Please discuss with your nurse any questions or problems you may have during your hospital stay.

**Figure 18-25**
*Information sheets on drainage precaution procedures can be distributed to patients and their families.*

ENTERIC ISOLATION

You have an infection that may be contagious, so you will receive special care to prevent the spread of infection to others. Children will have a private room and must stay inside unless given permission to leave it or escorted by staff. There are usually no restrictions for adults.

The germs that cause your infection are so small that they cannot be seen, but they can be spread on hands, clothing, or even some of the things that are used to care for you. Personnel will wash their hands before and after doing something for you or touching anything in your room. They will probably wear gowns and gloves when caring for you. You can help the nursing staff by asking them to take care of as many of your needs as possible when they are in your room.

Your condition can be transmitted by bowel or bladder excretions, so wash your hands carefully after using the toilet.

*Personal Belongings*

In general, you should send all unnecessary clothes and supplies home. For certain illnesses, your relatives will be given instructions for washing these items. Only toilet articles may be kept in your room. However, special appliances such as hearing aids or orthopedic devices may be kept in your room.

*Patient Care Supplies*

The nursing staff will take special precautions in handling articles contaminated with urine and feces, including instruments and linen.

*Visitors*

Your visitors should consult with nursing personnel when visiting you in isolation so that they can be shown what precautions to take. Visitors should not sit on your bed, drink, or eat in your room. They should not bring food without permission. Visitors may be asked to leave the room temporarily while you are receiving treatment.

Visitors should be limited to two at a time and should keep your condition in mind in determining the length of their visits. If visitors are making you overtired ask a nurse to limit the number of visitors allowed and/or the length of visits. Visits should be made only by family members; your friends should wait until you are better. No children under the age of 12 are allowed.

These precautions are enforced to ensure that infections are not spread throughout the hospital. Please discuss with your nurse any questions or problems you may have during your hospital stay.

---

**Figure 18-26**

*Information sheets on enteric isolation procedures can be distributed to patients and their families.*

236

Your have an illness that may be contagious, so you will receive special care to prevent the spread of infection to others. The germs that cause your infection are so small that they cannot be seen, but they can be spread through the air in small drops or moisture from your nose and mouth. Personnel will wash their hands before and after doing something for you or touching anything in your room. You can help the nursing staff by asking them to take care of as many of your needs as possible when they are in your room.

You will probably be in a room by yourself, and the door will remain shut as much as possible. You should stay inside your room, unless given permission to leave it or escorted by staff. You will be asked to wear a mask when you leave your room. Please remember to cover your mouth with a tissue when coughing and to put tissues in the waste receptacle.

*Personal Belongings*

You should send all unnecessary clothes and supplies home and keep only toilet articles in your room. You may, however, keep special appliances such as hearing aids or orthopedic devices in your room. Anything soiled with secretions from your mouth or nose may be handled in a special manner by the nursing staff.

*Visitors*

Your visitors should report to the nursing station before visiting you in isolation so that they can be shown what precautions to take. They will probably have to wear masks and be especially careful when they come to see you. Visitors should not sit on your bed, drink, or eat in your room. They should not bring food without permission. Visitors may be asked to leave the room temporarily while you are receiving treatment.

Visitors should be limited to two at a time and should keep your condition in mind in determining the length of their visits. If visitors make you overtired ask a nurse to limit the number of visitors allowed and/or the length of visits. Visits should be made only by family members; your friends should wait until you are better. No children under the age of 12 are allowed.

These precautions are enforced to ensure that infections are not spread throughout the hospital. Please discuss with your nurse any questions or problems you may have during your hospital stay.

---

**Figure 18-27**
*Information sheets on respiratory isolation procedures can be distributed to patients and their families.*

single-use equipment, cleaning, disinfection and sterilization of supplies, and handwashing are a few of the many policies and procedures used in hospitals to prevent infections from occurring and to minimize the risk of transmission. Isolation techniques are most useful if thought of in terms of a continuum of practices designed to prevent, detect early, and appropriately isolate communicable diseases for the protection of patients and personnel within the hospital setting.

# REFERENCES


1. Jackson M, Lynch P: Isolation practices: A historical perspective. *Am J Infect Control* 13(1): 21, 1985.
2. Public Health, *Encyclopedia Americana,* vol. 22. Americana Corporation, New York, 1960, p 763.
3. Top FH: *Control of Infectious Disease in General Hospitals.* American Public Health Association, New York, 1967, pp 71–76.
4. Centers for Disease Control: *Isolation Techniques for Use in Hospitals.* U.S. Department of Health, Education and Welfare, Public Health Service, Atlanta, Centers for Disease Control, 1970.
5. Schaffner W: Infection control: Old myths and new realities. *Infect Control* 1(5): 330, 1980.
6. Garner JS, Simmons BP: CDC guidelines for isolation precautions in hospitals. Hospital Infections Program, Atlanta, Centers for Disease Control, 1983.
7. Weinstein RA, Kabins SA: Strategies for prevention and control of multiple drug-resistant nosocomial infection. *Am J Med* 70: 449, 1981.
8. Centers for Disease Control: Recommendations for preventing transmission of infection with human T-lymphotropic virus type III/Lymphadenopathy-associated virus in the workplace. *Morbidity and Mortality Weekly Rep* 34(45): 682, 1985.
9. Castle M: Isolation: Precise procedures for better protection. *Nursing 75* 5: 51, 1975.
10. Maki DG: Double bagging of isolation items unnecessary—a comparative study of surface contamination. 25th Interscience Conference on Antimicrobial Agents and Chemotherapy, Abstract No. 935, Minneapolis, October 1985.
11. Steere AC, Mallison GF: Handwashing practices for the prevention of nosocomial infections. *Ann Intern Med* 83: 683, 1975.
12. Garner JS, Favero MS: Guideline for handwashing and hospital environmental control. Hospital Infections Program, Atlanta, Centers for Disease Control, 1985.
13. Ehrenkranz JN: Nosocomial infection: It's in your hands. *Infect in Surg* June: 421, 1985.
14. Barry MA, Craven DE, Goularte TA: *Serratia marcescens* contamination of antiseptic soap containing triclosan: Implications for nosocomial infection. *Infect Control* 5(9): 427, 1984.
15. Nauseef WM, Maki DG: A study of simple protective isolation in patients with granulocytopenia. *N Engl J Med* 304(8): 448, 1981.

16. Bodey GP: Isolation for the compromised patient. *JAMA* 233(6) : 543, 1975.
17. West KH: Physicians should wash their hands more often. *J Operating Room Research Institute* January : 26, 1983.
18. Albert RK, Condie F: Hand-washing patterns in medical intensive-care units. *N Engl J Med* 304(24) : 1465, 1981.
19. Larson E, Killien M: Factors influencing handwashing behavior of patient care personnel. *Am J Infect Control* 10(3) : 93, 1982.
20. Hyams PJ, Ehrenkrahtz NJ: The overuse of single patient isolation in hospitals. *Am J Epidemiol* 106(4) : 325, 1977.

# 19

# High Risk Areas and Equipment in the Hospital

There are a number of areas and procedures in the hospital that present special or additional infection control risks to the patients themselves, to other patients, or to personnel. These risks are discussed in more depth in this chapter. Infection Control Practitioners may spend most of their time dealing with these special areas or procedures because of the higher risks involved.

## INTENSIVE CARE UNITS AS HIGH-RISK AREAS

By definition, patients in intensive care units (ICUs) are more severely compromised than those on general nursing floors. In addition to the severity of illness that requires more frequent close nursing care, these patients may have therapies that include drugs or equipment that further increase their susceptibility to infection (1). And last, when a patient has an infection in an ICU or becomes colonized with a virulent or resistant microorganism, the open structure of the ICU allows transmission to occur more readily; therefore, the most compromised hosts are in a setting that, although it allows them to be monitored safely, actually adds to their risk of infection by virtue of its open structure and the nature of the other patients in the same unit. Nursing and other personnel caring for these patients must be aware of the infection risks associated with intensive care.

### Infection Control in General Medical–Surgical Intensive Care

The control of infections in general medical–surgical ICUs involves measures discussed previously with respect to the care of IVs, respiratory therapy equipment, and urinary catheters (2). Patients with infections should be isolated, according to hospital policy; patients with gram-negative rod pneumonia may also need isolation, depending on the structure of the unit, the ability to separate patients physically, and the degree of susceptibility of other patients in the unit. When transmission of infection is contact and not airborne, an isolation area in the ICU can be defined by the use of cubicle curtains and whatever barrier precautions interrupt transmission. When the infection is spread by airborne transmission, the patient should be transferred out of the ICU and placed in a single room with appropriate intensive care nursing and barrier precautions. Strict attention to general nursing policies and procedures with respect to handwashing and patient care is essential in any critical care unit.

The physical structure of the unit is important, if only because some geographic separation helps to minimize transmission. It is easy to move from one patient to another without washing hands, and the contact route of transmission is most significant in this setting. A cubicle with windows for good visibility, each with handwashing facilities, is a reminder that even in a centralized location, each patient should be considered as isolated and precautions should be taken between each patient contact.

The ventilation should be positive-pressure with respect to the hall. There should be isolation cubicles that can be closed off completely from the rest of the unit. Ideally, the ventilation of an isolation cubicle (for protection or for isolation of infection) should be separate from the ventilation of the rest of the unit.

Other general measures for ICUs include the judicious use of antibiotics, identification of those patients at high risk for sepsis and mortality, and appropriate, meticulous care of invasive devices (3). Reduction in the number of possible sources of infection in the environment, limiting the number of visitors and helping them carry out appropriate isolation procedures as needed, and improvement, through medical and nursing intervention, in the host defenses are other general measures.


## Infection Control in the Nursery

Newborn and premature infants are at high risk of infection, especially if critically ill, because of their immature defense systems. Newborns become colonized after birth with the mother's normal flora, but they can also pick up microorganisms endemic in a nursery, passed from baby to baby via the hands of personnel. Newborns become colonized with *Staphylococcus aureus* at a variable rate from less than 10% to greater than 75%. Of these, a small number will become infected. Busy neonatal wards, high census with overcrowding of babies, and subsequent understaffing contribute to the spread of these organisms from one baby to another (4). Another organism of concern in the nursery is Group B *Streptococcus* (5), which colonizes 3–26% of new-borns (6). The two clinical syndromes of Group B disease are early onset and late onset. Colonization at the time of labor and delivery can lead to early onset disease within the first few days of life; this syndrome is characterized by fulminating septicemia and respiratory insufficiency, with a mortality rate as high as 50%. Late-onset disease may follow nosocomial acquisition of the organism. This syndrome involves the central nervous system and shows a lower mortality (15–20%), but it is associated with neurologic sequelae in newborns who have meningitis.

Other organisms of concern in the nursery are enteropathogenic *Escherichia coli, Streptococcus pneumoniae* (7), viruses, and other gram-negative bacilli. Organisms acquired from the mother can be transmitted to other babies in the open nursery setting; the prevention of transmission of potentially life-threatening pathogens is complex and presents a challenge to the ICC and the ICP.

The physical design of the nursery should be given the same considerations as the general adult intensive care area: easy accessibility, handwashing facilities, and geographic separation (30 ft$^2$ per bassinet is suggested) (4), with isolation facilities available. The location of the nursery in the hospital should be chosen carefully: it should be near the obstetric ward and delivery suite to minimize the number of contacts with people in transit; it should be away from laundry chutes, trash collection areas, or dirty utility areas; and it should be far from areas where patients with communicable diseases are housed (8).

### *General Precautions in the Nursery*

Handwashing is especially important in preventing or minimizing the transmission of organisms from baby to baby. The use of an antiseptic for handwashing is generally recommended because of its residual bacterial activity. Single-use equipment and the use of supplies for one baby only will minimize transmission by inanimate objects; using a clean towel to cover the scales, for example, minimizes the chance of transmission of infection when babies are weighed. Outbreaks of infection have been traced to inanimate objects such as blood pressure cuffs, indicating the potential for transmission by common equipment (9).

Personnel should wear special clothing in the unit. Scrub outfits should be donned when personnel begin the workday; people from outside the unit should wear clean gowns. Personnel who have direct contact with babies should wear bibs that can be discarded after contact with each baby. When leaving the unit during the day, personnel should wear protective gowns. The ICP can help by stressing the reasons for the special clothing: first, since personnel don and wear clean scrub suits in the unit, and these suits have not been worn anywhere else, wearing protective gowns while outside the unit preserves this "unit-only" outfit. Second, direct contact with each baby requires a clean surface; therefore, a new bib is worn for each baby for feeding, holding, or other contact with the uniform.

Ideally, cohorting of all infants and personnel in a nursery should minimize transmission of infections. With this method, all babies born within a 48-hour period, for example, are housed together and share nursing personnel. Babies born earlier and later are in their own cohorts, with their own nurses. Contact is limited to members of one group, and members of one cohort only are exposed to infections, with little possibility of secondary cases of infections; that is, the index case would expose and possibly infect only those in the cohort, and those infected would not, in turn, have the opportunity to infect others. This method of isolation is frequently not feasible, but any efforts toward cohorting of patients or personnel help to minimize transmission.

Isolation of newborns with suspected infections is mandatory in a nursery because of the difficulty in diagnosing certain infections and the speed with which infections can spread in this setting. Any infant with signs or symptoms of infection should be promptly isolated. In the event that two or more cases of seemingly related infection occur, control measures and an investigation must begin immediately. Often, the measures that are adopted are 24-hour rooming-in (the baby stays in the mother's room) or discharge. There should be some mechanism, however, for detecting cases of infection that may occur after discharge, so that these infants can be adequately treated (8).

In cases of maternal herpesvirus infections, isolation precautions must be taken, because of the risk to her infant as well as to the other infants in the nursery. Neonatal herpes (Type 2) infection is generally acquired during birthing from mothers who have genital lesions; a cesarean section may be recommended if the mother is known to be infected and her membranes have not ruptured. Herpes (Type 1) infection may be acquired by the infant by direct contact with the person who has an oral lesion, whether the mother or nursery personnel. Isolation procedures, involving both the mother and the baby, follow (10).

1. Babies born to mothers with genital herpes infections are considered at risk if they are delivered vaginally or if rupture of membranes occurs 4–6 hours prior to delivery, and should be isolated from other babies.

2. Babies born to mothers with oral herpes infections are not considered at risk until they have been to the mother's room or have had contact with her after delivery.

3. Isolation for mothers with genital herpes infections include:

   a. Private room

   b. Gowning, gloving, and double-bagging of linen and dressings

   c. Baby may be with mother for feeding; mother must use good hand-washing techniques and wear a clean gown

4. Isolation of mothers with oral herpes infections include:

   a. Private room if severe

   b. Gowning, gloving, and double-bagging of linen and dressings

   c. Baby may be with mother when lesions have crusted or if lesions are covered or mother is instructed in transmission

5. Isolation of babies exposed to herpes or with active infection:

   a. Private cubicle or room

   b. Gowning, gloving, and double-bagging of linen and dressings

   c. Baby may be with mother; mother uses precautions as outlined above

Babies of mothers with genital herpes infections should be considered exposed during vaginal delivery. They should be isolated from other babies but not from the mother, although precautions should be taken for the mother as outlined above.

The isolation of babies from mothers with oral lesions, and the removal of employees from nurseries when they have oral herpes lesions, are controversial measures that are not carried out consistently. One report showed a wide discrepancy in policies with respect to these two issues in various institutions, and called for more research in order to show the nosocomial risk more clearly (10).

Prenatal and perinatal transmission of HIV virus can occur (11), and these infants require isolation for blood and body fluids from birth. Most infants born to mothers with hepatitis B are exposed at birth rather than in utero. Isolation in the nursery is not required because they do not become $HB_SAg$-positive for 3 months. They should receive passive–active immunization with hepatitis B immune globulin (HBIG) and hepatitis B vaccine (12).

Other general precautions are based on isolation techniques for specific infections; information on such precautions is available elsewhere (13).

### *Role of the Infection Control Practitioner in Infection Control in the Nursery*

The ICP should monitor the nursery as a special area because it is unique in that the patients leave the unit and have the potential of bringing in and taking out disease-producing microorganisms. The ICP should be aware of the special circumstances and potential problems in this area and be prepared to intervene if an outbreak is suspected. The hospital should have a policy for the authority and responsibility for control measures, from culturing through closing the unit, for this and other ICUs.

The ICP also has a role in educating nursing and medical personnel about the control of infections. Frequently medical and nursing programs address the individual care of the neonate, ignoring the epidemiology of nursery infections and their control. The ICP can encourage a high level of awareness of infection risks in this setting, so that problems will be prevented or detected and controlled early.

## Infection Control in the Burn Unit

Another ICU of concern in infection control practice is the burn unit. A burned patient is highly susceptible to infection, since many of the normal host defenses such as the skin, mucous membranes, normal bacterial flora, and granulocyte activity (14) have been disrupted.

During the first 24 hours, the burn wound is sterile or may have some superficial colonization. Two to three days after the burn the wound becomes colonized with gram-positive organisms, mainly staphylococci. Four to five days after the burn, the wound is colonized with gram-negative organisms, usually from the patient's bowel. It is thought that infections that complicate burn therapy are caused by the patient's own normal flora (15). At any time during the hospitalization the burn patient can become colonized with organisms from other patients, personnel, or the environment.

Prevention or control of infections is based on the promotion of host defenses, including the judicious use of antibiotics, the reduction of reservoirs of infectious organisms in the environment, and the prevention of cross-transmission. The value of burn units has been questioned because of the increased infection risks among burn patients housed together and selective antibiotic pressures resulting in resistant organisms (16) and because of studies suggesting that special burn unit facilities may not improve burn outcome (17). The design of the burn unit should involve the same considerations as other ICUs: physical separation if possible, with good accessibility and visibility; isolation; and handwashing facilities.

Protective isolation for burn patients remains a controversial issue; the use of a completely isolated environment, the Bacteria Controlled Nursing Unit (BCNU), showed good results in terms of lowered infection rates when compared to single-room isolation and isolation techniques on an open burn ward (18). The patient's bed is surrounded by a plastic curtain, and all personnel and equipment function outside the unit. Sleeves built into the curtain enable workers to handle the patient, and bacteria-free air continuously flows into the unit.

Many institutions do not have the funds or personnel to construct bacteria-free isolation islands of this kind; furthermore, the data are not conclusive about the overall patient morbidity and mortality rates in these burn units compared with open units, and with burn patients cared for in nonburn unit areas. In units without benefit of this special apparatus, general precautions are needed. Burn units, as do other intensive care areas, provide many possible reservoirs of organisms, in equipment and people, both patients and personnel. Methods to reduce the number of reservoirs of infectious organisms include the following:

1. Isolate infected patients in separate rooms. Patients with pneumonia, UTIs, or burn wound sepsis should be physically separate from other patients. Air is probably not significant except possibly in ICUs, where patients may be 3 ft or less apart. Ideally, separation of infected patients, with cohorting of personnel, should minimize possible transmission of organisms to noninfected patients. Strict adherence to gowning and gloving techniques as well as handwashing are most important.

2. Adhere to strict Foley catheter care. The CDC has suggested that patients with Foley catheters should not be housed in the same room with each other. The Foley catheter bag, especially in patients with UTIs, can be a reservoir for organisms, particularly gram-negatives, that can be transmitted to other patients. Measures to prevent infection, including Foley catheter care, removing the catheter as soon as possible, and good handwashing after handling the catheter and emptying the bag will minimize the Foley catheter as a potential reservoir for infecting organisms.

3. Exclude infected personnel or visitors from contact with burned patients. The hospital should have a policy stating this and a means of enforcing it through education of nursing personnel in screening themselves and visitors to the unit. Nursing personnel with active infections should stay at home or should care for other patients until they (the nurses) are well, and visitors should stay away if they are ill or should protect the patient by wearing appropriate isolation clothing, if the visit is necessary for other medical and nursing reasons.

4. Ensure that there is regular, effective disinfection of floors, furniture, and sinks. Housekeeping plays a part in helping to remove reservoirs in the unit, through general cleaning of the environment. The use of a regular cleaning agent, such as a quaternary ammonium chloride, with good mechanical cleaning of floors and adequate terminal disinfection of beds between each patient use and the next are important housekeeping techniques.

5. Eliminate open or opened containers of water or saline. Since *Pseudomonas* organisms are frequently found in tap water, open containers, including flower vases, drinking water, and cups for rinsing suction

tubing, should be removed from the burn unit or burn patient's bedside. Sterile solutions for irrigation, soaking dressings, or respiratory therapy equipment should be labeled and discarded after 24 hours. Saline or medication reservoirs in respiratory therapy equipment should be rinsed before being refilled, and this equipment should be changed at 24–48-hour intervals.

6. Minimize the use of multiple-use vials that might become contaminated and serve as a common source of infection for several patients.

7. Make sure that there is prompt and effective disinfection of soiled equipment and instruments. Instruments and equipment left soaking can be a source of infecting organisms if they are not handled properly. Instruments should be bagged and sent to central supply for processing. If processed in the unit, they should be washed immediately to mechanically remove blood, tissue, or other material; the instruments should then be sent for sterilization. Equipment that is disinfected must be thoroughly cleaned first, since most disinfectants are inactivated or overwhelmed by the presence of protein such as blood, pus, or tissue.

8. Specify the use of sterile instruments only and clean, packaged, and freshly laundered linen.

9. Make sure disposal of trash and linen is prompt and appropriate. Because of the high number of gram-negative microorganisms colonizing the burn wound, and the likelihood that much of the linen will be moist, linen from burn patients or burn units should be double-bagged and marked "isolation"; trash should be handled the same way, especially soiled dressings. Again, prompt removal of this material by housekeeping personnel is important.

10. Hands must be washed before and after each patient contact. Before invasive procedures or direct contact with the burn wound, during which sterile gloves are worn, scrubbing with an antiseptic soap solution is recommended. It is important to remember, however, that personnel with dermatitis or adverse reactions to soap solutions may be reluctant to wash and may harbor huge numbers of organisms on their hands. Therefore, the use of a mild soap and good technique may be far more important and successful in minimizing transmission than the use of a strong and irritating antiseptic solution.

11. Gowns, gloves, and masks should be worn when caring for infected patients in isolation and for direct contact with the burn wound itself. These barriers will provide protection for this patient and for other patients against organisms carried by personnel from one patient to another.

12. Impervious gowns should be worn during wound care and hydrotherapy, since organisms can move through wet protective clothing and contaminate uniforms or scrub suits, providing a means of transmission to other patients.

13. Adhere to strict intravenous catheter care, including changing entire tubing and solutions every 24 hours, sterile technique during IV site dressing changes, and, when possible, rotating the IV site every 48–72 hours.

14. Use sterile techniques during wound care or invasive procedures.

15. Equipment must not be shared by patients, except for fixed equipment such as that used in hydrotherapy. This equipment must be cleaned and disinfected immediately after each use. The use of disposable plastic liners in hydrotherapy equipment eliminates the need for between-patient cleaning, except when there are breaks in the liner; plastic liners may be economical in larger burn units.

16. Transportation of the burn patient should be minimized. When transportation is necessary, the stretcher or wheelchair should be covered with clean sheets, and the patient should also be covered. Personnel in the department that receives the burn patient should treat this patient immediately, using appropriate isolation clothing; the stretcher or wheelchair should be wiped with a disinfectant, if soiled.

### *Role of the Infection Control Practitioner in Infection Control in the Burn Unit*

Prevention of cross-infection in burned patients begins with hospital policies and procedures that involve all areas and departments having contact with the patient. Personnel education should include preemployment orientation for infection control, with continuing formal and informal education. Inspection and evaluation of techniques are the responsibility of the ICP but are also carried out on a continuing basis by the head nurse and surgeon in charge of the burn unit. Surveillance of patient infections, with prompt detection and control of outbreaks of cross-infection, are successful preventive measures in minimizing the risk of cross-infection among burned patients.

## INFECTION CONTROL IN THE DIALYSIS UNIT

In addition to intensive care areas, there are other units and areas that present special infection risks to patients and personnel; the dialysis unit is a source of such risk. There is a risk of bacterial as well as viral infections among dialysis patients, who are usually immunosuppressed. In a survey conducted from 1967 to 1970 by the CDC, the incidence of hepatitis in dialysis units was 4.4% for patients and 3.4% for personnel; nearly 70% of the infected patients were anicteric, whereas 85% of the infected personnel were jaundiced (19). A survey conducted in 1974 showed attack rates of over 6% for patients and almost 6% for staff (20). Because of the documented risk associated with this area and procedure, the ICP should be aware of the recommended infection control practices to minimize risks of hepatitis. The HTLV-III virus causing AIDS is also transmitted by infected blood, and the same precautions should be followed (21).

Once introduced into a dialysis unit, hepatitis B, NANB, and HTLV-III virus can be spread from person to person through direct contact or through a variety of inanimate objects such as dialyzers, forceps, needles, and other patient care equipment and inanimate surfaces (22). Infection control measures are based on limiting the number of sources of virus and preventing transmission from a positive patient to a negative patient or employee.

Information about control measures is available from the CDC (23). All personnel and patients in a dialysis unit should be immunized against hepatitis B. The hepatitis B vaccine (HeptaVax) was licensed in November, 1981. Large studies demonstrated antibody response in 90% of persons vaccinated. Many institutions have initiated vaccine programs without follow-up for antibody production based on results of these studies. Follow-up by the manufacturer shows antibody response of 88% when injections were given in the arm and only 73% response rate for buttock injections (24). Guidelines for administration of the HeptaVax are outlined by the ACIP (25). All vaccine recipients should have a hepatitis B virus antibody (anti-HBV) titer to determine antibody response to vaccine. Those who show no response to vaccine should be revaccinated and checked again for antibody response.

Patients who have demonstrated immunization to hepatitis B should still be routinely monitored with serum glutamic oxaloacetic transaminase (SGOT) and serum glutamic pyruvic transaminase (SGPT) for exposure to NANB hepatitis. Nonresponders, patients, and personnel who refused vaccine should continue a routine surveillance testing schedule as shown in Figure 19-1.

The CDC further recommends infection control practices that include the geographic separation of $HB_sAg$-positive patients and the selected assignment of $HB_sAg$-positive or anti-$HB_s$-positive personnel to care for them. Personnel with the best technique or the most experience can also be preferentially assigned to these patients; a change of gloves, lab coat, or gown and handwashing are necessary if both $HB_sAg$-positive and $HB_s$-negative patients are cared for by the same person.

Other recommendations include personnel practices such as wearing protective clothing, handwashing, eating, smoking, and drinking policies, and the

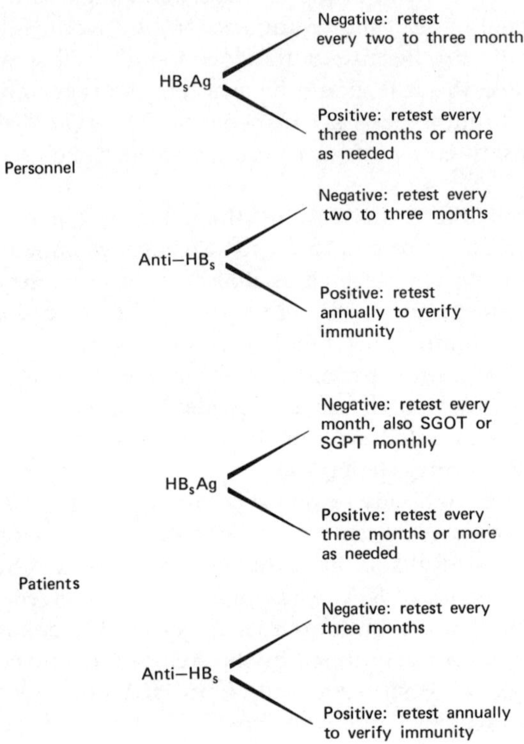



*Figure 19-1*

*A suggested schedule for testing personnel and patients for HB$_s$Ag, anti-HBs, and SGOT/SGPT, as recommended by the CDC.*

handling of equipment and patients in the unit. The ICP in a hospital with a dialysis unit must be familiar with these recommendations and must monitor test results and personnel practices and give in-service instruction to personnel on a regular basis.

## INFECTION CONTROL IN THE LABORATORY

Special attention should be given to other areas of the hospital where the infection risk to patients or personnel is high. Laboratory personnel, microbiologists in particular, are at risk of acquiring a variety of diseases because of the infectious agents they handle. Laboratory workers who are involved in blood collection and laboratory testing of blood specimens are at greater risk of exposure to hepatitis viruses (B, NANB) and HIV that causes AIDS. Laboratory personnel should be vaccinated against hepatitis B and educated in good infection control when handling blood and body fluids (26). Other infections reported among laboratory personnel include tuberculosis, tularemia (27), and Rocky Mountain spotted fever (28). The majority of infections are probably transmitted by aerosol, although exposure and infection by accidental needlestick, spraying or spilling, and mouth pipetting have also been suggested (27).

The ICP may be involved in developing infection control policies and procedures for the laboratory (29). The ICP may teach personnel infection control practices regarding mouth pipetting; drinking, smoking, and eating; handwashing; protective clothing; surface decontamination; or other subjects and may also become involved in the workup of any laboratory-associated disease. Periodic skin tests for tuberculosis should be available to microbiology personnel.

## EQUIPMENT AS A SOURCE OF INFECTION

New types of equipment, especially those meant for use in intensive care, are being developed at a fast rate. Unfortunately, some of this highly sophisticated machinery presents problems in infection control practice because of its invasiveness and fragility, making it difficult to clean, disinfect, and/or sterilize. In recent years pressure-monitoring devices and endoscopy equipment have tremendously improved medical and nursing care and, at the same time, presented additional infection hazards for hospitalized patients.

Pressure-monitoring devices are used in a variety of clinical settings to monitor vascular, intracranial, and intrauterine pressures in patients; a review of the indications and infection problems is available elsewhere (30). Outbreaks of blood infections with bacteria, viruses, and fungi have been reported to be related to the use of these devices. Recommended precautions include: (1) the use of this equipment only when clinically indicated, (2) surveillance and monitoring of infections related to these devices, and (3) periodic evaluation of procedures and training of personnel in the handling and care of this equipment.

Also recommended in the same review (30) are the use of sterile, preassembled, and packaged systems that remain closed; the use of disposable components, especially domes; proper cleaning and sterilization according to the manufacturer's directions; replacement of the system every 48 hours, with adequate site care for the catheter insertion site; and the use of solutions that do not contain glucose for flushing the system. In a recent study, disposable pressure transducers were left in place for 96 hours (31).

The ICP should become familiar with each type of pressure monitor in use in the hospital; their techniques, handling, and storage. Additional attention has been given fiberoptic endoscopy equipment and its role in the transmission of infections. Fiberscopes are used to visualize a variety of body cavities, including joints, the gastrointestinal and respiratory tracts, and peritoneal cavity, thus eliminating the need for exploratory surgery.

Because of the complex design of this equipment, conventional methods for cleaning, disinfection, or sterilization are difficult. Guidelines for cleaning and disinfecting gastrointestinal endoscopic equipment have been published (32). The risk of transmission of hepatitis B via this equipment has not been shown, in spite of inadvertent exposure (33), but additional guidelines are available for minimizing this risk (34). Outbreaks of infections related to this equipment have thus far been associated with faulty cleaning procedures (35); contamination of the equipment with resulting false-positive cultures from subsequent patients have also been reported (36), again related to inadequate cleaning procedures.

The ICP should become familiar with this equipment, the level of disinfection required, and the manufacturers' recommendations for cleaning.

There are more high-risk areas and equipment being developed that will present infection control problems; some ICPs are becoming involved with manufacturers during the development of this equipment, before the problems arise in the clinical setting. The ICP should identify and monitor high-risk patients, areas, and equipment in the hospital, and intervene quickly to minimize infection risks to patients and personnel.


## REUSE OF DISPOSABLES


Many institutions, in an effort to reduce costs, are reprocessing and reusing patient care items and medical devices labeled by the manufacturer as single-use only. At present there are no guidelines for the safety of reprocessing these items or how many times a disposable item may be reprocessed and still be safe to use. The FDA Compliance Policy Guide, 1981 states that the institution or practitioner who resuses a disposable medical device should be able to demonstrate that (1) the device can be adequately cleaned and sterilized, (2) the process will not change the physical characteristics or quality of the device, and (3) the device will remain safe and effective for its intended use. Any institution or practitioner who resterilizes and/or reuses a disposable device must assume the responsibility for its safety and efficacy (37). The

CDC in its 1985 Guideline for Hospital Environmental Control endorses this policy and states if this cannot be accomplished or results in residual toxicity the device should not be reprocessed (38). In 1984 an International Conference on the Reuse of Disposable Medical Devices in the 1980s was held to discuss legal, ethical, and technical issues of reprocessing, resterilizing, and reusing disposable devices. The reasons for addressing reuse of disposables is to control or decrease the costs of medical care. The recommendations of the conference were to find out the scope of reuse of disposables through a national survey, assess the safety and cost-effectiveness of this practice, and recommend funded research on this issue (39).

The 1986 Infection Control Standards of the Joint Commission on Hospital Accreditation state that an institution shall have written guidelines for the selection, storage, handling, use and disposition of disposable items (40). Each ICP and ICC shall establish their own policy for disposable items based on the findings of the 1981 FDA *Compliance Policy Guide.*

## REFERENCES


1. Wenzel RP, Thompson RL, Landry SM, et al: Hospital-acquired infections in intensive care unit patients: An overview with emphasis on epidemics. *Infect Control* 4(5):371, 1983.

2. LaForce FM, Eickhoff TC: The role of infection in critical care. *Anesthesiology* 47:195, 1977.

3. Meakins JL: Infection control in the surgical intensive care unit. *Can J Surg* 21(2):78, 1978.

4. Haley RW, Bergman DA: The role of understaffing and overcrowding in recurrent outbreaks of staphylococcal infection in a neonatal special-care unit. *J Infect Dis* 145(6):875, 1982.

5. Baker CJ: Group B streptococcal infections: Is prevention possible? *South Med J* 69(12):1527, 1976.

6. Speck WT, Driscoll JM, Polin RA, et al: Natural history of a neonatal colonization with group B streptococci. *Pediatrics* 60:356, 1977.

7. Bortolussi R, Thompson TR, Ferrieri P: Early-onset pneumococcal sepsis in newborn infants. *Pediatrics* 60:352, 1977.

8. American Hospital Association: *Infection Control in the Hospital,* ed 4. Chicago, American Hospital Association, 1979, p 149.

9. Myers MG: Longitudinal evaluation of neonatal nosocomial infections: Association of infection with a blood pressure cuff. *Pediatrics* 61:42, 1978.

10. Kibrick S: Herpes simplex infections at term: What to do with mother, newborn and nursery personnel. *JAMA* 243(2):157, 1980.

11. Centers for Disease Control: Recommendations for assisting in the prevention of perinatal transmission of human T lymphotropic virus type III/lymphadenopathy-associated virus and acquired immuno-deficiency syndrome. *Morbidity and Mortality Weekly Rep* 34(48):721, 1985.

12. Stevens CE, Toy PM, Tong MJ, et al: Perinatal hepatitis B virus transmission in the United States. *JAMA* 253(12): 1740, 1985.

13. American Academy of Pediatrics: *Report of the Committee on Infectious Diseases,* ed 18. Evanston, IL, American Academy of Pediatrics, 1977.

14. Craig C: Infection control in the burn unit. *Infect Control Urol Care* 2(6): 3, 1977.

15. Moncrief JA: Topical antibacterial therapy of the burn wound. *Clin Plast Surg* 1(4): 563, 1974.

16. Vilain RC: Is the burn center a septic ghetto? *Plast Reconstr Surg* May 1977, p 733.

17. Linn BS, Stephenson SE, Bergstresser PR, et al: Are burn units the best places to treat burn patients? *J Surg Res* 23: 1, 1977.

18. Burke JF, Quinby WC, Bondoc CC, et al: The contribution of a bacterially isolated environment to the prevention of infection in seriously burned patients. *Ann Surg* 186(3): 377, 1977.

19. Garibaldi RA, Forrest JN, Bryan JA, et al: Hemodialysis-associated hepatitis. *JAMA* 225(4): 384, 1973.

20. Center for Disease Control: Hemodialysis-associated hepatitis in the United States, 1974. *J Infect Dis* 135(4): 687, 1977.

21. Favero M: Recommended precautions for patients undergoing hemodialysis who have AIDS or non-A, non-B hepatitis. *Infect Control* 6(8): 301, 1985.

22. Snydman DR, Bryan JA, Dixon RE: Prevention of nosocomial viral hepatitis, type B (hepatitis B). *Ann Intern Med* 83: 838, 1975.

23. Centers for Disease Control: Hepatitis-control measures for hepatitis B in dialysis centers. Viral Hepatitis Investigations and Control Series, Atlanta, November 1977.

24. Centers for Disease Control: Suboptimal response to hepatitis B vaccine given by injection into the buttocks. *Morbidity and Mortality Weekly Rep* 34(8): 105, 1985.

25. Centers for Disease Control: Recommendations for protection against viral hepatitis. *Ann Intern Med* 103(3): 391, 1985.

26. Centers for Disease Control: Recommendations for preventing transmission of infection with human T lymphotropic virus type III/lymphadenopathy-associated virus in the workplace. *Morbidity and Mortality Weekly Rep* 34(45): 681, 1985.

27. Pike RM: Past and present hazards of working with infectious agents. *Arch Pathol Lab Med* 102: 333, 1978.

28. Oster C, Burke DS, Kenyon RH, et al: Laboratory-acquired Rocky Mountain spotted fever. *N Engl J Med* 297: 859, 1977.

29. Centers for Disease Control: Prevention of laboratory-acquired infection. *National Nosocomial Infections Study Report* Annual Summary 1976, issued February 1978.

30. Simmons BP, Hooton TM, Wong EG, et al: Guidelines for prevention of infections related to intravascular pressure-monitoring systems, Atlanta, Centers for Disease Control, 1981.

31. Luskin RL, Weinstein RA, Nathan C, et al: Extended use of disposable pressure transducers. *JAMA* 255(7): 916, 1986.

32. Committee on Infection Control in the Handling of Endoscopic Equipment: Cleaning and disinfection of flexible fiberoptic endoscopes (FEE) used in gastrointestinal endoscopy. *Assoc Pract Infect Control J* 6(4): 8, 1978.

33. Moncada RE, Denes AE, Berquist KR, et al: Inadvertent exposure of endoscopy patients to viral hepatitis B. *Gastrointest Endosc* 24(5): 231, 1978.
34. Bond WW, Moncada RE: Viral hepatitis B infection risk in flexible fiberoptic endoscopy. *Gastrointest Endosc* 24(5): 225, 1978.
35. Beecham HJ, Cohen ML, Parkin WE: *Salmonella typhimurium:* transmission by fiberoptic upper gastrointestinal endoscopy. *JAMA* 241: 1013, 1979.
36. Kellerhals S: A pseudo-outbreak of *Serratia marcescens* from a contaminated fiber-bronchoscope. *Assoc Pract Infect Control J* 6(4): 5, 1978.
37. Food and Drug Administration: Reuse of medical disposable devices. Compliance Policy Guide 7124.16, 1981.
38. Garner JS, Favero MS: Guidelines for handwashing and hospital environmental control. Hospital Infections Program, Atlanta, Centers for Disease Control, 1985.
39. Reuse of Disposable Medical Devices in the 1980s. Washington, DC, The Institute for Health Policy Analysis of the Georgetown University Medical Center, 1984.
40. Infection Control. *Manual on Accreditation of Hospitals 1986,* Joint Commission on Accreditation of Hospitals, Chicago, 1985, p 76.

# 20

# Investigations of Epidemics

Infection control programs are designed in part to detect and quickly control outbreaks of infections among patients or personnel. Surveillance is done to determine baseline endemic levels of infection, in different areas and services in the hospital, and for different sites and pathogens. Ongoing surveillance detects changes in the baseline rates or numbers, so that the ICP can recognize problems.

An outbreak, or epidemic, of nosocomial infections is defined as two or more people with the same infection, or infections with the same organism, generally from a common hospital source, which reflects an incidence clearly greater than the expected number of cases of that infection (1). In some instances an investigation will begin when one case occurs, if that infection is unusual, is nosocomial in origin, and the ICP would not expect to see any cases at all in the particular situation. Additionally, an investigation would be called for if the reported infection is easily transmitted; in other words, if the ICP suspects that more cases will quickly follow.

Outbreaks of disease have probably increased in frequency in hospitals during the past several years because, through improved medical technology, more severely immunocompromised patients are surviving; because medical equipment and devices have become more sophisticated but also more dangerous; and because more advanced drug and other types of treatment have altered host susceptibility. Also, the development of infection control programs has increased the awareness of the transmission of infections within hospitals.

Outbreaks of nosocomial disease can occur among healthy persons as well as among critically ill patients. Often, however, a situation occurs in which an opportunistic pathogen is allowed to colonize and infect, and is then transmitted among, compromised hosts. If undetected, the outbreak may end without intervention, because of small changes in nursing procedures, patient discharges, or other events that end the transmission or the ability of the organism to infect. The ICP and the ICC may, however, be able to intervene and prevent disease or even death associated with outbreaks; both should be prepared for this possibility.

# AUTHORITY AND RESPONSIBILITY FOR INVESTIGATION OF EPIDEMICS

The ICC must determine as one of its first priorities the authority and responsibility of those involved in an outbreak investigation. The ICC under most circumstances cannot convene at the time an outbreak is recognized. Therefore, it is most important to determine, before problems arise, the appropriate person or people involved in an outbreak investigation, the steps needed to close a unit or area of the hospital, and how decisions will be made.

In most hospitals, the two key people involved in outbreak investigations are the ICP and the chairperson of the ICC. Others in the investigation include the surgery representative to the ICC in the event of a surgery-related outbreak, or the member representing the affected service or area, and the infectious disease service representative, if the hospital provides that service.

Key decisions, such as closing a unit, must be made by the principal investigators and the nursing service, administration, and medical board. The authority to institute control measures, including closing wards or areas of the hospital, in the event of an outbreak, must be very clear in the institution's policies. Only then can those with clinical knowledge and epidemiologic expertise investigate the problem and institute appropriate controls to interrupt the outbreak and thereby decrease morbidity or mortality.

The primary goal of an outbreak investigation is the prompt control of the spread of disease. Time is the key factor in determining the success of an investigation in terms of decreasing or preventing morbidity and mortality. The methodology and specific activities that will ensure the most efficient use of time in effective investigation and control of a hospital outbreak are discussed below.

# METHODOLOGY

## Recognition of a Possible Epidemic

There are several ways that an outbreak may be brought to the attention to infection control personnel. Microbiology personnel may detect an increase in a certain isolate or a cluster of isolates from an area of the hospital. A physician or other hospital worker mày send several cultures to the laboratory because of a suspected problem. The infectious disease service (if the hospital has one) may receive consultation requests that indicate a cluster of infections. The ICP may recognize a problem through routine surveillance of the hospital for nosocomial infections.

## Preliminary Activities and Investigations

Generally, the ICP is called when there is suspicion of an outbreak and must gather some preliminary data and discuss the situation with some key people before beginning a full investigation. Included in these preliminary discussions are the committee chairperson, the microbiology laboratory director, the ICP, and a member of the infectious disease service, if there is one in the hospital.

Once the appropriate people have discussed the possibility of an outbreak, a preliminary investigation should be started by the ICP to confirm the presence of a problem and to organize and initiate the investigation. First, there must be agreement among those involved as to the person responsible for the investigation. At first, this is the ICP, who will gather the necessary data to determine the presence of a problem. Then, however, a principal investigator should be named as the person to coordinate activities and to receive and disseminate pertinent information. This person need not be the sole decision maker concerning the outbreak during investigation and control, but rather serves as a coordinator of activities and is the central person to whom and from whom information and decisions can be communicated. Often, this person is the ICP, since the ICP is responsible for infection control activities and is free to transcend departmental and physical barriers to investigate the institution as a whole if necessary.

Next, it must be determined whether an outbreak is present. This involves a decision as to whether a true outbreak exists or whether the apparent outbreak is the result of a change in the name of an organism, new microbiology personnel or procedures, or a change in surveillance or reporting methods that might falsely indicate a cluster of cases. Assuming no such artifacts, determination of the existence of an outbreak (and preliminary evaluation if there is) is carried out using the following procedure, which many epidemiologists refer to as a "quick-and- dirty" (preliminary and not detailed) investigation (1).

1.  Develop a working definition of a case. Most often, such a definition is derived from a combination of clinical and laboratory data. An example of a case in a specific situation fulfilled the following time-place-person criteria.

The patient involved

- was an inpatient in the surgical ICU from June 1 to June 14
- developed at least two of the following:
- temperature higher than 38.5 °C
- purulent sputum
- new infiltrate that was apparent in x-ray films
- had a sputum or blood culture positive for *A. calcoaceticus*

The case definition must include all possibilities in the determination of cases in an epidemic. In other words, it must be sensitive, so that all cases that seem to be related will be included. It must also, however, be specific, so that cases that are actually unrelated will not be included.

2. Conduct preliminary casefinding. Data should be collected on all those who fit the time-place-person criteria defining the case. The data collected should be demographic and should depend, in part, on the epidemiology of the disease involved in the outbreak. To continue the example used for the case definition, some of the data collected on cases should include the following:

- demographic (age, race, sex, identifying number)
- use of respiratory therapy equipment
- length of time in the unit before infection appeared
- surgical procedure
- anesthesia
- underlying diseases
- antibiotic therapy before disease

The preliminary information can be gathered by chart review, patient examination, review of laboratory records, discussions with nursing personnel, and so on.

3. Evaluate previous hospital experience. There must be documentation that the problem observed is new; therefore, information on past experience should be gathered. A review of the past year's experience with an organism can best be accomplished through a review of laboratory results. If the outbreak is related to a type of infection (rather than a specific organism), past nosocomial surveillance reports and baseline infection rates should be assembled for comparison with the current problem.

4. Prepare a line listing of cases. The information collected on the cases in the presumed outbreak should be presented in the form of a chart or line listing, as shown in Figure 20-1, for rapid analysis of variables associated with the disease.

LINE LIST FORMAT

| Name | Ward | ID # | Date of Admission | Date of Onset | Service | Site | Culture/ Antibiogram | Comments |
|---|---|---|---|---|---|---|---|---|
|  |  |  |  |  |  |  |  |  |
|  |  |  |  |  |  |  |  |  |
|  |  |  |  |  |  |  |  |  |
|  |  |  |  |  |  |  |  |  |
|  |  |  |  |  |  |  |  |  |
|  |  |  |  |  |  |  |  |  |

**Figure 20-1**
*A sample line listing for recording data during a possible outbreak.*

5. Draw an epidemic curve (Fig. 20-2). The cases can be plotted by date of onset to give more information to the investigator. It is helpful to include information from the review of past experience with the organism or the infection; it is also helpful to plot both the suspected cases and similar infections (presumably not related to the current outbreak) for comparison purposes. In addition to a time curve, it may be useful to plot geographic location by using a map and plotting cases by dates. This may help the investigator to scan the time, person, and place of the outbreak quickly.

6. Compute attack rates. In order to compare past experience with the present problem, rates, rather than numbers, must be used. An increase in the number of isolates of a certain organism may be the result of an increase in the number of patients in a certain area. For example, during the previous month, if there were four patients with a certain infection in a unit of 10 beds, then eight patients with the same infection may not reflect an outbreak if an additional 10 beds had been opened: 4 of 10 compared to 8 of 20. Attack rates are calculated as the number of cases divided by the number of patients at risk.

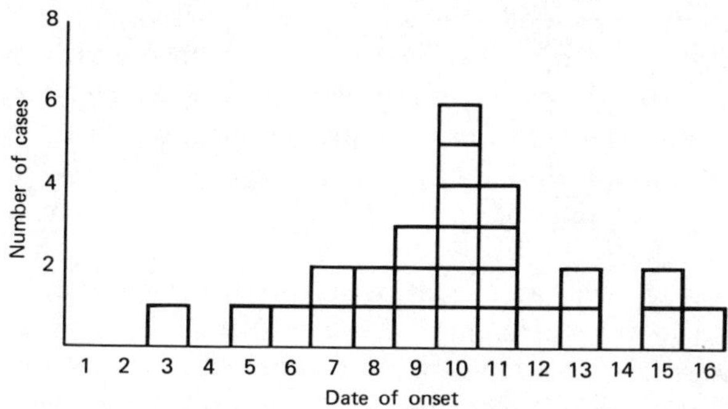

*Figure 20-2*
*A sample epidemic curve of cases over time.*

7. Compare "epidemic" to endemic occurrence of cases. Epidemic attack rates can now be compared to endemic, or usual, attack rates to verify that an outbreak is likely.

These steps may seem to be time-consuming and tedious. They are all necessary, however, in order to avoid a "wild goose chase" for a problem that may not exist. If at this point a comparison of attack rates shows that an outbreak is highly unlikely, active investigations can end until further information indicates otherwise. If the ICP feels that "something is going on," an investigation is warranted, but following these steps will in most cases rule out outbreaks that are simply the result of changes in nomenclature, personnel, procedures, reporting, or physical operation of the institution.

The next step is to develop a presumptive hypothesis. The results of the "quick-and-dirty" investigation may warrant further probing. At the time it is decided that an outbreak may exist, a presumptive hypothesis about the likely reservoir, source, and mode of transmission should be formed, based on the preliminary data collected. The ICP then investigates in an attempt to prove (or disprove) the hypothesis. In the example previously used, the hypothesis may be that respiratory therapy equipment is being contaminated with *Acinetobacter,* since the organism survives well in standing solutions, and that this contamination has resulted in an outbreak of nosocomial pneumonia after respiratory assistance was given using this equipment. An outbreak of postoperative nosocomial infections apparently caused by the same staphylococcal or streptococcal organism could be hypothetically traced to a shedding carrier or to a person with a frank infection who is part of the operating room staff, rather than to an inanimate source.

The ICP should immediately begin reasonable control measures. At the same time that it is decided that an outbreak exists, certain control measures are indicated to stop the spread of disease. In the surgical ICU example, control measures might include isolation of cases, changing respiratory equipment at more frequent intervals, and cohorting staff so that personnel handling proven cases would not handle noncases and vice versa. Geographic isolation of ill babies and cohorting of babies and staff might be initiated in a nursery outbreak.

The microbiology laboratory will be deeply involved in any investigation of transmission in the hospital. It is essential that the person in charge of the microbiology laboratory have a clear understanding from the start of the nature of the outbreak and the role or possible role of the laboratory in the investigation. The director and the ICP must maintain close communication. The principal investigator should be informed immediately of all new isolates that might be outbreak-related, and all isolates must be saved if the outbreak is apparently due to one organism (as opposed to general breaks in technique, where multiple organisms might be involved, as for example, might accompany poor care of IV catheters and infusion sites).

The scope of the problem should be estimated by the principal investigator, so that the laboratory workers can estimate media and personnel needs for environmental or people sampling or culturing, based on preliminary data concerning the number of patients and the type of organism(s) involved. Other decisions specifically related to the role of the laboratory include what kinds of cultures should be taken, by what methods, and by whom; who is to screen unauthorized cultures (presumably the principal investigator); the extent of identification and characterization of isolates, and whether antibiotic sensitivity testing will be done; and whether isolates should be referred to a reference laboratory.

Depending on the scope of the problem, a hospital outbreak may become a matter of common knowledge in the community. When questions from the community arise, particularly through public-information media, an information coordinator should be chosen (1). A representative from the office of the hospital administrator could best provide information to the community.

## Continuing Investigation

The preliminary investigation often is all that is necessary not only to indicate the presence of an outbreak but also to prove a hypothesized source and mode of transmission, as well as to make clear what should be done to control the outbreak. At this point further investigation may be unnecessary, and the principal investigator or other infection control person need only make sure that appropriate control measures are carried out and a final report prepared.

However, the cause of some outbreaks, or effective control measures, sometimes are not found so easily, and more detailed investigation is indicated. Hospital personnel may elect to seek outside help, from their local or state health department, or through them from the CDC.

More detailed data should be collected on cases of disease. New and more complete line listings of detailed characteristics, including possible predisposing factors and records of various procedures used in actual and possible cases, should be prepared, generally based on a thorough review of patient charts. Common factors should be sought in cases, based on the epidemiology of the organism or the disease and one or more presumptive hypotheses of causation, in an attempt to determine a common source and/or break in technique. Often, the study of an uninfected temporal control group (similar patients who did not develop disease) or careful comparisons of matched cases and controls may be necessary to elucidate causation (2). Evaluations of statistical significance of comparisons between cases and controls often are necessary. Cultures taken of the environment or personnel, when appropriate, also may be necessary to confirm or reject an hypothesized cause of an outbreak.

Based on the tabulation and analysis of the data, new measures may be developed and instituted to control the epidemic and to prevent future cases. Continued surveillance is necessary to assure that control measures are being followed.

## Conclusion of the Investigation and Follow-up

Concluding an epidemic investigation and appropriate follow-up are necessary to ensure that more cases are not developing or that there is a return to a baseline rate and also so that the experience and knowledge gained can be used to minimize future problems. New data should continue to be gathered by the principal investigator until it is decided that no new cases are occurring or that the rate has returned to the previously established endemic rate.

All personnel involved must be made aware of the end of the investigation and its results. Sometimes the precise cause of an outbreak is not determined; nevertheless, a written report should be prepared and sent to appropriate heads of departments and wards, formally confirming the findings (or lack of findings) and recommendations. The ICC, during its regular meeting, should review all events and the final report.

It should be decided either to store the isolates already on hand or to discard them, and all concerned should be informed when new cultures are no longer necessary. The development of a laboratory protocol for outbreaks may be a simple way of alerting laboratory personnel as well as other hospital personnel of the steps in outbreak investigation. This protocol should be available to all

*I. Recognition of the Problem*
  A. Laboratory personnel notice an increase in a certain organism and bring it to attention of the ICP or the Infectious Disease Fellow.
  B. Personnel bring in cultures because of suspected problem.
    1. Laboratory personnel call the ICP.
    2. Laboratory personnel call the Infectious Disease Fellow or the resident on duty.
    3. Laboratory personnel accept and process cultures unless notified otherwise by the ICP (nights and weekends, by the Infectious Disease Fellow).

*II. Definition of the Scope of the Problem*
  A. The size of the problem is estimated, based on the information available.
    1. It is decided which type of culture—personnel, patient, or environmental—should be taken.
    2. The number of cultures to be taken is estimated.
  B. Laboratory personnel determine anticipated media needs.

*III. Initiation of the Investigation*
  A. The person in charge of the investigation is named by the ICP and the chairperson of the ICC.
  B. Culturing methods are determined, based on type of culture and organism sought.
    1. Persons authorized to take cultures are named.
    2. Laboratory personnel should not be asked to take cultures from staff, equipment, or patients.
  C. Extent of identification or organisms is determined.
    1. Nonsterile sites—suspected pathogen is sought; no organisms reported unless other known pathogen (i.e., *Salmonella* sought, *Shigella* seen and reported).
    2. Sterile sites– all organisms are reported.
  D. Decision is made concerning sensitivity testing.
    1. The need for sensitivity tests is determined.
    2. Method of sensitivity testing is decided.
    3. Which cultures and how many will be tested is decided.
  E. Laboratory personnel determine who in the laboratory is responsible for culture processing.

*IV. The Investigation*
  A. List of cultures taken from patients or personnel is given to the laboratory by the ICP or the Infectious Disease Fellow.
  B. If unauthorized cultures are submitted to the laboratory, inform the ICP, the person in charge of the investigation, or the designated substitute (weekends, nights).
  C. All significant isolates are kept on appropriate media and frozen.
  D. Laboratory personnel save all laboratory slips for the ICP, for investigation and billing purposes.

*IV. Conclusion*
  A. The ICP or person in charge of investigation will notify the laboratory of end of the investigation.
    1. Laboratory will stop stocking extra media.
    2. Laboratory will no longer notify ICP of new cultures.
  B. ICP will determine what is to be done with saved isolates.
  C. Final report of investigation and results will be given to the laboratory.

---

**Figure 20-3**

*A protocol for outbreak investigations can also be useful when problems arise on weekends or holidays.*

personnel and will be useful during weekends and nights should a problem come up, since the laboratory is often the first area hit by the confusion of an outbreak. An example of a protocol is shown in Figure 20-3.

In order to prevent future problems, administrative, nursing, and medical policies and procedures may need reevaluation and alteration. The ICP and the ICC should address these issues after the emergency measures have ended the outbreak.

An outbreak of nosocomial infections can arouse fear among patients, personnel, and the community. The concluding activities are critical, not only to wrap up the situation from the investigators' standpoint, but also to bring about education and changes in behavior whenever possible to prevent further problems and better prepare personnel against the panic that can occur during an epidemic. Changes can be in the form of major alterations in techniques or simply an increased awareness and therefore early detection of new problems in infection control. It is the responsibility of the ICC to disseminate conclusions of outbreak investigations as well as to follow up the changes instituted as a result of the epidemic.

# REFERENCES

1. Castle M, Mallison GF: Effective investigations of nosocomial outbreaks. *Assoc Pract Infect Control J* 5(2): 13, 1977.
2. Friedman GD: *Primer on Epidemiology.* New York, McGraw-Hill, 1974.

Portions of this chapter were adapted from the article listed as reference 1 at the end of this chapter.

# 21

# Cleaning, Disinfection, and Sterilization

Cleaning, disinfection, and sterilization are activities in which ICPs are frequently involved, from the selection of products to the development of specific procedures. Often, ICPs have little formal background or training in the concepts of cleaning, disinfection, and sterilization; yet they are viewed as experts in the use of antiseptics and disinfectants in a health care facility.

## Definitions of Useful Terminology

Some general definitions may be useful as an introduction. *Cleaning* is the physical removal of visible dirt and debris. *Sanitization* renders an item clean, generally by the use of a chemical agent. *Decontamination* refers specifically to the removal of potentially pathogenic microorganisms, using a process that renders the item safe for handling, usually before further treatment of the item is done.

*Disinfection* is defined as the reduction in the numbers of disease-producing microorganisms, or potential pathogens, by physical or chemical means. This process generally does not include the destruction or removal of spores. There are different levels of disinfection, both because of the different "potential pathogens" on pieces of equipment and the body sites the equipment contacts.

*Sterilization* can be defined as the complete destruction of all microorganisms, leaving no viable microbial forms, including spores. In reality, this is most difficult to achieve, and a more practical definition is that the possibility of any microorganisms surviving the process is remote, and that those subsequently found on the item will be nonpathogenic.

In general, the level of disinfection selected will depend on three factors:

1. The type and amount of contamination suspected.

EXAMPLE. The countertops in a hemodialysis unit laboratory area may be disinfected with an agent thought to be effective against hepatitis viruses. By contrast, the countertop in the nursing station of a general medical floor may be cleaned with a general housekeeping agent, such as a quaternary ammonium chloride. It is likely that a hemodialysis unit will have blood spills in the laboratory area that may be contaminated with the hepatitis virus. Therefore, the use of a strong agent to remove or kill these organisms is warranted. By contrast, a nursing station is an unlikely place for heavy contamination with the hepatitis virus or any other pathogen, therefore the use of a general disinfecting agent is adequate.

2. The type and degree of contact the object has with the potential host.

EXAMPLE. Instruments that enter a sterile system, such as the bloodstream, should be rendered sterile. Objects having contact with skin or mucous membranes, such as thermometers and respiratory therapy equipment, require a high level of disinfection.

3. Susceptibility of the host who will have contact with the object.

EXAMPLE. For certain patients with combined immunodeficiency diseases and who are thus highly susceptible to infection, attempts are made to sterilize everything that enters the patients' closed environment.


## SOLUTIONS AND PROCEDURES FOR CLEANING, DISINFECTION, AND STERILIZATION

The ICP should understand some basic characteristics about the various solutions available for cleaning, disinfecting, and sterilizing the environment, both animate and inanimate. The most common of these solutions are discussed briefly below (1–3).


### Soap

Soap is made by combining animal or vegetable fats and a caustic agent such as lye. Its action is based on the splitting of molecules into electrically charged ions when dissolved in water. These particles then cause the formation of lather that emulsifies fats, lifting off dirt and other material from the area washed. Soap's action is mainly mechanical.

## Alcohol

Isopropyl alcohol in 70–90% concentrations will kill many vegetative gram-positive and gram-negative bacteria, including *Mycobacterium tuberculosis.* Isopropyl alcohol is more effective than ethyl alcohol in its ability to degerm the skin. With constant friction, the skin can be adequately prepped by this antiseptic, but the effect is transient. Alcohol evaporates quickly and leaves no residual effect. It is not sporocidal or virucidal.

## Tincture of Iodine

Tincture of iodine is a combination of iodine and isopropyl or ethyl alcohol; the solution is used as an antiseptic. Iodine is highly active against microorganisms and continues to be one of the best antiseptic agents. It is effective against both gram-positive and gram-negative organisms and is tuberculocidal, sporocidal, and fungicidal.

When used as an antiseptic skin prep, however, it must be washed off after 30 seconds with alcohol; otherwise, burning and chapping of the skin results. Additionally, patients with allergies to iodine cannot come in contact with this solution. It may also stain the skin and fabrics.

## Iodophor

Povidone-iodine, known as *iodophor,* is a widely used antiseptic; it is a polyvinyl–pyrrolidone–iodine complex. Povidone is a polymer that, when combined with iodine, has the following qualities: it retains the germicidal activity of iodine; it liberates iodine slowly, thereby prolonging its activity; and it has a lower toxicity than free iodine.

Although allergic reactions to iodophor are possible, they are greatly reduced compared to those resulting from the use of tincture of iodine. An iodophor is not generally washed off; it remains on the skin and has some residual effects.

## Hexachlorophene

Hexachlorophene is a halogenated bisphenol that acts as a bacteriostatic, preventing growth, rather than a bacteriocidal agent; it is more effective against gram-positive than gram-negative organisms. Its minimal effect against gram-negative organisms is shown by the fact that gram-negative organisms can grow in hexachlorophene preparations. Peak bacteriostatic effect occurs after multiple washings; this effect can be interrupted by the use of alcohol.

Hexachlorophene bathing was once widely used as an effective prophylactic measure in nurseries to prevent outbreaks of staphylococcal skin infections.

In 1971, a study of 50 newborns showed blood levels of 0.009–0.646 $\mu$g/ml at the time the babies were discharged from the hospital, following daily bathing with a 3% hexachlorophene product (4). In December 1971, the FDA and the American Academy of Pediatrics (AAP) concluded that routine bathing with hexachlorophene was not recommended, because of the possible neurotoxicity resulting from absorption through the skin of infants, burned or denuded skin, or mucous membranes (5).

Following this recommendation and the termination of the use of hexachlorophene, staphylococcal outbreaks in nurseries occurred, and the FDA, CDC, and AAP suggested that, in addition to other control measures, a once-daily prophylactic bathing with 3% hexachlorophene, followed by through rinsing, be considered. In March of 1973, based on further data, the CDC recommended that this temporary use of hexachlorophene be restricted to personnel handwashing and infants weighing more than 2500 g, for two washings only. Other recommendations to control staphylococcal infections in the nursery did not include the use of hexachlorophene (6). Currently, hexachlorophene solutions of 0.75% or greater concentration require a prescription, and solutions containing 0.75% or less hexachlorophene must have precautionary labeling.

### Chlorhexidine Gluconate

Chlorhexidine gluconate is an antiseptic that is effective against both gram-positive and gram-negative organisms. It has persistent residual activity, increasing its effectiveness after repetitive use. Skin reactions may be rare, but the product is relatively new in the United States and data are not available. Currently chlorhexidine gluconate's use in the United States is restricted to handwashing and surgical scrubbing; it is not used at this time as an antiseptic wound care product, although it has shown good results abroad for this antiseptic use.

### Mercurial Compounds

Mercurial compounds are poor antiseptics that are only weakly bacteriostatic and are inactivated by protein. These compounds are generally not recommended for use in the hospital as antiseptics.

### Quaternary Ammonium Compounds

There is one quaternary ammonium compound (quat) that was widely used as an antiseptic, benzalkonium chloride. Because of the ability of gram-negative organisms, *Pseudomonas* in particular, to grow in these solutions, the CDC recommended in 1974 that aqueous benzalkonium chloride be replaced by other solutions for antisepsis (7).

The other quats are used for general housekeeping as disinfectants; they are cationic, anionic, or nonionic groups of detergents. Their activity covers a wide range, depending on the specific chemical composition of each agent in each group. In general, however, they are ineffective against *M. tuberculosis* or spores, are relatively nontoxic, and can be inactivated by soap.

## Phenolic Compounds

Phenolics other than hexachlorophene are used as disinfectants and are broad-spectrum germicides that kill *M. tuberculosis,* viruses, and, sometimes, spores. Generally they are relatively irritating and toxic to the skin but are relatively stable and are not inactivated by organic matter or soap. Reports of cases of hyperbilirubinemia related to the inappropriate use of phenolics in bassinets led to their discontinuation in the nurseries in many hospitals (8).

## Chlorine Compounds

Sodium hypochlorite, a common chlorine product, although corrosive can be useful as a disinfectant in dialysis areas because of its reported activity against the hepatitis virus (9). It is, in addition to being corrosive, irritating to skin and mucous membranes.

## Glutaraldehyde

Aqueous activated glutaraldehyde is an effective solution for achieving high-level disinfection or chemical sterilization. It has the ability, when used over the appropriate time period, to kill all vegetative bacteria, fungi, viruses, and spores. It has low protein coagulability and can be used when steam or ethylene oxide is not possible or practical. However, it is toxic to the skin and mucous membranes.

## Pasteurization

Pasteurization is a disinfecting process whereby heat is used to kill certain microorganisms and reduce the numbers of others, so that bacteria are kept under control within acceptable limits. The item is heated to a certain temperature for a certain period of time; this method has been suggested as a process for the disinfection of certain pieces of respiratory therapy and anesthesia equipment (10), although it does not guarantee sterility or even cleanliness if the equipment is not washed first.

A hot-water bath at 60–70 °C for 20–30 minutes is thought to be effective against gram-positive, gram-negative, and tubercle bacilli but not against spores (11).

## Ethylene Oxide

Ethylene oxide (EO) is a colorless gas used to sterilize (or to achieve high-level disinfection) equipment that would be harmed by moisture or heat. Ethylene oxide can penetrate plastic, rubber, cotton, and other substances but cannot sterilize liquids because it is absorbed and not released by them. Products that have absorbed EO must be aerated before they can be used; this includes rubber products, plastic, muslin, and paper. Aeration times differ based on the temperature and air flow. A heated aeration cabinet, used according to manufacturer's recommendations, will result in the fastest aeration times.

The Environmental Protection Agency (EPA) expressed concern for the health of workers constantly exposed to EO, and in January 1978, released a report outlining the potential problems (12). Data are not available on long-term effects of exposure to this agent, which is widely used as an alternative to steam sterilization.

## Steam

Steam under pressure remains the most effective means of destroying microorganisms on a piece of equipment. High-vacuum and gravity-displacement sterilizers are in use throughout hospitals. Although this is the best and quickest means of sterilization, it cannot be used on an increasing number of delicate pieces of equipment being developed for health care today. Its efficacy, in addition, is based on care in following manufacturer's instructions, including time, temperature, pressure, wraps, load size, and load placement, variation in any of which can affect the results.

Acceptable solutions for selected patient care equipment and procedures are shown in Figures 21-1 and 21-2. Information on appropriate solutions and contact times are available elsewhere (13) or from the manufacturer.

## CLEANING

There are many areas of the health care facility that must be rendered clean, for esthetic as well as infection control reasons. They include, in the general

*SUGGESTED DISINFECTANTS AND PROCEDURES FOR PATIENT CARE AREAS AND EQUIPMENT*

Bedpans and Urinals
- Quaternary ammonium chloride
- Iodophor
- Phenolic
- Sodium hypochlorite
- Boiling water

General Housekeeping
- Quaternary ammonium chloride
- Phenolic
- Iodophor
- Sodium hypochlorite

Thermometers
- Tincture of iodine (1 percent iodine in 70 to 90% ethyl or isopropyl alcohol)
- Iodophor
- Ethylene oxide
- Activated glutaraldehyde

Respiratory Therapy Equipment
- Steam autoclave
- Ethylene oxide
- Activated glutaraldehyde
- Pasteurization

***Figure 21-1***

*SUGGESTED ANTISEPTICS FOR PATIENT CARE PROCEDURES*

Routine Handwashing
- Soap

Handwashing Before Invasive Procedure or in Special Care Area
- Iodophor
- Chlorhexidine gluconate
- Antiseptic with hexachlorophene

IV Catheterization
- Tincture of iodine (1 or 2 percent iodine in 70% alcohol), followed by 70% isopropyl alcohol after 30-second drying time
- Iodophor
- 70% isopropyl alcohol

Urinary Catheterization
- Iodophor

***Figure 21-2***

environment, walls, floors, countertops, and furniture. Additionally, cleaning must precede any disinfection or sterilization of an object. All practical methods for disinfection or sterilization can be overchallenged by grossly dirty and heavily contaminated materials. Also, certain chemical disinfectants are inactivated by protein. Therefore, cleaning is essential in nearly all areas of the hospital, whether or not further steps are taken to achieve disinfection or sterilization.

Perhaps the most important component of the cleaning process is friction. In order to physically remove protein material such as blood, tissue, pus, and dirt, mechanical rubbing or scrubbing is necessary.

## Cleaning the Inanimate Environment

Floors, walls, and furniture in a health care facility may be cleaned with a disinfectant germicide solution and cloths or mops for scrubbing. Wet mopping and dusting are more efficient than dry and are the preferred techniques. Quats, phenolics, or iodophors can be used. The environment should be kept aesthetically clean; those areas in direct contact with patients or patient secretions need additional attention and more specific procedures.

In a typical patient room, the bed mattress and pillow should be covered with plastic, since these items are difficult to clean if they become wet with secretions. Since the patient has prolonged contact with the bed, it should be cleaned between patient use with fresh solution and cleaning cloths. Next, surfaces that receive less patient contact, such as overbed tables, and other pieces of furniture are rendered visibly clean, and walls are spot cleaned as necessary. Such cleaning is best done, either concurrently (during a patient's stay in the room) or for terminal cleaning (after the patient has been discharged), with a spray bottle of cleaning solution, so that the solution does not become dirty from rinsing out the cleaning cloth. The bathroom should be cleaned last, since the toilet and sinks are likely to be the most contaminated, and the moisture in these areas will harbor or even foster the growth of microorganisms. The cleaning cloths used in this area should not be used subsequently on a patient bed mattress or overbed table. Separate cleaning supplies for bathrooms are best.

Mopping also should be done often enough to keep the patient's room or general environment visibly clean. Methods for cleaning the floor include a spray-down, wet-vacuum pick-up machine, which can be used in larger open areas such as hallways, or mopping by hand. There is no evidence that floors contribute directly to infections in hospitals, but they may contribute in an indirect way: a generally dirty environment may be a subtle encouragement to personnel to be lax in their patient-care techniques, or it may reflect a general problem in adherence to good techniques. A visibly clean environment is certainly a better place to work and will probably make most patients more comfortable during their stay.

All areas of the hospital should be maintained as needed; specific procedures for the Housekeeping Department are available elsewhere (14). Cleaning isolation rooms is the same as any other area, except that the materials used should not be used in another area afterward. Additionally, personnel may need to use isolation techniques while in the area. Disinfectant fogging has been shown to be ineffective and is not recommended as part of the cleaning procedure for terminal and isolation cleaning (15).

## Cleaning the Animate Environment

The patient's skin, as well as the hands of nursing and other personnel, must be cleaned regularly. It is important to remove secretions and keep the skin dry to prevent skin breakdown in the immobilized patient. Removal of dirt or contamination from the hands is important to prevent transmission of possible disease-producing microorganisms from a patient to an employee or from one patient to another via the hands of health care personnel.

A soap with the following characteristics should be used for handwashing: it should be mild to avoid irritation; it should make a good lather, since emulsification of surface oils is part of the action necessary to remove contamination. It is best to wash the hands with warm, running water, so that the material is rinsed away with the soap lather. Friction, as with cleaning of other materials, is probably the most important aspect of the procedure of handwashing.

Mallison and Steere have summarized and presented detailed information on handwashing techniques and the appropriate solutions to use (16). Although bar soap has been shown to become contaminated with microorganisms, it has also been shown that personnel do not pick up these microorganisms on their hands after the procedure has been done. A soap dish that allows water to drain freely and the use of small (hotel size) bars will minimize microbial growth and ensure frequent change of soap. Soap solutions and powders are acceptable and should be chosen for ease of use, nonirritability, and cost. The specific handwashing procedure for general cleaning of the hands is outlined in Chapter 18, **Isolation Techniques.**

Hands should be washed between the routine care of patients, before eating, and after using the bathroom. Often, nursing personnel admit that it is impossible to wash each and every time they make a patient visit. Handwashing is not necessary, for example, when patient trays are delivered (except as needed before the process of delivering starts), if the patient and the immediate environment will not be touched. There are several instances when health care personnel have little direct contact with the patient; when contact does occur, however, hands should be washed.

Similar considerations apply to keeping the patient clean; the product used should be a nonirritating soap, and the skin should be cleaned as often as necessary to prevent maceration of the tissues from secretions or soilage.

# DISINFECTION

Certain pieces of equipment and areas of a health care institution require more than cleaning or sanitization. There are several ways to disinfect the inanimate environment. Similarly, in certain cases disinfection of skin or tissue is needed during patient care; antiseptics are chemicals used to disinfect live tissue.

## Disinfecting the Inanimate Environment

Objects that have extensive contact with patients or areas where survival and transmission of pathogens could occur may need disinfection in addition to cleaning to ensure that potential pathogens are not transmitted. Countertops in dialysis units and laboratories, for instance, need a higher level of disinfection than those at a nursing station. For disinfection to be successful, the object must have been adequately cleaned earlier and the contact time must be long enough for the solution to work. To minimize the growth of microorganisms, equipment such as bedpans, urinals, and thermometers should be stored dry between patient uses; in addition, a thermometer used for one patient should be washed carefully before and after each use and stored dry in the patient's room. Fiberoptic endoscopy equipment should be disinfected according to manufacturers' directions.

## Disinfecting the Animate Environment

Antisepsis of the hands is recommended before performing invasive procedures such as IV catheterization or surgery. The handwashing procedure is the same in terms of running water and friction; the scrub may be required for 2 minutes or longer, and the handwashing solution may differ. Antiseptic soaps such as those containing hexachlorophene, in iodophor, or chlorhexidine gluconate have a certain amount of residual bactericidal action that may be helpful in lowering the number of microorganisms on the hands. Since it is nearly impossible to produce a glove without minute holes in it, this action may reduce the number of microorganisms on the skin that could penetrate a glove and contaminate a sterile body area.

Similarly, the skin of patients going into surgery is treated with an antiseptic scrub. The prolonged action of the solution, as well as its bactericidal activity during the scrub, may eliminate more microorganisms and prevent recolonization during the surgical procedure.

## STERILIZATION

In most cases, pieces of equipment that are invasive and that enter sterile body cavities require high-level disinfection or sterilization. This process can be done by steam autoclave, ethylene oxide, boiling water, or chemicals such as activated glutaraldehyde. Items that should be sterilized range from IV fluids, which enter the bloodstream directly, to surgical instruments, which disrupt blood flow and the integrity of skin and body tissues, to the sterile environment created for certain patients with combined immunodeficiency diseases.

## ROLE OF THE INFECTION CONTROL PRACTITIONER IN CLEANING, DISINFECTION, AND STERILIZATION PRACTICES

The ICP alone, as a member of a products committee, or as a screen for the ICC, may make many decisions about product selection and the determination of appropriate procedures to render a patient care item safe and reusable.

The ICP must understand fully the type of procedure and equipment in question and be able to determine the level of cleaning or disinfection necessary. Thus the ICP must not only understand the nature of the procedure or contact a patient or employee will have with an object but also realize the limitations and frailties of the piece of equipment itself, since in many cases very fragile equipment requires high-level disinfection.

The choice of an antiseptic for skin or tissues can be based on these ideal characteristics (17):

1. It should be effective against resident and transient microorganisms on the skin.

2. It should be applied quickly and have effects that last throughout a procedure.

3. It should be effective against all microorganisms.

4. It should be able to be used on any part of the human body, at any age, without toxic effects.

5. It should not be inactivated by protein such as organic matter, by soaps, or by other materials.

The ICP must consider these ideal characteristics when considering a product for use on patients or personnel in the hospital.

Spaulding (18) set up criteria for the ideal disinfectant, and these still stand as useful considerations in the selection of a product. An ideal product

- produces rapid killing of microorganisms, including vegetative bacteria, spores, and viruses
- will not corrode metal, damage rubber parts, or dissolve cement in lens systems
- will not discolor or stain
- is not inactivated or coagulated by the presence of body proteins such as secretions, tissue, or blood
- is nonirritating to the skin and is nontoxic
- is tasteless and odorless
- is heat stable
- is stable over a wide pH range
- does not alter electric conductivity
- remains active over a long period of time
- can be diluted without losing its activity
- is inexpensive
- is a good wetting agent
- is miscible with water in any proportion
- will not produce a residue or buildup after use

Each of these characteristics must be considered by all those involved in the purchase of disinfectants. The ICP will be called upon to address those criteria that pertain to the killing of microorganisms, in-use life, and use factors that might affect the product's ability to perform as a disinfectant. With information about the desired level of disinfection and the characteristics of the product, the ICP can recommend acceptable alternatives that can be considered from other standpoints, such as cost and toxicity.

## Product Selection

The EPA evaluates labels on products that are classified as pesticides. Disinfectants come under this classification, and the product label must include the following: brand name; chemical formula, including all active ingredients and the proportion of inert chemicals; name and address of the manufacturer; information to alert user to toxic side effects; first aid; warnings; disposal of container; directions for use; EPA registration number; and establishment number.

Any other information on the label is the choice of the manufacturer, but it must be approved by the EPA. Included might be results of the Association of Official Analytical Chemists (AOAC) Use-Dilution Confirmation Test. This test is based on the product's ability to kill selected organisms, *Salmonella cholerasuis, S. aureus,* and *P. aeruginosa.* Although this testing must be true, it is done under laboratory conditions and may not be exactly the same as that of the hospital environment.

Manufacturers frequently supply brochures with test results that stimulate in-hospital use. However, since the label claims are carefully controlled by the EPA and the additional information in brochures may come from a variety of sources, the ICP may choose to look at the label only for determining the qualities of a product. Some manufacturers encourage in-use microbiologic testing of products. This is not recommended for the selection of a product for use in the hospital, since the tests when done correctly are costly, time-consuming, and difficult to control (19). Certainly the ICP can elect to test a product as a specially designed study, but simple culturing of solutions or equipment to test the efficacy of a product is not a reliable or cost-effective means of evaluation.

In summary, the ICP can in most cases get all the needed information from the product label. He or she should understand the desired level of disinfection, as well as characteristics of different groups of disinfectants. Other considerations, then, will be cost, toxicity or irritation, and personnel preference. Sometimes discussing products with another ICP whose institution uses the product in question may supply additional information that will help in the selection process.

## REFERENCES

1. Kretzer MP, Engley FB: Effective use of antiseptics and disinfectants. *RN* 32 : 48, 1969.

2. Laskowski LF: What the purchasing agent should know about hospital cross-infection. *Hosp Prog* October 1964.

3. Centers for Disease Control: Properties of germicides. Atlanta, Centers for Disease Control, 1966.

4. Curley A, Hawk RE, Kimbrough RD, et al: Dermal absorption of hexachlorophene in infants. *Lancet,* 2(1) : 296, 1971.

5. Hexachlorophene in newborns. *FDA Drug Bulletin.* December, 1971.

6. Centers for Disease Control: Control of nursery-acquired staphylococcal disease: Present status of use of hexachlorophene. Atlanta, Centers for Disease Control, 1973.

7. Centers for Disease Control: Hazards of infection associated with the use of aqueous benzalkonium chloride. Atlanta, Centers for Disease Control, 1974.

8. Neonatal hyperbilirubinemia. *Morbidity and Mortality Weekly Rep* 24(35):222, 1975.

9. Bond WW, Pattison CP: Control of hepatitis B virus in environmental contamination. *JAMA* 231:700, 1975.

10. Nelson EJ, Ryan KJ: A new use for pasteurization. *Resp Care* 16:97, 1971.

11. Nelson EJ: Sterilization and disinfection of respiratory therapy and anesthesia equipment. *Techniques of Infection Control in Respiratory Therapy and Anesthesia.* Seattle, Wash, Olympic Surgical Co Inc, 1, 1973, series 1, p 1.

12. *Federal Register* (6560-0), January 27, 1978.

13. American Hospital Association: *Infection Control in the Hospital,* ed 4. Chicago, American Hospital Association, 1979, p 120.

14. Craig CP, Reifsnyder DN: *Departmental Procedures for Infection Control.* New Jersey, Medical Economics Company, 1977.

15. Centers for Disease Control: Disinfectant fogging—an ineffective measure. Atlanta, Centers for Disease Control, 1974.

16. Steere AC, Mallison GF: Handwashing practices for the prevention of nosocomial infections. *Ann Intern Med* 83:683, 1975.

17. Joress SM: A study of disinfection of skin. *Ann Surg* 155(2);296, 1962.

18. Spaulding EM: Chemical disinfection of medical and surgical materials, in Reddish GF (ed): *Antiseptics, Fungicides, and Chemical and Physical Sterilization.* Philadelphia, Lea & Febiger, 1957, p 642.

19. Mallison GF: Viewpoint. *APIC Newsletter* 3(3):15, 1975.

# 22

# Infection Control: In-Service Education

Perhaps one of the most challenging aspects of infection control practice is the orientation and continuing education of virtually all personnel in a health care institution. With one common goal in mind, to minimize infection risks to patients and personnel, the ICP must work with people in many disciplines and educational levels, with differing individual and group motivations.

The ICP is rarely an educator by formal training but usually enjoys teaching. The JCAH requirements for teaching can be so overwhelming, along with the other duties, that the ICP may develop several classes at different educational levels and give them periodically simply to fulfill this rule. Most ICPs would prefer, however, to conduct meaningful classes and to measure the positive results of teaching in terms of lowered infection rates.

There is much written on the subject of the education of the adult learner, and it is well beyond the scope of this book to cover all the modern theories and methods. The remainder of this chapter outlines some basic principles about adult learning, as well as suggestions for the ICP for the development of inservice programs and more formal conferences. Education is a large part of infection control practice, and the careful design, implementation, and evaluation of educational programs will, hopefully, be reflected in lowered infection rates in health care facilities.

## STEPS IN DESIGNING EDUCATIONAL PROGRAMS FOR INFECTION CONTROL

The overall educational component of the infection control program can be planned using the same steps as those taken in preparation of a single course

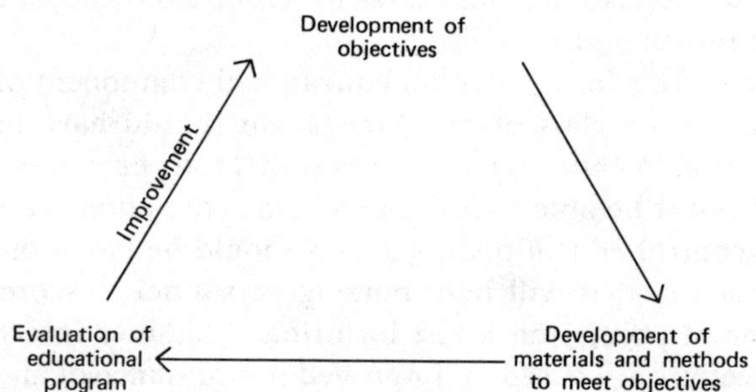



*Figure 22-1*

*The design, implementation, and evaluation of an educational program forms a cycle;
once the cycle is completed, objectives can be improved and the cycle is repeated.*

for a specific group. These steps are the development of objective; the development of materials and methods to meet the objectives; and the evaluation of the program (1). The process should be viewed as a cycle (Fig. 22-1), with the evaluation leading to changes and improvement in the educational program in infection control for health care personnel.

## Development of Objectives

Infection control practitioners must determine what goals they want to achieve in the institution through education of personnel in infection control.

An objective is a description of the performance the person will be able to do after receiving the instruction (2). An objective is important because it can show whether the instruction was successful, it gives the desired result or outcome, and therefore it is useful in helping determine what kind of course to plan, and it helps the student understand and work toward the same accomplishment.

The JCAH requires all personnel to be educated in infection control; therefore, an objective of the infection control program should be to satisfy the JCAH regulation. Still another objective is to increase the knowledge of infection control of personnel in a health care facility. The target population to be educated must also be determined at the time objectives are developed. Since regulations exist and all groups must be educated, the ICP can determine target populations based on specialty, educational level, department, or geographic area. The population selected (i.e., mixed group, such as all the people working in a nursing unit, including aides, orderlies, and RNs; or a homogeneous group, such as registered medical technologists) will influence the kind of objectives chosen, since personnel of varying backgrounds and with different job descriptions may have different motivations; the results desired from the instruction may also vary.

As well as objectives for the overall educational component of the infection control program, each class or program taught should have objectives. The important criterion in choosing objectives is that they be measurable; in other words, the ICP must be able to find out whether the objective was met.

In infection control education, objectives should be based on behavior; for example, instruction that will help nursing personnel to score higher (by a certain number of points) on a test on urinary catheter insertion and care. Often, the objectives are based on improved performance of an activity rather than the demonstration of increased knowledge of the subject itself: the nursing personnel not only learn to label and discard solutions of sterile saline after 24 hours but actually do so in practice.

To determine what objectives are appropriate for each group in the health care facility or for each class to be given, the ICP may have to assess and analyze those personnel groups most in need of instruction in infection control. The JCAH requires education for all health care personnel, and there is a certain amount of peer pressure as well as requirements for continuing education among some professional groups. This does not tell the ICP, however, what each group needs to know, or what behavior must be altered to minimize infection risks. Need can be assessed by looking at abnormally high infection rates or the occurrence of an outbreak due to a slip in nursing or medical technique. Or the ICP can formally or informally assess the knowledge level and motivation of a group to determine an appropriate objective.

Objectives, then, should be formed for the overall educational component of the infection control program; they should be measurable, have a time element built in, and outline a specific desired result. An example of an overall objective is: classes in isolation technique will be offered to personnel in all departments that have patient contact; the classes will be documented in the *Infection Control Manual.* This is a measurable objective, since a list can be made of all such departments, and the ICP can see whether the classes were given; it has a time element–all the classes are to be given during a 1-year period. The desired result is the list of inservice courses in the manual.

Objectives are necessary for each specific educational program and may be based on observed (by the ICP) or expressed (by the target population) need.

EXAMPLE. The ICP reads the charts of surgical patients during a study of wound infections and finds that the nursing personnel have written little in the nurses' notes to describe the wound. These notes should be the means by which the physician or other nurses become aware of the need for isolation precautions and the need to alter wound care. However, even wounds that had begun to drain heavily were not well described in the notes. As a result, in determining objectives for a class on wound infections, the ICP sets one objective as: nursing personnel on this unit will describe the amount and characteristics of drainage in patient wounds in the nurses' notes.

In this example, the objective is measurable and the desired result is the demonstration of the ability to evaluate wounds in written nurses' notes. The time interval was set by the duration of the class; based on knowledge gained in the course, nurses could begin appropriate charting immediately after instruction.

Infection control practitioners can choose courses and target populations to teach randomly throughout an institution and still satisfy JCAH requirements. It is most useful, however, to determine objectives for teaching and have the results affect personnel behavior, which should ultimately be reflected in lowered infection rates.

## Development of Materials and Methods for Infection Control Instruction

Once the ICP has determined whom to teach and the desired result of the instruction, it is easy to determine how best to achieve the result. Many aspects of the actual instruction will affect the ultimate success of the program.

### *People, Place, and Time*

The target population has been defined, but the participants for each class must be specified further. For example, a class for nursing personnel in surgical units (target population) might be given only once, to all those able to attend, at 2:00 PM on a weekday, in a large auditorium. Alternatively, classes could be given during all three shifts to smaller groups, in the conference room of each unit.

### *Teaching Tools*

The principles of adult learning have been described, and the specific methods used in educational programs should be designed with these principles in mind. These principles are (3):

- Learning depends on motivation.
- Learning depends on capacity to learn.
- Learning depends on past and current experience.

- Learning depends on the active involvement of the learner.
- Learning is enhanced by problem solving.
- Learning effectiveness is dependent on feedback.
- Learning is enhanced by an informal atmosphere and the freedom to make mistakes.
- Learning is augmented by novelty, variety, and challenge.

Instruction can be given in a variety of ways, and the ICP may find each useful at different times:

1. Formal instruction in a classroom setting
2. Seminar or workshop, including group discussion, case presentation, problem solving, and role playing
3. Informal consultation–coffee break

There are also many instructional aids and program materials that can be used in formal or informal settings:

1. Audiovisual aids such as slides, filmstrips, movies, chalkboard, overhead or opaque projector, real models, or dummies
2. Handouts
3. Self-instructional equipment

The ICP may use any combination of methods and materials to meet the objectives. Much more information is available on the development and use of each specific program aid, in terms of best audience size and seating arrangement, making slides, lighting, and other aspects of program preparation (3).

## Evaluation of the Program

Each educational program should be evaluated. First, the ICP should evaluate whether the original objectives were met, based on the measurement tool stated in the objective. In the example cited earlier, the evaluation may show that the instructional program did not result in nurses writing more specific notes about surgical wounds, and another approach may be needed.

Second, the education program itself should be evaluated by the participants and by the ICP. Most in-service education programs in health care facilities are not evaluated, perhaps affecting the amount of learning achieved, because of potential solvable problems in the methods used. Also, denying the participants a chance to evaluate the program may make them feel relatively unimportant, thus violating one of the learning principles listed earlier, that is, that learning depends on active involvement of the learner.

Evaluation should begin at the planning stage of the program, when needs are determined and objectives are set. The evaluation process should be specific and include some means of measuring results. In most cases, participants fill out an evaluation sheet. An evaluation by participants should include a reaction to the meeting itself, the facilities, and the time allotted to the course(s); comments on the speaker (interest, knowledge, communication) and on the subject (applicability). The evaluation can be in the form of a multiple choice:

Did the subject meet your needs and interests?
_ No _ To some extent _ To a large extent _ Yes

where participants rate their answers to various questions on a scale. Others have open-ended questions:

List the benefits this program has for your particular job.

Evaluations may also have lists of possible answers; the participants may check one or more that they believe is correct:

What aspects of the program on urinary care were most important for you to learn about?

__________ reasons for catheterization
__________ insertion technique
__________ catheter care
__________ interpreting culture results
__________ outbreaks related to urinary catheters

An evaluation should also be done by the ICP or the person instructing, as a guide for the next educational endeavor. Results immediately following an educational program can be compared with later performance of participants; problems recognized in the program may account for any adverse results and vice versa.

Tests and quizzes are also a means of evaluation. Pretests and posttests to assess the knowledge level of participants are useful in measuring the success of a program. One program objective may be an improved score, by a certain number of points, from a pretest to posttest. The pretest can also be used as a focus for discussion, which may be less threatening to adult learners. The use of testing outside the formal classroom is difficult for some adults, especially in an in-service type of setting.

The ICP is required to teach infection control principles and practices to all personnel within the health care facility. Although education techniques are not generally part of his or her background, the ICP should recognize the need for education and the potential role it can play in lowering infection rates. (See the list of additional readings at the end of the chapter.) Most ICPs have experienced the frustration of planning an inservice course and having few or no people attend; the realities of hospital life must be recognized, among them the difficulty in finding free time for personnel to attend classes. Careful assessment of need and design of objectives, teaching tools, and evaluations will optimize the participants' motivation. The result of the time and care spent in planning will be success in meeting the stated objectives of the educational aspect of the infection control program.

## REFERENCES

1. Mager RF, Beach KM: *Developing Vocational Instruction.* California, Fearon Publishers Inc, 1967, p 3.
2. Mager RF: *Preparing Instructional Objectives,* ed 2. California, Fearon Publishers Inc, 1975, p 5.
3. Hospital Research and Educational Test: *Training and Continuing Education.* Chicago, Hospital Research and Educational Trust, 1970, p 87.

## ADDITIONAL READINGS

1. Bischof L: *Adult Psychology,* ed 2. San Francisco, Harper & Row, 1976.
2. Knowles M: *Modern Practice of Adult Education.* New York, Associated Press, 1970.
3. Kidd JR: *How Adults Learn.* New York, Associated Press, 1969.

# 23

# Infection Control Regulations

In the practice of infection control, there is more than one agency governing the activities and monitoring the results of program efforts. Some of these agencies, briefly discussed or referred to previously, will be covered in more depth here to give the ICP a view of the overall responsibility for infection control within an institution and between the institution and the community.

Health care institutions must be accredited or licensed in order to receive Medicare and Medicaid funding and to participate in other federal programs. Most hospitals are accredited by the Joint Commission on Accreditation of Hospitals (JCAH). Extended care facilities, including rehabilitative and psychiatric institutions, are generally licensed by state health departments. Additionally, departments within an institution may be reviewed and approved by other agencies, such as the review of a microbiology laboratory by the College of American Pathologists. Because the JCAH regulations are broad in scope and affect the majority of ICPs in the country, they will be described in more depth; although state regulations for licensure tend to parallel JCAH standards closely, pertinent regulations should be obtained by those individuals reviewed and licensed by state health department officials.

## JCAH STANDARDS

The JCAH is a private agency that reviews and accredits hospitals at each hospital's invitation. Generally, a JCAH team reviews all aspects of the hospital's governing structure and functioning, makes a report, and accredits qualified hospitals for up to a 2-year period. The team usually includes representatives of the nursing, medical, and administrative fields of hospital operations. The guidelines given to JCAH-reviewed institutions cover many subjects, including an infection control section (1). The standards listed in this section are divided into two areas: a description of the elements of the infection control program itself, and infection control activities throughout the facility.

The revised JCAH manual is written to be used for self-assessment of the infection control program as well as the survey report form that surveyors will use for their on-site visit. Key items are asterisked to indicate they are essentials of the infection control program. The rating scale of the standards includes six rankings that report the level of compliance of the infection control standards. Rankings range from substantial compliance to no compliance at all (1). The use of the standards as a self-assessment tool allows the ICP to assess strengths and weaknesses of the infection control program and, with the ICC, make appropriate changes.

## Infection Control Program Elements

### *Surveillance, Reporting, and Analysis of Infections*

The JCAH requires that each facility have written definitions of nosocomial infections as well as a surveillance system to collect and review data and to perform follow-up studies as needed. The JCAH also requires input into the employee health program relating to infections. In addition, there must be a system for monitoring and following up problems identified in the inanimate environment of the hospital. All these systems must be in writing and carefully outlined to show that patients, personnel, and the environment are being monitored adequately.

### *In-Service Education*

Education in infection prevention and control must be provided to all personnel in the health care facility through orientation and continuing education programs. Documentation of this educational program must be available to the review team.

### *Laboratory Support*

The infection control program must include written evidence that there is microbiologic and serologic support for any activities related to the surveillance, prevention, and control of infections within the hospital.

### *Policies and Procedures*

There must be hospitalwide or facilitywide policies and procedures regarding the handling of patients in isolation. These rules should cover any personnel having contact with a patient in isolation. There should be documentation that the hospital will provide safe and adequate patient care that will not be compromised by the need to isolate the patient. These policies and procedures should be available in every department and area of the hospital as hospitalwide documents; they should not form part of a specific department's manual, such as that used only in the nursing service.

### Approval of Adequate Patient Facilities

The JCAH-accredited hospital must provide adequate facilities to house infectious patients, including negative-pressure rooms for respiratory isolation.

### Infection Control Committee

The JCAH requires that a standing committee of the medical staff be responsible for the infection control program and activities in the facility. Required membership includes representatives from the medical staff, administration, nursing service, microbiology laboratory (if available), and the ICP or any person responsible for the implementation of the infection control program. The chairperson of the committee must be a person with knowledge or special interest and experience in infection control, preferably a physician. Meetings must take place at least bimonthly. Documentation of the existence of the committee, its members and meeting dates, its minutes, and the scope of its authority in routine and emergency situations within the administrative structure must be available for review.

The ICC must design and direct the infection control program, including the determination of the kind of surveillance and reporting program that is needed and the approval of definitions and criteria related to surveillance. Activities of the ICC required by the JCAH include the review of the results of any pertinent studies or collection of data, including nosocomial surveillance data, findings from reviews of antibiotic use, and special studies of infections or related procedures. The committee must document these reviews, as well as the ongoing review and approval of policies and procedures for all hospital areas.

## Infection Control Activities

As stated, the ICC directs the activities of the ICP and therefore determines the structure and functioning of the infection control program. Some specific activities are required by the JCAH and are spelled out in their guidelines. These activities include the provision of documented policies and procedures, as well as the inservice orientation and continuing education for all departments within the hospital. Specifically named departments are:

- Nursing service
- Anesthesia and postanesthesia care units
- Blood bank
- Cafeteria, coffee shops, canteens
- Food service
- Emergency service
- Nuclear medicine
- Newborn nurseries
- All obstetric services–labor, delivery, and postpartum
- Outpatient areas and services
- Pathology
- Pharmacy
- Physical medicine
- Radiology
- Respiratory care service
- Special care units
- Central service
- Housekeeping
- Linen and laundry
- Engineering and maintenance
- Operating rooms

In addition to policies and procedures regarding the handling of isolated patients in these areas, the JCAH requires documentation of policies for handling waste, use of disposables, and all personnel and equipment procedures that are associated with the occurrence of nosocomial infections. These policies and procedures must be specific for the area, patients, and personnel involved and must be available for review and accessible to people working in the department. The ICC must review and, if needed, revise these policies and procedures on an annual basis. Suggested departmental policies and procedures for infection control are available commercially (2) and offer at least a base from which modifications can be made to fit individual facility specifications.

Additionally, certain procedures in patient care that transcend departmental or area lines, such as intravenous catheter and Foley catheter insertion and care, and the selection, handling, and disposal of disposable items must be documented and reviewed annually by the ICC.

In summary, the JCAH requires that any hospital seeking accreditation have an active infection control program, designed and monitored by an ICC. It suggests that an ICP implement the program directly. The committee must report directly to the executive committee of the medical staff and must have the authority to intervene as necessary in infection control emergencies such as outbreaks. The committee, by its authority and through its review functions, ensures that all areas and departments within the hospital are covered by adequate infection control policies and procedures and can show proof of their ongoing educational programs in infection prevention and control.

## OTHER STANDARDS FOR INFECTION CONTROL

Other standards for infection control in health care facilities are similar to or parallel those of the JCAH. The requirements for reporting communicable diseases to health departments, for example, may vary from state to state but must be followed within each facility. The ICC must follow state laws regarding these areas.

## ROLE OF THE INFECTION CONTROL PRACTITIONER IN ASSURING COMPLIANCE WITH REGULATIONS

The ICP is generally the expert in infection control in the facility and takes the main responsibility for implementing the infection control program. Therefore, the ICP is usually responsible for making sure that all the necessary requirements for JCAH accreditation or other licensing boards have been met.

### Infection Control Program

It is usually the ICP who drafts the statement of authority and the descriptions of the surveillance program, the ICC, and other structural and administrative parts of the hospital's *Infection Control Manual.* These documents should be available in the Infection Control Department (or where the ICP works) as well as in the hospital administration office, along with other sections of the hospital manual.

### Infection Control Activities

Departmental policies and procedures for infection control are the combined responsibility of the ICC and the individual department head. Both sets of JCAH standards, the section on infection control and the section for each department, will state the requirement for information on infection control.

In reality, the responsibility for writing the infection control portion of a departmental manual often rests with the ICP, who has the most knowledge and can at least begin by providing pertinent information to the department head. Again, commercially available manuals can serve as a starting point. These sections must appear in each department's own manual and must be available for review in the *Infection Control Manual* as well. Annual review of the infection control policies and procedures is generally a responsibility of the ICP, to ensure that all materials receive the needed review before the JCAH accreditation team's visit.

Similarly, the responsibility for implementing the standard for inservice education is often given to the ICP. Documentation of at least yearly in-service courses for each department, as well as input into the overall hospital orientation program, is necessary; this information is compiled in the Infection Control Department and is available for review. In larger institutions it may be more reasonable for the ICP to put together a videotape presentation for orientation purposes or to provide department heads with information on infection control that they can give their own personnel. The JCAH standards do not require that every in-service course be given in person or directly by the ICP, as long as documentation is available that classes were indeed held.

The ICP will in most situations be asked to meet with one or more members of the JCAH review team to go over the infection control program. It is important to remember that evidence of efforts and progress in meeting a certain standard is often acceptable, so that complete compliance with every standard is not expected for the first review.

There has been considerable variation in the emphasis different teams have placed on different aspects of infection control practice; the best approach is for the ICP to have adequate documentation of the structure and functions of the infection control program, to relax, and to be open-minded and willing to learn from a discussion of what priorities an accrediting agency sets in infection control practice.

## REGULATIONS AND THE LAW

All the standards required by the JCAH and other regulatory agencies are legally important in the event of a malpractice suit associated with an infection. These regulations become the standard of care the courts will use to determine the probability of negligence in cases involving both patient infections and personnel infections (3). The ICP may be called as a witness or named in a suit as a codefendant. The complete documentation of an infection control program, covering the surveillance, policies and procedures to prevent infections, isolation procedures, and authority to intervene to control infections, with documentation of in-service education, will serve to show the court that the hospital is striving to meet and maintain the accepted standard of care in infection control.

# REFERENCES


1. *Accreditation Manual for Hospitals: Infection Control.* Chicago, standards adopted by Joint Commission on Accreditation of Hospitals, 1985.
2. Craig CP, Reifsnyder DN: *Departmental Procedures for Infection Control Programs.* New Jersey, Medical Economics Company, 1977.
3. Dornette WHL: Legal aspects of hospital-acquired infections. *Leg Aspects Med Pract* May–June, 1973, p 37.

# 24

# Special Studies in Infection Control

There are two prevalent attitudes in infection control practice regarding its current status; both were expressed at an infection control workshop in 1972 and still are evident today (1). One view is that there is an adequate knowledge base in infection control to lower nosocomial infection rates significantly. More time spent in communication with and teaching health care professionals would result in a decrease in nosocomial infection rates (2).

The other viewpoint is that there are some areas where factors directly involved in infection risks are known, but there are many more areas where significant variables are not clear. The second group believes that further research is needed to clarify significant risk factors before intervention can effectively lower infection rates. Both views are true in part, and examples can be found to illustrate each (3,4).

EXAMPLE.  It has been well documented that a closed system for urinary tract drainage is accompanied by a lowered infection rate. Teaching nursing personnel to handle this equipment correctly, as in needle aspiration of specimens, would probably result in lowered nosocomial urinary tract infection rates.

There are nursing and medical procedures designed to lower the risk of a patient acquiring bacterial pneumonia in the hospital. The exact mechanisms of colonization and infection are not clear, nor are prevention and control measures. Specific research into the epidemiology of pneumonia caused by gram-negative organisms is needed before intervention can significantly alter the level of risk to hospital patients.

The ICP may become involved in various research projects in infection control. The amount of time spent and the degree of involvement will depend on the personnel, time, and money available beyond the required infection control activities and the experience and education of the ICP in research methodology.

## SURVEILLANCE OF ANTIBIOTIC USE

The overuse and misuse of antibiotics has been well documented in recent years. Reports have shown increased health care costs, use of antimicrobials without evidence of infection and some of the suspected reasons for the inappropriate use of antimicrobials (5–8 ). The public has become aware of this problem and in recent years has demanded accountability of appropriate antibiotic usage with lowered costs (9,10).

The JCAH requires that antibiotics be monitored in the hospital and that the ICC be responsible for coordination with the medical staff on action relative to the findings from the regular review of the clinical use of drugs and the results of any antimicrobial susceptibility—resistance trend studies (11).

The medical staff may elect to monitor antibiotic use through a committee-of-the-whole or may delegate this function to a standing committee, such as the ICC, Medical Audit, or Pharmacy and Therapeutics. Or the medical staff may create a separate, multidisciplinary group to monitor the use of antimicrobials. The medical staff in each hospital will decide the role of the ICP in an antibiotic audit through the determination of the responsible committee.

In the course of traditional surveillance activities, the ICP will collect data on antibiotics (10). Figure 24-1 is a schematic representation of the subgroups of antibiotics. It should be noted that the representation is not to scale; that is, the groups are not accurately proportional to one another or to the population as a whole. In traditional surveillance, the ICP looks for patients with nosocomial infections from among the entire hospital patient population. In certain institutions the ICP may also collect information on patients with community-associated infections. In both these groups the ICP can calculate the proportion of patients with infections who are also receiving antimicrobials. However, there is no way to discover the number of patients who receive antibiotics during hospitalization among those who were neither admitted with an infection nor acquired one.

Therefore, surveillance of antibiotic use in a hospital cannot be considered part of the total infection control surveillance system as it has been defined. If total-hospital antibiotic surveillance is made part of the ongoing infection control program, additional personnel, time, and money must be allocated by the hospital administration. Certainly, the surveillance program includes collecting, tabulating, and analyzing data on antimicrobial use among patients

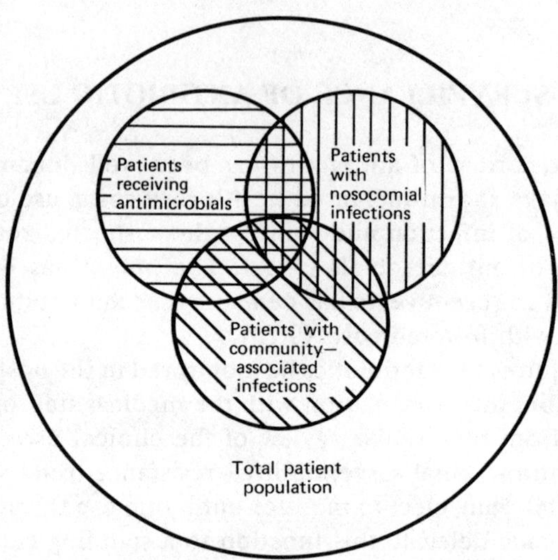


*Figure 24-1*

*Groups investigated in surveillance of infections and antimicrobial use. Of the total patient population, three groups overlap in the areas of infection control and antibiotic audit. The ICP studies patients with infections (nosocomial and, sometimes, community associated); antibiotic audit focuses on patients receiving antimicrobials. During normal surveillance activities, the ICP does not get a full picture of antimicrobial use in the hospital.*

with infections. This information may be extremely useful as an indication of the need for further study of a specific patient group or of an antimicrobial. Such data should not, however, be viewed as an audit of antibiotic use for the entire facility, since patients with infections comprise a select group in the hospital population.

Infection control practitioners can, however, become involved in an audit of antibiotics as a special project; the extent of involvement will depend on that ICP's available time, education, and experience in research methodology.

## Steps in a Review of Antibiotic Use

Counts in 1977 suggested the following steps as an approach to antibiotic review and control (12):

1. *Obtain use and cost data.* These data will provide a baseline for further activities.

2. *Establish criteria for antibiotic use.* These guidelines must be agreed on by prescribing physicians in the institution.

3. *Review antibiotic use.* Once guidelines have been set and agreed upon, a study can be designed to examine any variable: all antibiotic use and appropriateness, therapy for certain diseases or procedures, or nosocomial infection rates in patients with or without antibiotic therapy.

4. *Intervene.* Based on the findings of studies, the medical staff takes action through educational programs or controls.

5. *Review antibiotic use after controls are imposed.* Studies should be carried out to determine if problems have been corrected by intervention.

The ICP can become involved in antibiotic reviews in a special project directed by the ICC. The review is the responsibility, however, of a multidisciplinary committee, since the ICP's role will be limited to study design and data collection activities. The ICP can provide or assist in the provision of baseline antibiotic use data. The development and approval of criteria for appropriate antibiotic use, as well as any direct intervention based on the results of use data, should be the responsibility of the medical staff.

There are three kinds of studies to determine antibiotic use: prevalence, retrospective, and prospective. The role of the ICP will vary in each study.

### Prevalence Survey

A prevalence survey, as previously described, is the study of a certain characteristic in a population group at a given point in time.

EXAMPLE. The overall prevalence of antibiotic use in a hospital can be calculated by using the equation below.

$$\frac{\text{Number of patients receiving antibiotics at one point in time}}{\text{Number of patients in hospital at the same point in time}} \times 100\% = \text{prevalence}$$

The prevalence survey is a good way to make a quick assessment of antibiotic use in an institution; the survey provides detailed, descriptive information on the patients and the antibiotics used.

The ICP can take much of the responsibility for the design of a prevalence survey. The ICP has a good understanding of data sources in the hospital, as well as of methods for collecting, analyzing, tabulating, and reporting this information. The ICP can also be the data collector, alone or with others. Patient name and hospital ID number, diagnosis, service, ward, antibiotic drug, dose, and route are data that the ICP is accustomed to reviewing during traditional surveillance and other activities. The tabulation of the information on antibiotic use and the sorting of data by ward, service, antibiotic, or other variable are also within the area of expertise and experience of the ICP.

The ICP can participate in reporting antibiotic use data to the medical staff, but this report is handled best by the ICC (or whatever committee is responsible for antibiotic review) as a whole. Any further studies or action, based on the results of a prevalence survey, should be recommended by the ICC in conjunction with the medical staff. The ICP participates in these decisions as a member of the ICC.

### Retrospective Survey

Like the prevalance survey, a retrospective study can give baseline information on antibiotic use in institutions. This study is retrospective, that is, it looks at the past, and therefore it can be carried out at a comparatively leisurely pace, since it is the completed medical record that is reviewed. A review of the charts of patients who received antibiotics and who were discharged at a particular time, or a review of all patients discharged at a certain time, both of which determine use patterns, can provide more information than a prevalence survey. A review of all or a random sampling of the completed medical records will provide data on the results of antibiotic and other types of therapy from which the appropriateness of antibiotic therapy can be assessed.

The ICP can provide input for the study design, including data collection methodology. Any assessment of the appropriateness of antibiotic use, however, must be designed in conjunction with other committee members, the physicians in particular. The criteria for acceptable use must be determined and agreed upon by the medical staff in order to make the results of the study meaningful to prescribing physicians. Kunin's (10) suggested guidelines for antibiotic use can be modified for the study. He states that "it was unfair to audit and arrive at judgements concerning use of antimicrobials by physicians without first providing them with the opportunity to review and criticize the criteria and make appropriate revisions that meet the special needs of practical problems in the management of their patients."

The ICP may collect data for a retrospective review of antibiotic data, but those whose responsibility it is to assess therapy should also be involved in data collection. It would be very difficult for a physician to interpret antibiotic use without having access to the full medical record. The physician members of the audit team should analyze and report the results of a retrospective assessment of antimicrobial use and should also take any action indicated by the results. The ICP can participate, but only as a member of the committee, and should not be responsible for the interpretation of this information or any action taken because of it.

### *Prospective Study*

Studies that provide baseline information on the magnitude of antibiotic use and possible problems that are discovered because of a review of this use may indicate to the medical staff a need for a current, ongoing review of antibiotic therapy as it is being administered. Although the design and data collection activities can be done in part by the ICP, physicians must be responsible for the evaluation and any intervention in medical therapy in a review of this kind. The ICP can provide the physicians responsible for the monitoring program with information about patients receiving antibiotics or about breaks in agreed-upon criteria for antibiotic use.

Infection Control Practitioners may become involved in various ways in the review of antimicrobial use as a special project. Working in conjunction with the medical staff, ICPs can supply their expertise in the review process and, in turn, learn a great deal about the relationship between antibiotic use and nosocomial infections in the institution. The interpretation and the direct action based on these data, however, must be provided by the medical staff.

# RESEARCH IN INFECTION CONTROL

There are a number of areas in infection control practice in which research is needed. The ICP, working alone or with members of the ICC or others, can provide meaningful data to improve practice in this new field.

## Studies of Risk Factors

Careful epidemiologic studies are needed to define areas of risk in the hospital. The ICP can study the risk of acquiring an infection associated with certain procedures, diseases, or conditions. There are host risks (susceptibility factors), environmental risks (placement in a certain area of the hospital; private versus semiprivate versus ward, for example), and medical and nursing risks (procedures) that contribute to nosocomial infection rates. When risk factors have been defined and quantified, through controlled prospective studies, then mechanisms that lower risk or increase host resistance to infection can be studied.

## Cost-Effectiveness Studies

The Study on the Efficacy of Nosocomial Infection Control (SENIC) conducted by the Centers for Disease Control proved that a well-designed infection control program that included surveillance, infection prevention, and physician feedback on nosocomial infections rates could reduce the incidence of nosocomial infections in hospitals by 32% each year (2).

Isolation practices have changed to use articles as barriers judiciously and only articles (gown, mask, gloves) necessary to interrupt disease transmission (13). Cleaning procedures, and other commonly used procedures for environmental control, need evaluation; some of these procedures may be costly and may not contribute to lowering infection rates in the hospital. The ICP can look at any of a number of infection control procedures to determine their cost and their value in preventing infections.

## Funding and Research Design

Infection Control Practitioners may receive funding for research from the institution in which they are employed. In other settings, research may need to be funded from outside sources. Just as the success of a research project is based on the care with which the study is designed, success in obtaining funding is based on the care with which the grant proposal is written.

Sources of funding include the National Institutes of Health, the Public Health Service, other government sources, and private sources such as industry. Most medical libraries can help beginning researchers find lists of funding sources; many large teaching hospitals, university-affiliated medical centers, and nursing and medical schools employ people whose job is to help in obtaining grants. Any ICP interested in obtaining outside funding for research should seek help from this employee, who is experienced in dealing with the details of grant proposals. Additionally, many universities offer continuing education seminars in the art of writing grant proposals.

Any research carried out in the hospital should be approved by all necessary administrative persons and groups. There should be adequate facilities available, and permission should be obtained from appropriate departments to conduct the research. Any experiment involving patients or employees must be submitted for approval to a Human Subjects Committee of the institution, and acceptable methods for obtaining informed consent, if necessary, must be available. The grants officer should be able to help to interpret the Department of Health and Human Services regulations regarding human subjects in research.

There will be different forms and information requested based on the funding source, but the same basic components of a good research design are required for all.

1. *Define the problem clearly.* A literature review will provide information on what has been done on the subject and is the basis for a good research design. The problem must be stated clearly, along with the purpose of

the proposed study. The depth of the review of the subject area will depend on the background and expertise of the reviewers; members of the funding committee who are involved in infection control will need less explanatory evidence than those in unrelated fields (14). This introduction should show the review committee the importance of the subject and the need for research in the area.

2. *Describe your project.* The study design must be spelled out in detail: what is to be accomplished, how, when, where, and by whom. In any good research project, the more complete the design the better the project. Details must be provided to the reviewers on the methodology, including such information as the choice of data collector, the time frame, the data collection tool, the population to be studied, how the sample will be selected, and how the data will be collected, tabulated, analyzed, and reported (Table 24-1) Potential problems in the study should be brought up and discussed in the design.

3. *Describe your qualifications.* In addition to a good proposal, reviewers require that the principal investigator be qualified to conduct the study. Therefore most proposals will require that all those involved in the study be described in terms of background and education. The reviewers must be convinced that, in addition to a good idea for a research project, the people involved in the research have the needed skills to carry it out.

4. *Outline how the money will be spent.* Perhaps the most difficult part of the grant proposal is the budget. The protocol should include all the anticipated costs, such as salaries and supplies, realistically estimated. The calculations must be complete and accurate (16). It is important to include all the possible costs, such as secretarial, telephone, or laboratory expenses, but it is equally important not to pad the estimates to cover unanticipated costs. The proposal most likely to be accepted will be simple, accurate, and realistic.

**Table 24-1**
STEPS IN RESEARCH DESIGN

---

1. Describe the problem
2. Review the literature
3. Make hypotheses
4. Define variables
5. Determine how variables will be quantified
6. Define the target population
7. Develop method of collecting data
8. Develop method of analyzing data
9. Determine how results will be interpreted
10. Determine methods of communicating results

---

Other guidelines for grant proposals can be found in medical libraries. Research in infection control is badly needed, and ICPs can do simple, inexpensive studies to show cost-effectiveness or evaluate infection control practices to increase the knowledge base in this field. The ICP should get help as needed, however, to do valid research that will be meaningful to infection control practice.

# REFERENCES


1. Sanford JP, Hewitt WL: Workshop on hospital associated infections. *J Infect Dis* 130(6):680, 1974.

2. Haley RW, Culver DH, White JW, et al: The efficacy of infection surveillance and control programs in preventing nosocomial infections in US hospitals. *Am J Epidemiol* 121(2):182, 1985.

3. Feeman J, McGowan JE: Methodologic issues in hospital epidemiology. III. Investigating the modifying effects of time and severity of underlying illness on estimates of cost of nosocomial infection. *Rev Infect Dis* 6(3):285, 1984.

4. Haley RW, Culver DH, Morgan WM, et al: Identifying patients at high risk of surgical wound infection. *Am J Epidemiol* 121(2):206, 1985.

5. Castle M, Wilfert CM, Cate TR, et al: Antibiotic use at Duke University Medical Center. *JAMA* 237:2819, 1977.

6. Kunin CM, Tupasi T, Craig WA: Use of antibiotics: A brief exposition of the problem and some tentative solutions. *Ann Intern Med* 79:555, 1973.

7. Klimek J, Ajemian E, Hryb K, et al: Patterns of antibiotic usage in a surgical intensive care unit. *J Hosp Infect* 5(Suppl A):129, 1984.

8. Sutherland RD, Martinez HE, Guynes WA: Antibiotics and coronary artery bypass operations: An 11-year experience. *Infect Surg,* August 1985, p 585.

9. Anderson J: Some new antibiotics: overprescribed, lethal. *The Washington Post.* January 27, 1974.

10. Kunin CM: Evaluation of antibiotic usage: A comprehensive look at alternative approaches. *Rev Infect Dis* 3(4):745, 1981.

11. *Accreditation Manual for Hospitals 1986: Infection Control.* Chicago, standards adopted by Board of Commissioners, Joint Commission on Accreditation of Hospitals, 1985.

12. Counts GW: Review and control of antimicrobial usage in hospitalized patients. *JAMA* 238(20):2170, 1977.

13. Garner JS, Simmons BP: *CDC Guidelines for Isolation Precautions in Hospitals,* Hospital Infections Program, Atlanta, Centers for Disease Control, 1983.

14. McGowan JE Jr: Research proposals: Guidelines to dueling for dollars. *Assoc Pract Infect Control Newsl* June 6, 1976.

15. Abdellah FG, Levine E: *Better Patient Care through Nursing Research.* New York, Macmillan, 1965.

16. Nash DB: The power of protocol. *Med Dimensions,* March 1977, p 44.

# 25

# A Cost-Effective Infection Control Program

Nosocomial infections cause considerable morbidity and mortality to approximately 5% of all hospitalized patients, for an annual cost of several billion dollars. The emphasis during the 1960s and 1970s was infection reduction without regard to cost. Many infection control practices were initiated without well-defined studies to prove their effectiveness. Costs of these practices were of little concern, to either the hospital administrator or the infection control group, because most of these charges were passed directly to the patients and inevitably to the third-party payers.

The spiraling costs of health care and the increased elderly population prompted Medicare to look at the cost of health care, as well as the quality. For example, a new method of payment for Medicare payments was begun in October 1983. This prospective payment system pays hospitals a fixed rate for patient services according to diagnosis-related groups (DRGs) (1). This method of payment allows a uniform payment system for Medicare rather than an individual cost–payment system.

Therefore, if the actual charges are less than the fixed fee for the DRG, the institution is permitted to keep the money. If the actual patient charges exceed the DRG reimbursement, the hospital must absorb the extra cost. This same type of payment system is being adopted by some insurance groups and state health care cost commissions. These recent changes in conditions for payment have forced hospital administrators to evaluate costs of hospital programs, including infection control programs.

Some ICPs have become concerned their programs would be trimmed by administrators as cost-saving measures. One infection control group, concerned with this possibility of reduction, set out to quantify and justify their program. They calculated that 26 nosocomial infections cost their institutions more than $43,000, of which only $1696 was reimbursable in accordance with the DRG system of payment. This was so effective in this institution the program was expanded rather than reduced. The hospital expects to more than recover the cost of the expanded program (2).

Most nosocomial infections are not reimbursable under the DRG system of payment, or the amount recoverable for a nosocomial infection listed as a complication is so much less than fees for other complications that institutions rarely seek payment for them.

These recent changes in methods of payment and the high costs of nosocomial infections have forced hospital administrators to consider infection control programs more seriously. This is an excellent time to show hospital administrators that an efficiently run infection control program committed to infection reduction will more than save the cost of the program. In order to accomplish this objective, the ICP must be able to calculate the costs of nosocomial infections, the costs of infection control practices that prevent these infections, and show a cost-effective program.

Haley states in the SENIC report that a high-intensity infection control program, which includes a trained hospital epidemiologist, a surveillance nurse for every 250 beds, a well-defined surveillance system, and feedback to the surgeons about the surgical infections rate, will reduce nosocomial infections by one-third (3).

## CALCULATING THE COSTS OF NOSOCOMIAL INFECTIONS

A major priority in developing any cost effective infection control program is determining the costs of nosocomial infections. Various studies, using several methods, have been done to measure the costs of nosocomial infections (4–8). The three basic methods used in these studies are direct assessment, comparison, and matched comparison. The ICP trying to determine the cost of nosocomial infections should be aware that all of these study methods have bias and that no study method yet designed approximates the absolute cost of nosocomial infections.

The direct assessment method determines the cost of a nosocomial infection by tabulating all the charges incurred during the hospitalization of a patient with a nosocomial infection. A designated person, usually a physician, reviews the record and determines which charges are attributable to the nosocomial infection. This is a subjective assessment and frequently a review by a physician underestimates the cost of a nosocomial infection. This method is the easiest and most accurate for the majority of infection control programs. The ICP can work with the accounting department and obtain the charges for a patient with a nosocomial infection. The hospital epidemiologist or the chairperson of the ICC can determine charges attributable to the nosocomial infection. Costs not recoverable through reimbursement are actual costs to the institution.

The comparison method measures the total hospitalization costs incurred by a patient admitted for a specific surgical procedure, or for a primary diagnosis and who develops a nosocomial infection and compares it with the costs incurred by a patient with a similar surgical procedure, or primary diagnosis and who does not develop an infection. The difference between the two figures is the cost of the nosocomial infection. This method of determining the cost of a nosocomial infection does not take into consideration that patients with underlying diseases are usually more ill and at a greater risk for developing a nosocomial infection than are patients without these underlying diseases. The matched comparison method was initiated because of the bias in the method of matching patients by surgical procedure or primary diagnosis. The matched comparison method, besides matching for surgical procedure or primary diagnosis, matches for age, sex, and underlying disease. The difference between the costs of the matched pair is the cost of the nosocomial infection. Both of these comparison methods tend to overestimate the cost of a nosocomial infection. The matched comparison method requires a very large patient population to obtain accurately matched controls. One study revealed that even when 3800 controls were available to match 240 patients with nosocomial infections, the infected patients and their controls were not totally matched (4).

Hospital administrators must be educated to the fact that nosocomial infections can cost their institutions money. These methods of determining costs of nosocomial infections provide the infection control group with a vehicle for demonstrating this. Even small decreases in the incidence of nosocomial infections will save hospitals money.

## COST-EFFECTIVE INFECTION CONTROL

Some infection control costs, such as the infection control budget, which includes salaries, supplies, journal subscriptions, and conference fees, are evident. Other costs, such as those for surgical dressings and masks, gowns, and gloves for isolation, may be hidden in routine room charges. The cost of tubing used for intravenous or respiratory therapy may be included in the procedure charge. Also, cost savings, using appropriate but less expensive antibiotics, will show up as savings in the pharmacy budget.

Infection control practices should be evaluated continually and continued only when they are shown to have a positive effect on the control of nosocomial infections. Some practices, which have been discontinued because they proved to be ineffective in controlling nosocomial infections, are antiseptic solutions for daily meatal care for patients with Foley catheters and placing hydrogen peroxide in the urinary drainage bag (9,10). Routine environmental culturing is both costly and ineffectual in preventing nosocomial infections. Environmental culturing should be done only when a situation, such as an outbreak, warrants it (11). Practices that have been shown, by well-designed and controlled research studies, to reduce nosocomial infections should be continued. These practices are stated as "category 1 items" in the nosocomial prevention guidelines published by the Centers for Disease Control.

Other practices, that historically have been done for the prevention of nosocomial infections, but have not proved to directly effect the incidence of nosocomial infections, are shoe covers in the operating room and cover gowns in the well-baby nurseries (12,13).

The use of protective isolation–masks, gloves, and gowns–for direct contact with severely immunocomprised patients had no effect on the incidence of infection, but organisms carried on the hands of personnel because they did not wash their hands often enough, had a direct bearing on the incidence of infection (14,15).

Spending money for educational conferences and journal publications is money effectively spent, if it informs the ICP of new research that allows for cost-effective changes in infection control practices. For example, research showed that there was no increased incidence of infection if respiratory or intravenous therapy tubing was changed at 48-hour intervals or every 24 hours (16,17).

Chapters 8–12 discuss in detail the causes and prevention of nosocomial urinary, respiratory, surgical wound, and bloodstream infections. Prevention of different kinds of nosocomial infections will result in vastly different cost savings to the institution. In one study, nosocomial urinary tract infections occurred most frequently but incurred only 15% of the overall costs of the nosocomial infections. However, surgical patients who developed a post operative wound infection accounted for 48% of the overall costs of the nosocomial infections but were only one-third of the total infections. The most expensive site per infection was the lower respiratory tract, with 13% of the total infections accounting for 29% of the total costs (8).

It is stated that proper handwashing is the single most important infection control practice and can reduce nosocomial infections by 50%, when done appropriately (18). Yet, studies show it is the least practiced infection control measure in most hospitals (19,20).

The primary objective of any infection control program should be nosocomial infection reduction. The second objective should be decreased patient costs for nosocomial infections through the judicious use of effective infection control practices. The first objective will decrease patient morbidity and mortality, and the second will decrease the hospital operating budget and save money. Commitment to these objectives will show hospital administrators that a cost-effective, efficiently run infection control program is a vital component of a fiscally sound institution.

## REFERENCES


1. Inglehart JK: Medicare begins prospective payment of hospitals. *N Engl J Med* 313(19):1201, 1983.
2. Beyt BE, Troxler S, Cavaness J: Prospective payment and infection control. *Infect Control* 6(4):161, 1985.
3. Haley RW, Culver DH, White JW, et al: The efficacy of infection surveillance and control programs in preventing nosocomial infections in US hospitals. *Am J Epidemiol* 121(2):182, 1985.
4. Haley RW, Shaberg DR, Von Allmen SD, et al: Estimating the extra charges and prolongation of hospitalization due to nosocomial infections: A comparison of methods. *J Infect Dis* 141(2):248, 1980.
5. Haley RW, Shaberg DR, Crossley KB, et al: Extra charges and prolongation of stay attributable to nosocomial infections: A prospective interhospital comparison. *Am J Med* 70:51, 1981.
6. McGowan JE Jr: Cost and benefit in control of nosocomial infection: Methods for analysis. *Rev Infect Dis* 3(4):790, 1981.
7. Freeman J, McGowan JE Jr: Methodologic issues in hospital epidemiol. III. Investigating the modifying effects of time and severity of underlying illness on estimates of cost of nosocomial infection. *Rev Infect Dis* 6(3):285, 1984.
8. Pinner RW, Haley RW, Blumenstein BA: High cost nosocomial infections. *Infect Control* 3(2):143, 1982.
9. Burke JP, Garibaldi RA, Britt MR, et al: Prevention of catheter-associated urinary tract infections. Efficacy of daily meatal care. *Am J Med* 70:655, 1981.
10. Thompson RL: Catheter associated bacteriuria: Failure to reduce attack rates using periodic instillations of a disinfectant into urinary drainage systems. *JAMA* 251:747, 1984.
11. Garner JS, Favero MS: Guidelines for handwashing and hospital environmental control 1985. Hospital Infections Program, Atlanta, Centers for Disease Control, 1985.
12. Hambraeus A, Malmborg AS: The influence of different footwear on floor contamination. *Scand J Infect Dis* 11:243, 1979.
13. Cloney DL, Donowitz LG: Overgown use for infection control in nurseries and neonatal intensive care units. *Am J Dis Child* 140:680, 1986.
14. Nauseef WM, Make DG: A study of simple protective isolation in patients with granulocytopenia. *N Engl J Med* 304(8):448, 1981.
15. Garner JS, Simmons BP: CDC guidelines for isolation precautions in hospitals. Hospital Infections Program, Atlanta, Centers for Disease Control, 1983, p 81.
16. Craven DE, Connolly MG Jr, Lichtenberg DA, et al: Contamination of mechanical ventilators with tubing changes every 24 or 48 hours. *N Engl J Med* 306:1505, 1982.

17. Josephson A, Gambert ME, Sierra MF, et al: The relationship between intravenous fluid contamination and the frequency of tubing replacement. *Infect Control* 6(9):367, 1985.

18. Steere AC, Mallison GF: Handwashing practices for the prevention of nosocomial infections. *Ann Intern Med* 83:683, 1975.

19. Albert RK, Condie F: Handwashing patterns in medical intensive care units. *N Engl J Med* 304:1465, 1981.

20. Preston GA, Larson EL, Stamm WE: The effect of private isolation rooms on patient practices, colonization and infection in an intensive care unit. *Am J Med* 30:614, 1981.

# 26

# Future Trends in Infection Control

Although measures to prevent or control infections have been attempted for as long as there have been nosocomial infections, formal infection control practice is really just beginning. In just a few years, infection control programs have been developed and already changes in activities and objectives have been made.

The results of the Study on the Efficacy of Nosocomial Infection Control (SENIC) project indicated that 83% of the hospitals surveyed had some kind of surveillance program for nosocomial infections; in 1965 only 16% of the responding hospitals had these programs (1). The SENIC report demonstrated the effectiveness of the ICP and the infection control programs throughout the United States. Hospitalwide surveillance, utilization of the knowledge and skills of the ICP, and a program of feedback of surgical wound infection rate to physicians could reduce nosocomial infections by 32% (1).

The infection control programs in hospitals throughout the United States are fairly consistent with one another, since most hospitals have adopted the guidelines and recommendations of the CDC and the JCAH for setting up and running infection control programs. The SENIC study also showed that about three-fourths of the ICPs, in hospitals that have that position, spent more than half their time in surveillance activities (1). The future of infection control practice depends on the other activities performed and the uses to which the surveillance data is put. Changes will occur in three areas: infection control practice, education, and research.

## INFECTION CONTROL PRACTICE

For the purpose of evaluating programs as well as educating ICPs and other health care personnel, standards of care for infection control practice must be determined. The future of infection control practice depends on the continuation of these standards. In hospitals that decreased surveillance or practices to decrease nosocomial infections and infrequently reported surgical wound infection rates to the surgeons, the overall nosocomial infection rate reduction was only 9% and reduction in surgical wound infection rates showed a decrease of only 13%; by contrast, hospitals where surgical infections were followed and reported to physicians showed a decrease in wound infection rates of 35% (2). Since nosocomial surgical wounds account for one-half of all nosocomial infections costs, this practice should be continued. In the future, these measures and activities, as well as those that are unproven but are thought to be appropriate, should be included in standards for infection control practice.

## EDUCATION

The education of the ICP and the hospital epidemiologist is not standard. Once standards for practice are more clearly defined, educational programs can be designed that will meet those standards. Educational programs are now being developed that have different bases and offer different emphases, fragmenting the field even more. Programs in nursing schools, graduate schools of public health, and colleges of basic sciences are developing programs with different admission requirements and varying curricula. A consistent educational approach, based on specific standards for care, is needed (3).

Certification of ICPs to confirm their knowledge base has been established. There may be different levels of practice, with different educational backgrounds required and different job descriptions. An example is a person responsible for data collection, tabulation, communicable disease reporting, and monitoring sterilizer tests, and another person who is responsible for analysis of data, interpretation, determining preventive or control measures, and teaching. There are groups as well as single consultants who oversee infection control programs, aid in problem solving, and direct outbreak investigations. Again, the development and education of the ICP, whether this title remains one position or becomes several levels of positions, are based on clear definitions of appropriate infection control practice.

Changes will also take place in the education of all other health care workers. As there is more awareness in general about risk management, educational programs in other fields will include more information on infection control, especially preventive measures. The ICP now may be more an advisor and trainer, who makes direct decisions on infection control matters, educates, and supervises practices. However, this current role may not foster independence among other health care workers. The ICP is the expert (largely because of the others' deficient educational background in infection control) and therefore is called upon for advice and decisions.

The ICP will continue to need more management skills to accomplish this task of decision-maker. These practitioners must select programs for self education in management as they have done in the past on infectious disease and microbiology.

In the future, the position may shift toward that of observer and counselor–facilitator, as described by Axnick and Yarbrough (4). In this position, the ICP fosters independence among health care workers and helps them to clarify and make their own decisions. Ultimately the improved education of all health care workers in infection control will end the stereotype of ICPs as detectives and finger-pointers. Until this happens, and the ICP is no longer directly or indirectly providing the main infection control education to hospital personnel, the ICP will continue to fight the same brush fires and will be more crisis-oriented than prevention-oriented.


## RESEARCH

Infection control practitioners have been involved in research on efficacy of infection control practice rather than continuance of practices because of historical precedent. Infection control measures cost money; therefore, in the area of cost containment, the efficacy of practice should be documented. In 1985 APIC established the APIC Research Committee to promote and foster quality, innovative research. The first two actions of the committee are to provide the ICPs with a list of infection control issues needing research and a list of funding agencies pertinent to the discipline of infection control. Much research has been accomplished on device-related nosocomial infections but little on patient risk factors. More research is needed in this area.

Until the minimal unavoidable rates of nosocomial infections are determined, ICPs and ICCs will not be able to know where best to spend their time and efforts to lower infection rates.

Cost-effectiveness studies are also being done by practitioners to show the methods and activities that lower hospital costs without increasing risks to patients or personnel. The lowest risk of nosocomial infection is in a situation where the patient is totally isolated from other patients and has contact with personnel or equipment through a sterile barrier of some sort. Obviously this situation is impossible and economically unfeasible, but there may be some infection control rituals that are just as costly and yet do not significantly decrease infection risks. Research is needed to find the best methods of patient care with the lowest possible infection risks, in balance with the least possible cost.

The cost-effectiveness of infection control programs themselves have been determined. Infection control programs are lowering infection rates and risks and therefore saving money for patients, third-party payers, personnel, and hospitals by lowered morbidity and mortality, shorter hospitalizations, and fewer lawsuits. Infection control practitioners and ICCs must continue to document savings and evaluate the programs they have set up in these areas.

## FUTURE ROLE OF THE INFECTION CONTROL PRACTITIONER

Infection control practitioners are involved in the future of the field through their actual practices and by influencing the hospital and community to improve the image and status of the position within hospitals. Individually and as a group, ICPs, along with ICC chairpersons, can improve the quality of care in hospitals through education, research, monitoring, and prompt intervention in infection control problems.

As more emphasis is placed on preventive health care, infection control practice in hospitals may become more important and therefore may receive more administrative and financial support. The ICP and the ICC chairperson should be aware of health care legislation as it affects infection control practice, so that sound decisions are made on the goals, objectives, and requirements of infection control programs in hospitals.

## REFERENCES


1. Haley RW, Culver DH, White JW, et al: The efficacy of infection surveillance and control programs in preventing nosocomial infections in the US hospitals. *Am J Epidemiol* 121(2):182, 1985.
2. Haley RW, Morgan WM, Culver DH, et al: Update from the SENIC project: *Am J Infect Control* 13(3):97, 1985.
3. Yarbrough MG: Training needs of the infection control nurse. *Ann Intern Med* 89 (Part 2):815, 1978.
4. Axnick KJ, Yarbrough M: *Infection control: An integrated approach* St. Louis, Mosby, 1984.

# Index